Coming Full Circle

Coming Full Circle

Spirituality and Wellness among Native Communities in the Pacific Northwest

SUZANNE CRAWFORD O'BRIEN

University of Nebraska Press Lincoln and London

Sections of chapters 5 and 6 originally appeared as "Healing Generations in the South Puget Sound" in Suzanne Crawford O'Brien, *Religion and Healing in Native America: Pathways for Renewal*.
Manufactured in the United States of America

∞

Library of Congress Cataloging-in-Publication Data
Crawford O'Brien, Suzanne J.
Coming full circle: spirituality and wellness among native communities in the Pacific Northwest / Suzanne Crawford O'Brien.
pages cm
Includes bibliographical references and index.
ISBN 978-0-8032-1127-8 (hardback: alk. paper)
1. Coast Salish Indians—Religion. 2. Coast Salish Indians—Health and hygiene. 3. Coast Salish Indiains—Medicine. 4. Indigenous peoples—Ecology—Northwest, Pacific. 5. Traditional medicine—Northwest, Pacific. I. Title.
E99.S21C73 2013
305.897'0795—dc23 2013020789

Set in Sabon Next by Laura Wellington.

Contents

Illustrations

Preface

As a fourth generation Oregonian I identify deeply with the landscape, culture, and history of the Pacific Northwest. My most vivid childhood memories are of hiking, camping, and canoeing in the Cascade Mountains and along the Oregon coast. And my most powerful moments of being spiritually awake always took place on a ridge top, after a good hard climb: an updraft drying sweat, the inspiration of an amazing view. From an early age I was drawn toward religious traditions rooted in natural places and had a curiosity about Native traditions of the region. As a small child I was introduced to the people and culture of the area through the usual modes of tribal museums and art galleries. And I went to school with Native students, though within the Portland public school system of the 1970s and 1980s such students were rarely inclined to talk about their cultural identity, and I did not know enough to ask. My grandfather, a depression-era migrant to the Northwest from Oklahoma, told us what little he knew about his own Native heritage, and it fed my initial scholarly interest in the subject. As an undergraduate at Willamette University and later as a graduate student in comparative religions I was repeatedly drawn to Native traditions, both because of my own heritage and because of a deep commitment to social and ecological justice, concerns that I felt were exemplified in the history and contemporary experience of Native Americans.

This particular project began on an afternoon in Santa Barbara, California, when I opened a newspaper to read about the Shoalwater Bay tribe on the Washington coast, who were confronting a medical and spiritual crisis on their reservation. From 1988 to 1999 the Shoalwater people had been experiencing staggeringly high rates of pregnancy loss, some years as high as 89 percent. In such a small community, each loss was a collective tragedy. In the fall of 2000, with the support of my graduate advisor Inés Talamantez, I traveled to the Shoalwater reservation. There I volunteered at the tribal wellness center and spoke with tribal leaders, clinic staff, and community members. I wondered how the community was coping with the losses, what forms of religious practice or traditional healing they were drawing upon, and how they were making sense of their experiences. Two people provided vital guidance during this time: then tribal chairman Herbert "Ike" Whitish and community member and staff member Midge Porter. Tragically, both of these powerful individuals passed away before this book could be completed. Both devoted themselves to promoting health and wellness among their communities, and both offered me invaluable assistance as I began this project.

As I spoke with community members and clinic staff, my project took a very different turn. By this time the pregnancy loss crisis was behind them, and most community members did not want to discuss it: the memories were simply too painful. And after a decade of struggling with the tragedy, seeking federal aid, and grieving as a community, most tribal members were weary of the topic. Instead they encouraged me to look at how the community had responded to the crisis, at what they had accomplished and what more remained to be done. As one woman told me quite bluntly, "Let's talk about the healthy babies. We have a lot of babies here now—more than we've had in a long time."

While I was very interested in the community's responses to the pregnancy loss crisis, I was equally committed to crafting a project that would help meet tribal needs and concerns. As a result, I began to shape a different set of questions: What did it mean to be "healthy"? How can that best be achieved? What cultural and spiritual resources is the community drawing upon to get there? Such questions framed the issue of health more broadly and were guided by the desire of the community to focus on how healthcare could be (and was being) improved, rather than dwelling upon tragedy.

Midge Porter soon introduced me to the staff of the Women's

Wellness Program at the South Puget Intertribal Planning Agency (SPIPA). SPIPA is a coalition of the Shoalwater Bay, Nisqually, Chehalis, Skokomish, and Squaxin Island nations who have joined together to address a wide range of tribal needs, including healthcare, domestic violence prevention, education and job training, and a variety of other social services. I spent the next five summers volunteering with the Women's Wellness Program at SPIPA and helping to facilitate their annual Women and Girls' Gathering, a four-day gathering of Native women and girls from throughout the region focusing on health, wellness, and traditional culture and spirituality. The more I learned, the more questions were raised, and the more I realized I needed to understand the cultural background and religious and political history of these communities in order to begin to make sense of their contemporary experience.

After 2003, when I was fortunate enough to be hired to join the faculty of Pacific Lutheran University (a relatively short drive from the tribal communities whom SPIPA serves), I continued to volunteer with the organization, and also facilitated the placement of two student interns with the Women's Wellness Program. These students worked alongside us on projects ranging from the annual gathering to traditional craft workshops and domestic violence prevention programs.

I also continued to pursue research through an examination of historical, textual, and ethnographic materials. I gathered information from previously published and archival resources, including documents from the tribes themselves, ranging from grant proposals, annual reports, flyers, and newsletters. Ethnographic work in the form of participant observation, formal interviews, and informal conversations was conducted intermittently between 2000 and 2005 with the Shoalwater Bay tribal community on the central Washington coast, and between 2001 and 2006 with the South Puget Intertribal Planning Agency's Women's Wellness Program. I worked to include tribal leaders and SPIPA staff within the writing process. Along the way, relevant chapters were submitted to tribal chairpersons and SPIPA staff for their comment and review.

During this time I was invited to attend various community and religious gatherings. One of the most memorable for me as a teacher took place on a chilly January morning when I was able to bring a class of twenty first-year Pacific Lutheran University students to attend a Sunday service at one of the original Indian Shaker churches. My students were keenly aware that it was an honor and privilege to be there, and I was proud of how they conducted themselves and how they learned from the opportunity. Such experiences have been invaluable as I have reflected on the texts and material that I consider here. For the most part however, I have chosen not make explicit reference to these experiences in the pages that follow. Many ceremonies and religious gatherings are considered private affairs. Unless a ceremony was open to the public, specific descriptions of religious practices in this text are drawn from previously published studies, works done with the permission and consultation of the people involved.

Acknowledgments

This book is the culmination of various journeys, both personal and intellectual. That it exists at all is due in no small part to the support and assistance of many people, too numerous to mention here. The work was possible because of generous funding from many sources: a Jacob K. Javitz Fellowship for Graduate Studies in the Humanities, a Dissertation Year Fellowship from the University of California Santa Barbara, a grant from the Wabash Center for Teaching and Learning in Theology and Religion, and grants from Pacific Lutheran University, including a much-appreciated sabbatical leave. Profound thanks are due to the South Puget Sound Native communities who have allowed me space to explore these questions and to learn from the remarkable ways in which they have addressed the very real concerns facing them. The South Puget Intertribal Planning Agency staff and volunteers have given generously of their time and welcomed my own small volunteer efforts within their important work. I am privileged to have known them and grateful for the opportunity to join in their efforts. To that end, proceeds from the sale of the book are being donated to the agency's Women's Wellness Program, in the hope that its work will continue to improve the lives of Native women in western Washington for generations to come.

Throughout the process of researching and writing I have been privileged to meet many amazing individuals. Few struck me as powerfully as did Herbert "Ike" Whitish (1955–2005), tireless and inspired tribal chairman of the Shoalwater Bay tribe. His vital leadership and commitment carried his community through a difficult and painful period in their history, and his work has resulted in dramatic improvements in the health and wellness of this community that will have a powerful impact for generations to come. I hope my studies honor his memory and help those outside his community to better understand the significance of his work.

Midge Porter (1951–2011) worked with SPIPA from 1991 to 2007, spearheading the Women's Wellness Program and tackling the monumental task of organizing the annual Women and Girls' Gathering. Her energy appeared limitless, and her commitment to creating healthy, vibrant tribal communities was an inspiration. She cherished her Chinook heritage and identified strongly with the waterways of southwest Washington. She took me under her wing in many ways, supporting my project and believing that it would make an important contribution. I am so very thankful for her and her work.

Many mentors, advisors, and colleagues have offered invaluable support throughout the years. I would like to thank Allan Siegel, one of those great teachers who change young people's lives, for inspiring in me a love for reading and writing and the confidence to believe I could succeed. For their support and guidance in this project, my sincere gratitude to my graduate advisors at the University of California Santa Barbara: Inés Talamantez, Laury Oaks, Wade Clark Roof, and William Powell. Particular thanks go to Dr. Howard Harrod of Vanderbilt University, who passed away before this book could be completed. I am also very grateful to my colleagues in the Religion Department at Pacific Lutheran University who have read drafts, offering valuable editorial advice, and who have created an atmosphere where the life of the mind has space for expression, in the classroom as well as within scholarly work. I am fortunate to have such loving, supportive, and brilliant colleagues. Profound gratitude as well to ChiXapkaid (D. Michael Pavel) for your support, encouragement, and the generous gift of artwork for he cover of this book. I value your friendship.

Profound thanks to my parents, Timothy and Jeanne Crawford, whose own sacrifices and support made it possible for me to complete my doctoral degree and begin the journey toward becoming a university professor. I could not ask for better role models of how to live well, how to think deeply, and how to cultivate compassion in the world. I treasure their presence in my life. Thanks as well to friends and loved ones who have surrounded me with empathy and encouragement over the past years. I offer my thanks to Carson Anderson, Kirsten Anderson, Tanya Barnett, my sister and friend Michelle Crawford-Thorla, Antonios Finitsis, Dennis Kelley, Megan MacDonald, Heather Mathews, Liz O'Dea, Marie Pagliarini, Brian Peterson, William Robert, Elijah Siegler, Linh Vu, and Wendy Wiseman. Thanks go to Kevin Brown for his valuable assistance with images. There are many others I should name as well, and I must ask their forgiveness for cutting this list so very short.

I want to thank my husband and dearest friend Michael Timothy O'Brien for his encouragement, patience, and countless small kindnesses that made this project possible. This is a collaborative effort in a great sense of the word: without his generosity and help I would never even have attempted such an audacious undertaking. And finally, this book is for my son Declan, whose arrival in my life has given me an entirely new perspective on what it means to live, to love, and to be delighted by Creation.

Introduction: The Case of Ellen Gray

Myron Eells was a missionary, scholar, and collector who worked among Native Americans in the Pacific Northwest, spending many years on the Skokomish reservation near Puget Sound. In 1883 he described the illness and death of a young Skokomish girl.

Death of Ellen Gray, 1883

> Ellen Gray was a school girl, about 16 years of age, and had been in the boarding school (at Skokomish) for several years, nearly ever since she had been old enough to attend, but her parents were quite superstitious. One Friday evening she went home, to remain until the Sabbath; but on Saturday, the first of January 1881, she was taken sick. . . . Her parents and friends made her believe that a bad tamahnous had been put into her, and no one but an Indian doctor could cure her. . . . The Agent and teacher did not like the way the affair was being maneuvered, took charge of her, moved her to a decent house near by, and placed white watchers with her, so that the proper medicines should be given and no Indian doctor brought in. . . .
>
> But the effect on her imagination had been so great that for a time she often acted strangely. She seldom said anything; she would often spurt out the medicine when given her as far as she could; said she saw the tamahnous; pulled her mother's hair; bit her mother's finger so that it bled; seemed peculiarly vexed at her; moaned most of the time, but sometimes screamed very loudly; and even bit a spoon off . . . one night she threw off the clothes, took cold, and would not make any effort to cough and clear her throat and on the twenty-second she died, actually choking to death. It was a tolerably clear case of death from imagination, easily accounted for on the principles of mental philos-

ophy, but the Indians had never studied it, and still believe that a bad tamahnous killed her.[1]

Eells's near-clinical account of the death of young Ellen Gray reveals a profound disconnect between Euroamerican and indigenous worldviews at the close of the nineteenth century. Eells understood his task to be the eradication of Native cultures and religions, and he firmly believed that it was vital for their spiritual and physical salvation. But a century later, perspectives would change dramatically. By the twenty-first century even federal officials would come to argue that indigenous well-being could be found within the revival of Native cultures. And Native people themselves would carve out a distinctly indigenous blend of Euroamerican biomedicine and Native American healing.

Shoalwater Bay Tribal Wellness Center Dedication, May 27, 2005

A crowd has gathered outside the new Wellness Center of the Shoalwater Bay tribal community. As my soon-to-be husband and I join the group, we pause to admire the new structure, its glass windows gleaming in the May sunshine, and we step into the line of people waiting to enter the tent erected for today's ceremony. As we arrive at the entrance to the tent, two young people put strings of trade beads and semiprecious stones around our necks, giving us red cloth pouches filled with sage and tobacco. The sound of drumming draws us under the shelter of the canopy, and shortly after we have taken our seats, Charlene Nelson, the tribal chairwoman rises to speak. She welcomes the assembled crowd to this dedication of the new Shoalwater Bay Tribal Wellness Center, going on to say that while this place is new, with the most modern of biomedical technologies, it is also a place for traditional things. She explains that their intention today has been to do things in a traditional way. This very new place, she says, is actually a place for making the past present. The drum, she points out, is traditional. It is the traditional way to call people, to welcome people to a place, and to invite them into the community. Long ago when visitors arrived on these shores, they were greeted by drums and by a welcoming song. With that, she invites a group of Chinook drummers and singers to offer an opening blessing.

The lead drummer rises to speak. "Today, we are bringing things full circle," he says. He goes on to explain that for millennia the Chinook and Chehalis people have made their homes on Willapa Bay, returning every year to fish and gather shellfish. And now, within this new wellness center, the traditions of their ancestors are being revived. He explains that the drums and the songs are traditional ways of honoring a place, and that earlier in the day, before the arrival of guests, the building had been smudged and prayed over in a traditional way. He offers a Chinook *wawa* prayer, asking that the ancestors come to those assembled, speaking to them in quiet places. He asks that within this new center, those ancestors will show people how to live in a traditional way. He then sings an honor song, a *syowen* song. This song too, he says, is a sign of things returning. His Chinook grandfather had given the song to a Yakama man, who had recently gifted it back to the Chinook. "Now, singing this song," he says, "we are bringing it full circle."

Following these dedications, Charlene stands to introduce the tribal council, honoring those present and also welcoming all those unseen elders "who have walked on." These ancestors, she says, she welcomes most of all. She then extends her welcome to members of other tribes present, representing nations from throughout the Pacific Northwest. "We are here," she says, "to celebrate the visions of our elders, their dreams, and their tenacity." She goes on to tell the assembled crowd about how the Shoalwater Bay tribal community built their first clinic, in 1995, but that even then the vision of their leaders was for something else, for a Wellness Center, a place for preventing illness, for building community, for meeting the needs of the whole person, where all these things could come together under one roof. This vision, and the spirit and determination that would ultimately make it possible, came from former tribal chairman Herbert "Ike" Whitish and his mother Rachel Whitish, for whom this center is dedicated. Further honoring their vision, it is now announced, the tribe has also established a medical scholarship, with the intent of sending a Shoalwater Bay tribal member to medical school, so that she or he, in turn, can come back and care for their community. As gifts are given to Ike, to his family, and to friends of the tribe, speakers explain that the Wellness Center was born out of a difficult time, a time of loss and pain, but a time that nonetheless gave birth to a renewed sense of purpose in this community, a determination to survive and to care for one another.

That determination is likewise celebrated through gifts to the Shoalwater community from other visiting tribal communities: gifts of song and kinship. A singer comes forward to offer a Bear Song, explaining that Bears are the Medicine People and that these songs are songs for strength and healing. The Squalliabs Drummers from the inland community of the Nisqually tribe step forward as well, performing a song that came to one of them in a dream, a song that removes fear, a song that represents the call of the eagle and is dedicated to Ike and Rachel, people who overcame their fears. They also sing a song from the Skokomish Nation (sung with their permission), to honor the place and the community. A Quinault tribal member stands to speak, sharing memories of Shoalwater Bay, his family's close ties to those present, and the relationships that bind them. Like the people of Shoalwater, the Quinault are a fishing people, even though, as he reflects, the Quinault River is closed to fishing: there are no fish this year. "We are poor in material wealth," he says, "but we are rich in relations." He brings his own spiritual offering of strength to the Shoalwater community, a song that comes from his father, a 1910 Shaker Church missionary, and from his grandfather, a spiritual leader in his community. The ancestors are present, he reminds us all, "and they are rejoicing, proud of the accomplishments of this community."

The heart of this gathering is Ike, and people's gratitude for his work, for his sacrifice, for his unfailing devotion to this community and its needs. People stand to share their memories with Ike and to thank him. Despite his own present illness, the collected crowd celebrates his many achievements, honoring his spirit and his determination. The day is joyful and sad—celebrating what fifteen years ago seemed impossible while also honoring the losses that have come along the way.

Central Questions

These two narratives are a good place to begin. They bookend the historical period that I will be considering. And they are in many ways a crystallization of the events described: a history of illness, displacement, disrupted families and communities, as well as a contemporary moment in which Native communities have regained local control of their medical care and are finding common ground with western biomedicine in ways that reflect and include their spiritual and cultural traditions. My work is about the intersection of health, healing, and spirituality in the experience of and resistance to colonization among Native communities of western Washington. As the dedication narrative pinpoints, it is about how Native people in these communities are indeed coming full circle: drawing upon traditional wisdom and practices to confront contemporary challenges to their health and well-being, while adapting to new contexts and creatively integrating elements of the dominant culture alongside their own.

The two stories also serve to identify some key questions and ideas at the heart of my research. The experience of Ellen Gray raises questions about indigenous healing traditions, about the impact of boarding schools and missionization, the cultural significance of families and kinship, and how the history of colonial encounters in the Northwest has affected Chinook and Coast Salish mental, spiritual, and physical well-being. The dedication, taking place more than 120 years later, raises a different but interrelated set of questions. In contrast to the first story, which appears to present two cultures dramatically at odds, the second attests to the ways in which contemporary communities have responded creatively to colonial history, integrating biomedicine alongside traditional worldviews and religious practices and working collaboratively with physicians.

The second story raises questions about *how* contemporary communities are integrating traditional healing practices into biomedical care. What does "traditional" mean in the contemporary context?

How can a clinic using the latest in western biomedical technology be a place for traditional Native culture to thrive? In our contemporary context, religion and science are typically presented as profoundly antithetical. Why then do we find prayers, songs and drums to honor a place focused on the biomedical treatment of disease?

One can also note in these narratives the central place of kinship within these Native communities; they are, as one speaker says, "rich in relations." These are the ties that bind people both across tribal lines and to those who have gone before. The relational ties are most noticeably given expression within songs, stories, and Indian names, all items of cultural property that are gifted and inherited, creating and sustaining kinship relationships throughout the region and across generations.

The voices present on the warm May day on the Washington coast also testify to the continued importance of religion and spirituality in these communities, particularly as they take shape in the Indian Shaker Church, in healing songs, and in dreams and visions. Spiritual practices remain central to Native identity, to strong communities, and to what it means to be well. What begins to emerge here is a sense of wellness strongly shaped by relationships—between individuals and their ancestors, between people and place, and within and between human communities.

I argue that illness, health, and healthcare in this region have acted as key locations of cultural negotiation throughout the past two centuries. To do this, I undertake a historical analysis of disease and disease etiologies in the region, analysis of previously published ethnographic works, and contemporary case studies among present-day descendents of these communities. The material suggests ways for thinking about how differing views of the body and the self have historically been the site of cultural conflict. In many ways and at many moments Native people have experienced their bodies as battlegrounds: sites of negotiation between conflicting notions of embodiment and the self. But bodily experience also becomes the site where such conflicts are reconciled and where individuals find spaces for wholeness, healing, and renewal. In the twenty-first century it is within the sphere of health and healing that Native communities continue to do the complicated work of sorting out what it means to be both Native and American, both traditional and contemporary.

Why Religious Studies?

It may not be immediately clear why a scholar of religion would undertake this focus on health and healthcare: my training is in religious studies, not public health or medical anthropology. But when one considers the profound connection between health and identity, healing emerges as a genuinely *religious* experience. At the core of much of religion is the making of the self and establishing the self in right-relation to the universe. If we think about healing as *self-making* (through communal ritual activities that reflect and reinforce beliefs regarding health and illness and meaning), then wellness and healthcare should be a central concern of scholars of religion. Without a clear understanding of a culture's perspective on the self and what it means to be well, the rituals, ceremonies, oral traditions, and basic belief systems of that culture remain elusive. And without an analysis of the ways in which competing systems of viewing the self and the body come into contact, the processes of missionization, colonization, and religious coercion cannot be fully understood.[2]

The value of thinking about healing and selfhood within Religious Studies is reinforced by anthropologist Clifford Geertz's definition of religion as "systems of symbols" that work to create moods and motivations within people, that teach them how they ought to live (ethos), and that facilitate and reinforce a general order of existence (worldview).[3] According to Geertz, religious symbols shape notions of selfhood, obligation, responsibility, and identity, which form the foundations for one's worldview and ethos. Likewise, theologian Paul Tillich's notion of religion as "the dimension of depth" found within all aspects of human culture is also useful here. Tillich argues that religion is "the state of being grasped by an ultimate concern," a state which "cannot be restricted to a special realm. . . . Religion as ultimate concern is the meaning-giving substance of culture, and culture is the totality of forms in which the basic concern of religion expresses itself." If religion is expressed throughout the totality of culture, then "religion" can happen in places that may not look "religious." Formal ceremonies and services are not the only places where ultimate concerns are sought and expressed.[4]

I would contend that the cultural understandings of what it means to be a whole and healthy self are at the heart of "religious" activity and symbol. Health, healing, and embodiment are locales of "depth" of "ultimate concern," where the very relationship between self and other is worked out. And as Geertz would attest, such understandings are culturally distinct. They can only be grasped through an interpretation of the symbolic language at hand, as viewed from within. How we construct, reinforce, and renew a sense of working identity—of the relationship between self, other, landscape, and universe—is fundamentally a religious question and central to the act of meaning making.

Because of this, questions of religious traditions and spirituality are often examined indirectly in this project, by looking at cultural, social, and symbolic activities as a whole. In part this is because many of the particulars of indigenous religious practice among Coast Salish communities are extremely private and are not meant to be shared with the outside world. I also take this approach because religious symbols and sensibilities must be understood as one piece of a larger cultural system, intertwined with other aspects of experience. Hence my approach is to consider religion as a system of symbols that are threaded throughout lived cultural experience and that act to reveal, challenge, and reinforce worldview, ethos, and sensibility, as they enable people to engage directly and indirectly with the Sacred. It is the collective process of meaning making and the construction of identity, particularly in terms of relationships with spiritual beings, both human and more-than-human. When I write of spiritual worldviews and sensibilities, I am often looking for these in unlikely places. They are certainly present in ceremony and prayer, but the work of meaning making can also be found within the very concrete ways in which communities organize themselves and respond to pressing needs.

My goal is to show how historical experiences of religion, illness, and healing have contributed to contemporary understandings of health and wellness, and how western Washington Native communities in the twenty-first century are responding to contemporary threats in ways that are both contemporary and "traditional." Given the questions I am asking, my approach is necessarily an interdisciplinary one. If one's goal is to consider culture as a whole, one must include a wide array of sources and methods, which may be disconcerting to those deeply rooted in particular methodologies. To a historian, this may not be "history enough." To an ethnographer, it may likewise not be "ethnography enough." A theoretician may find it "theory-light," while others may find it too "theory-heavy." But because scholars in Religious Studies recognize that religion as a cultural experience is intricately bound with all aspects of the human experience, an interdisciplinary approach can sometimes be the only way to understand what religious practice means for people and communities.

My analysis is also informed by postcolonial theory, and yet the term *postcolonial* does not necessarily apply to Native Americans, who are still struggling to preserve their cultures and political sovereignty. And it is informed by feminist theories and approaches to scholarship, keeping in mind Marie Annette Jaimes Guerrero's injunction: any scholarship "that does not address land rights, sovereignty, and the state's systematic erasure of the cultural practices of native peoples, or that defines native women's participation in these struggles as non-feminist, is limited in vision and exclusionary in practice."[5] Such caveats are important, not only theoretically but also practically, as they impact the way we work with and for Native communities. Thus while women's health and approaches to healthcare are the primary concern, I have sought to locate these women's experiences within the larger context of collective well-being and efforts to resist the multiple and complex processes of colonization.

Native communities today demand that researchers take part in cooperative efforts with the community and that their research address issues about which the community itself is concerned.[6] Participant action research is defined by Diane Wolf as research "guided by locally constituted needs," in which "subjects define the research agenda" and take part in "a more interactive process to define the terms, goals, and procedures of the project."[7] As Wolf acknowledges, such efforts are complicated and problematic. Still, the challenge stands, in part because of the standards that feminist and critical scholarship have set in recent years and in part because of what Native communities demand from those working with them.

Other scholars working with Coast Salish communities and cultures illustrate this commitment to community engagement, as they have shaped their work to contribute to ongoing legal battles, such as land claims cases in British Columbia.[8] Daniel Boxberger, for instance, has said he hopes to see scholarship shift toward "a politically motivated research agenda directed by the Fourth World State."[9] While I do not necessarily agree with Boxberger's outright rejection of all "interpretive" work as being without "practical application," I do agree that scholars writing in an era of land claims and legal battles need to be cognizant of the impact their work can have in the political arena and of shaping research questions in ways that reflect the needs and interests of the communities in question.

With that in mind, I have long made it a goal that any work I produce be something of theoretical *and* material benefit to the communities with whom I am working. I did my best to frame a project that might speak to the concerns and interests of those with whom I worked at SPIPA. By presenting two case studies of vibrant tribally led and community-directed programs promoting health and wellness, at SPIPA and at Shoalwater Bay, I aim to show that locally directed initiatives are indeed best suited for meeting the health and wellness needs of Coast Salish and Chinook people. I also aim to show that what it means to be a healthy self is culturally and locally distinct. The needs of Native people are complicated by a history of ongoing colonialism and cannot be adequately met by generic healthcare programs based on a Euroamerican biomedical model. Health and wellness are best achieved through community-controlled efforts that are informed by local worldviews, symbol systems, and ethos. For my work to buttress that work, I keep several questions in mind: what particular historical and cultural issues shape Native struggles for health and wellness? How are contemporary communities responding effectively to these issues? And what makes those efforts effective?

My hope is that this book contributes to theoretical conversations about the nature of the self, healing, and the body within comparative religious practices, symbols, and worldviews. My further hope is that it contributes materially to the betterment of contemporary efforts toward Native health and wellness. I would argue that theory detached from material reality is scarcely worth doing. And at the same time, I believe that thinking deeply and carefully about the how and why of our cultures and belief systems can have genuine material consequences. Theory matters. Hence it is my belief that both theoretical and practical concerns can benefit from this conversation. To that end, I begin by venturing into theoretical territory. Chapter 1 describes the current conversations within medical anthropology, religious studies, and feminist studies about the nature of the self and the body and the relationship between "my self" and "my flesh." A fundamental question explored in chapter 1 is how the meaning of being healthy is a culturally distinct experience, drawn from a people's understanding of what it means to be a whole, healthy self. Such understandings differ from place to place and moment to moment and are informed by religious, economic, social, and political realities. I bring Native American religious studies into this theoretical conversation, making the case that these philosophies have a great deal to contribute toward a more nuanced understanding of the nature of the self, the body and what it means to be healthy in a comparative context.

The People and the Place

My focus is the experience of Chinook and Coast Salish communities, with emphasis upon those communities inhabiting the South Puget Sound and lower Columbia River regions. At the beginning of the nineteenth century the Chinook lived along the lower Columbia River and northern Willamette Valley. Until the arrival of white settlers and their attendant epidemics, the Chinook were one of the most powerful tribes in the region, speaking distinct Chinookan languages and communicating with other tribes, such as the Coast Salish to the north, in a trade language that has become known as Chinook *wawa* (also known as Chinook jargon, which is distinct from Chinookan proper). They controlled the lower Columbia, the central highway for trade and travel in southern Washington and northern Oregon, and were exceptionally skilled at fishing, trade, and negotiation. They spent much of the year on the Columbia River, though many also migrated to the coast and Willapa (Shoalwater) Bay in particular, during peak fishing and shellfish gathering times. In the early to mid-nineteenth century epidemic diseases struck the Pacific Northwest, devastating communities with onslaughts of smallpox, measles, influenza, and malaria, among other ailments. During this time some Chinook fled to Shoalwater Bay, seeking refuge from the illnesses on the river. There they were joined by members of the Coast Salish lower Chehalis, with whom the people of Shoalwater Bay maintain close relational ties. Other Chinook survivors of the nineteenth-century epidemics, those living in the Willamette Valley and along the Columbia River, were gathered together on the Grand Ronde reservation in 1855. Still others remained where they were, keeping a sense of their distinct identity even as they integrated into the predominantly Euroamerican economy.

The precolonial territory of the Coast Salish extended from southern British Columbia through western Washington and Puget Sound and as far south as the Tillamook on the Oregon coast. I focus primarily on those in southern Puget Sound: the Squaxin, Skokomish, Nisqually, Chehalis, and those alongside the coast at Shoalwater Bay. I also draw heavily upon ethnographic studies of other related Coast Salish communities, such as the Puyallup, Upper Skagit, Nooksack, Tulalip, Cowlitz, and Klallam and the Sto:lo of British Columbia.

Using the overarching name Coast Salish runs the risk of creating an image of a monolithic group rather than portraying a large number of autonomous and distinct communities that shared common linguistic and cultural foundations. For instance, unlike in most other Northwest Coast culture groups that share a common language, there were fourteen distinct languages within the Coast Salish language family, some of which are as different from one another as German is from English.[10] The independent autonomous social structure of the precontact era is reflected in the contemporary political situation: today there are dozens of distinct Coast Salish tribes and nations in Washington and British Columbia.

While they were in many ways independent, precolonial villages were also deeply connected through intermarriage, sharing religious and cultural systems and political and social affiliations. As the dedication of the Shoalwater Wellness Center attested, a sense of kinship is still strong among contemporary Native communities in the region. Recall that the ceremony included gifts to representatives of other tribal nations as well as honoring songs and prayers offered by guests from the Chinook, Quinault, Nisqually, and Skokomish, among others. This interrelatedness among tribes is a historical reality, stemming from strong intervillage networks of trade and kinship, but it has also been reinforced (and at times challenged) by their historical experience.

In part 2 I take an explicitly historical approach, reconstructing the course of events from 1800 to 2000 that impacted Coast Salish and Chinook health, healing, and religion. Chapter 2 examines the early years of settlement and missionization in western Oregon and western Washington (1800–1845), discussing the impact of epidemic diseases on Native people and on the missionaries who sought to evangelize them. Chapter 3 begins with the establishment of reservations in the 1850s. This era of reservation living put enormous stresses on indigenous communities as they struggled with poverty, racism, loss of traditional subsistence activities, and growing threats to health and well-being. The chapter goes on to examine federal policies and a second wave of missionary activity in the region in the late nineteenth century and how both were influenced by prevailing racial stereotypes of the day.

In part 3 I shift from a focus on Euroamerican policies, agendas, and perspectives concerning Native people toward a focus on Coast Salish and Chinook *responses* to this period of history. Chapter 4 explores the history of religious change among Coast Salish communities from 1800 until the 1970s. I argue that while religious and healing traditions transformed over time, many of the central philosophical foundations and understandings of what it means to be a whole and healthy self remained very much the same. Chapters 5 and 6 present two contemporary case studies that illustrate this point: the Women's Wellness Program at SPIPA and the story of the Shoalwater Bay tribal community.

Many of the challenges that contemporary American Indian communities face—alcoholism, depression, and abuse—have been the result of (at times well-meaning) federal policies. Reservation officials sought to clamp down on Native religion, healing traditions, potlatches, and gambling, imposing a "quasi-martial law," which prompted some people to leave reservations so as to continue such activities.[11] Indeed, many contemporary Native people locate the origin of chronic social problems with these and other U.S. and Canadian federal policies, particularly those that mandated the removal of Native children and their placement in residential schools. First person accounts describe scenarios where parents were refused the right to raise their own children, while the children themselves experienced abuse, neglect, and shockingly high mortality rates. Those who survived often emerged as adults suffering from anger, alienation, and depression and not equipped to care for children of their own, beginning a generational cycle of neglect and abuse.

Chronic social problems that emerged as a result have indeed carried on into subsequent generations. George Guilmet and David Whited noted in 1989 that some of the highest mortality rates in contemporary American Indian communities were attributable to "accidents, suicides, substance abuse, and violence—all expressions of the emotional stress experienced by individuals who have been stripped of their cultural traditions and forced into schizophrenically bicultural existence."[12] Statistics gathered in 1993 confirmed that alcohol-related deaths were 579 percent higher for American Indian and Alaska Natives than for the general population, while suicide rates were 70 percent higher, homicide rates 41 percent higher, and the rate of drug-related deaths was 18 percent higher.[13] Poverty rates among reservation communities range from 30 to 90 percent; unemployment ranges from 13 to 40 percent; accidental death rates are typically three times the national average, alcoholism rates are 30–80 percent higher, and domestic violence, teen pregnancy, child neglect, and suicide are often twice the national rate. By 1990 only 15 percent of Native adults had graduated from high school or received their GED, and the dropout rate of Native students in public schools was as high as 60–80 percent.[14] Healthcare providers note that spiritual and mental distress associated with the impacts of colonialism, poverty, and intergenerational violence are commonly expressed somatically among Native communities. A report from one Coast Salish medical clinic notes that "fatigue, headache, back pain and stomach upset" can be signs of "spiritual problems which sometimes create bodily symptoms," symptoms that often require referral to a traditional healer in order to be remedied.[15]

If the major threats to indigenous health prior to the reservation era were epidemic diseases such as smallpox, malaria, influenza, and measles, such statistics show that the twentieth century brought a new onslaught of ailments, often tied to the impacts of colonialism, including changes in diet and lifestyle. Throughout Native America a reliance on commodity issue foods and a loss of traditional subsistence activities has led to rising rates of obesity, diabetes, and heart disease. Heart disease remains the leading cause of death among the general American Indian and Alaska Native population. It is the number one cause of death for people over sixty-five (the same is true of the general population), but it is also the leading cause of death for people under forty-five.[16] Yvette Roubideaux has argued that diabetes was rare among Native communities prior to World War Two. As she points out, "There were no words in traditional languages for diabetes; pictures from the 1800s of [American Indians and Alaska Natives] show healthy, thin, fit individuals; and the messages of traditional Indian medicine include messages that encourage keeping active, eating healthy foods in moderation, and being mindful of the health of the community as well."[17]

Like diabetes, cancer appears to have been rare among previous generations of Native people, becoming increasingly common only since the 1940s. Cancer is now the leading cause of death for Alaska Native women, the second leading cause of death for Alaskan Native men, and the third leading cause of death for American Indian and Alaskan Natives overall.[18] Many scholars conclude that growing toxicity in the natural environment, poor detection and treatment availability, and poor diet and lifestyles have contributed to growing rates of heart disease, diabetes, cancer, and obesity.

The ability of Native people to engage in subsistence activities and eat traditional foods has been systematically undermined by centuries of federal policies designed to "free" Native lands for settlement. For instance, the Dawes Act of 1887 (also known as the General Allotment Act or Dawes Severalty Act) established a policy of assigning parcels of reservation land to Native individuals and thus freeing "surplus" land for white settlement. The result was the breaking up of collective ownership and resource management and the subsequent loss of enormous amounts of reservation land. In some areas Indian-held land was reduced by as much as 95 percent after the Dawes Act was implemented. A policy shift in the 1930s, led by John Collier and embodied by the Wheeler-Howard Act (also known as the Indian New Deal), established tribal governments and reversed many federal policies, moving away from the eradication of Native cultures and toward their preservation. However, termination and relocation policies of the 1950s and 1960s marked a return to some earlier policies, seeking to terminate tribal status and claims to tribal land by relocating Native people to urban centers.[19]

Such policies targeted at the removal of Native people from their ancestral land base had a particularly traumatic effect upon Native health and well-being. As contemporary tribal mental health workers have argued, land plays a key role in mental health because of its role in community and familial cohesion: "Each tribal group 'belongs' to a general area or tract of land which they hold in a sort of sacred trust, but which they do not 'own' per se." The division of tribal lands under allotment policies "did a great deal to destroy the basic foundation of the communal lifestyle of Indian people," while relocation to urban centers contributed to depression, isolation, poverty, and homelessness.[20]

This history took an important turn with the cultural revival of the 1970s. While what many have referred to as the "Red Power" movement had its roots in political and cultural organizations that had begun decades earlier, it was the nationwide American Indian political resurgence of the 1970s that brought the movement into full flower. These years saw a renewed sense of pride in Native heritage and a revitalized commitment to and engagement in religious and cultural traditions. This era also saw implementation of the Boldt Decision (1974), a pivotal moment for many Washington State tribes, which determined that Native communities had a legal treaty right to half the annual salmon harvest.[21] Salmon, which had been at the heart of traditional Native subsistence and spirituality, quickly became a central concern for many tribes in the region as they revived annual first salmon ceremonies and allied with other tribes to protect salmon habitat and restore salmon runs.

Legislation enacted during the 1970s also set key precedents for the decades to come. The Indian Self-Determination and Education Assistance Act (1975) granted federal support to tribes wishing to take local control of education, healthcare, and social service programs, and over the next thirty years more and more tribes would build their own schools, health clinics, and wellness centers. Likewise, the 1978 American Indian Religious Freedom Act (AIRFA) supported tribal autonomy and cultural cohesion through a declaration of Native people's legal right to practice traditional religions, formally ending centuries-long federal policies that actively suppressed Native religious practices.[22]

Spiritual revival, political mobilization, economic growth (due in part to the Indian Gaming Regulatory Act of 1988, making tribal casinos possible), and the return of subsistence activities under the Boldt Decision have all contributed to the present moment. Contemporary cultural renewal in the Pacific Northwest is powerfully illustrated by a growing revival of traditional canoe culture, within the annual intertribal canoe journey in which teams from coastal and Puget Sound tribes journey hundreds of miles in traditionally built canoes. Thousands of people participate in this month-long event, culminating in a week of ceremony and celebration.

Religious life in the region has also been transformed by a return of first salmon ceremonies and the revival of traditional winter spirit dances (also known as the longhouse or smokehouse tradition). First salmon ceremonies celebrate the return of salmon each year, affirming tribal communities' kinship with salmon and their commitment to preserving and restoring salmon runs for future generations. A fish is caught, ceremonially brought to shore, and welcomed with song and drumming. The fish is carefully filleted, and everyone present receives a single bite of it. Every bone is collected and ritually returned to the water, so that the fish might be reborn and return in future years. Winter spirit dancing has also seen a dramatic revival since the 1970s, with more and more individuals being initiated into the longhouse each year. In all-night ceremonies, participants sing and dance, honoring their individual spirit powers and singing the songs of their ancestors. Such religious and cultural revivals demonstrate how Native nations, while still struggling against the deep wounds of colonialism, are gathering cultural, economic, and spiritual resources to address those wounds.

Chapters 5 and 6 take place within this recent history, with two case studies of contemporary Coast Salish and Chinook communities exemplifying this movement toward cultural revival and local management of health and social services. I take a close look at two community-based wellness programs, examining them in light of the historical and cultural background earlier presented. Chapter 5 addresses the Women's Wellness Program of the South Puget Intertribal Planning Agency and how its efforts to promote health and wellness among Native women reflect traditional practices and beliefs about what it means to be a healthy individual. While identification with one's tribe and heritage remain strong, equally important in this part of Native America is a broader sense of kinship, and tribal groups continue to work together toward shared goals. This is well exemplified in the approach SPIPA takes. Within this organization, five relatively small tribes have joined together to work toward common goals of sustaining their communities and offering a variety of social services. SPIPA coordinates efforts among the tribes to meet the needs of the whole person and the whole community. Such collaborative intertribal efforts reflect Salish notions of community and kinship, adapting them to address contemporary challenges. In this chapter I argue that the program, while at first glance quite different from nineteenth-century approaches to wellness, is in fact building on traditional modes of approaching healing. While cultural expressions have changed, many of the core beliefs and values about the self, the body, and wellness have remained the same.

Chapter 6 brings us back to the Shoalwater Bay tribal community. I examine how this community has responded to the era of tragic pregnancy losses on the reservation by shaping a collective consensus of what it means to be "healthy," and applying this to community-led healthcare programs, support systems, environmental quality controls, and the Wellness Center dedicated in May 2005.

The final section of the book explores the ways in which Coast Salish and Chinook cultures understand the nature of the self and what it means to have a healthy working identity. While recognizing that Coast Salish traditions can vary widely from community to community and family to family, this section provides an overview of Coast Salish and Chinook perspectives on self and healing, tracing how traditional views and practices have survived into the contemporary era. Chapter 7 explores the relationship between self and community in Coast Salish and Chinook cultures; chapter 8 looks at the relationship between self and place; and chapter 9 lays out Coast Salish and Chinook understandings of illness and approaches to healing.

Concluding this discussion, I return to an analysis of the life and death of Ellen Gray in light of the historical and cultural data. Her poignant story provides a tragic illustration of how the body and the self act as locations of symbolic and material negotiations, the space wherein power relations are expressed, resisted, and experienced within the lives of Native people. My hope is that this project honors Ms. Gray and gives voice to stories as yet unheard, by contributing both to the ongoing conversation about the nature of embodiment and subjectivity and to the very material concern of improving healthcare for Native people.

One

Locations

1. Theoretical Orientation

Embodied Subjectivity and the Self in Motion

> The soul of sickness is closer to the self than the cell.
>
> —ROBERT HAHN, *Sickness and Healing: An Anthropological Perspective*

The two main questions addressed in this book are: what does it mean to be a healthy self in Coast Salish and Chinook communities, and how have these views changed over time? Before discussing the communities and cultures in question, in this chapter I set out to define some key terms and lay the philosophical groundwork for the project as a whole. For instance, what, exactly, do I mean by "healing," "wellness," and "illness"? Talking about these issues raises some tricky questions: what exactly do we mean by the "self"? How do people understand the relationship between the self and the body, or what I call the "embodied subject"? And how *should* we talk about bodies? As odd as it may sound at first, an entire philosophical and theoretical discussion has grown up around the question of whether we can even talk about bodies or, at least, what the best way to do so may be. This ongoing conversation has centered on a debate between those concerned with the semiotics of embodiment (how the body is constructed through language and culture) and those who see such reflection as working against materialist (political and economic) concerns.

The study of Native American traditions contributes to this conversation by providing models of thought that consider *both* the symbolic language used to construct and give meaning to bodily experience *and* the material consequences of those symbolic processes. This is particularly important in Indian Country, where language and symbol systems can have profound implications for people's material and spiritual well-being. Studies drawing on Native American epistemologies (ways of knowing) articulate indigenous philosophies that engage with the intersection of meaning and bodily experience. Overall, this chapter positions this project within larger theoretical conversations, discussions that extend beyond Native American studies, because I believe Native cultures and worldviews have something to contribute to such conversations. My assertion is not simply that these theories can help provide interpretive lenses for understanding Native cultures but that Native cultures have valuable insights to contribute as well.

Illness, Disease, and a Working Identity

In order to understand better the approaches to healing, illness, and disease among Coast Salish and Chinook communities, we first need to understand what it means to be a healthy self, how the self relates to the body (or the embodied subject). By *disease* I mean a discrete diagnosis or particular ailment that has been identified and categorized as such, typically by a biomedical physician. Such ailments are "cured" by locating and removing a particular cause and eliminating the isolated disease. In contrast, I understand *illness* to be a much broader term, reflecting "an inability to be one's self." When I talk about *healing*, I am talking about restoring what Jerome Levi has called a "working identity," the self that one is meant to embody within one's particular social and cultural context.[1] This involves wellness on a physical, spiritual, psychological, social, political, and economic level. It is fundamentally the *ability to be one's self.*

For present purposes, then, I define healing as the process of (re) constructing what Jerome Levi refers as a working identity and restoring a person to a sense of wholeness—a state of being that does not always entail doing away with the "disease" in question (although one certainly hopes it will). This, of course, immediately calls into question what one means by *working identity.* If it is "the self one is meant to be," as understood within one's culturally and individually specific locale, what is this *self* that has been compromised and needs to be re-created? This is important because the way healing is approached depends upon how this self is understood and, in particular, the way the relationship between self and body (the embodied subject) is understood. As various scholars and theorists have pointed out in recent years, both "self" and "body" are *culturally* specific notions, made up of factors that are geographical, social, economic, political, cultural, and spiritual. Selfhood is also *individually* specific, reflecting one's unique location within one's community and family. Among American Indian communities this becomes an even more complex scenario, where individuals may have to negotiate multiple working identities—those that meet the needs of their home community and that of the dominant culture.

As medical anthropologists Arthur Kleinman (1988) and Robert Hahn (1996) have shown, understandings of what it means to be healthy, the origins of disease, and modes of healing directly reflect particular social and cultural understandings of personhood. And as scholars of cross-cultural medical systems can attest, healing, religion, and philosophical worldviews are inextricably intertwined. The embodied self is shaped by religious, philosophical, political, economic, and medical worldviews and experiences. As Arthur Kleinman has argued, "To understand how symptoms and illnesses have meaning, therefore, we first must understand normative conceptions about the body in relation to the self and the world." Such understandings "inform how we feel, how we perceive mundane bodily processes, and how we interpret those feelings and processes. . . . Illness takes on meaning as suffering because of the way this relationship between body and self is mediated by cultural symbols of a religious, moral, or spiritual kind."[2]

Medical anthropologist Robert Hahn has likewise explored the nature of the self as revealed in cultural understandings of illness, arguing that different notions of the embodied self lead to different understandings of illness. Hahn defines illness as "an unwanted condition in one's person or self" and argues that healing is intrinsically connected to the creation and maintenance of that self.[3] To understand local definitions of illness it thus becomes necessary to grasp understandings of the embodied self within that community. "For example, whereas disturbances in the capacity for independence may be regarded as pathological in the West, disturbances in the capacity for interdependence may be regarded as pathological elsewhere."[4] As Hahn has argued, "the soul of sickness is closer to the self than the cell."[5] From this perspective, illness compromises one's ability to be the person one is meant to be, to fulfill one's healthy working identity.

Understandings of health and illness do not merely reflect the construction of individual identity but extend to the construction of community identity as well. For instance, Deborah Lupton has argued in her work on public health policies that "'health' has become a way of defining the boundaries between Self and Other, constructing moral and social categories and binary oppositions around gender, social class, sexuality, race, and ethnicity."[6] As we shall see later, communities define "health" in ways that reflect their sense of a proper life, well lived, and use this as a barometer by which to distinguish themselves from "others" who live differently. These culturally distinct modes of perceiving the body, and the unique religious expression that these perceptions take, have provided and continue to provide the foundations for healing and the perception of health within the communities explored in this text.

However, understanding what illness, selfhood, and embodiment mean to people is no simple matter. Kleinman calls for an ethnographic approach that allows individuals and communities to voice these "culturally salient illness meanings" within their social, political, and spiritual context.[7] By listening to individuals' illness narratives, we can gain a fuller picture of the way individuals understand illness and experience wellness. I return to this notion of illness narratives toward the end of this chapter. But first, it is important to locate the theoretical perspective that I bring to this project within broader comparative conversations about the nature of the body and the self.

Body Talk: Locating This Project

Talking about healing and wellness brings us into an ongoing theoretical debate about the nature of the body and how best to approach the body and embodiment within scholarly work. On one side of this seemingly endless debate are theorists who might be identified as "idealists." These writers are deeply committed to theorizing about and deconstructing the origins of language and culture—often in increasingly abstract language. At its extreme, bodies are purely the products of culture and language: they almost cease to exist. Like the bodies they talk about, the language of these theorists can also become almost entirely inaccessible, particularly to nonacademic audiences, and so is often considered unhelpful for those on the political frontlines. Critical of this approach are Marxist materialists, for whom anything that smacks of postmodern theorizing (or reflecting on the nature of culture and how we know things) is a distraction from time that should be spent talking about *real* material economic concerns. My aim it to chart a middle path between these extremes. I am primarily concerned with the material well-being of Native people; my topic is bodies—sick and healthy—and it is hard to get more material than that.

At the same time I believe that theory can make an important contribution to the discussion. If we do not take the time to think critically and analytically about why we see the world the way we do, it is that much more difficult to *change* the way we see and live in the world. This is important because the stories we tell ourselves about our bodies and our bodily experiences *matter*. These narratives fundamentally shape our sense of personal and collective identity. They shape our values and priorities and the ways in which we treat others. In the case of Native America, the stories that have been told about indigenous bodies and embodiment have had dramatic repercussions for the survival of Native people. To understand the implications of these issues better, it is helpful to explore this philosophical debate more fully.

BODIES AS CULTURAL SYMBOL

Those philosophers and theorists most strongly influenced by idealism have concluded that the body and the embodied self can only be accessed and analyzed through a study of symbolic (or *semiotic*) language and discourse. The embodied subject is seen as being inscribed or created by cultural, religious, economic, and philosophical systems that work to construct bodily experiences of gender, health, and wellness. Within this view, the body itself nearly vanishes, reduced to a culturally derived system of symbols that work to construct the body and our experience of the body.

The history of this theoretical approach within Religious Studies can be traced back to Marcel Mauss, who argued as early as the 1950s that bodily actions and embodied activities were not simply the natural or inevitable result of biology but that our basic bodily activities were culturally constructed and learned through socialization.[8] For Mauss, "the body is at the same time the original tool with which humans shape their world, and the original substance out of which the human world is shaped."[9] The work of Mary Douglas (1973) added to Mauss's description, as she discussed the use of the body in social symbols and the role of bodily purity in religious and cultural practice.[10] For Douglas and the emerging field of Religious Studies, embodiment raised the question of "how exactly corporeal practices mediate social meanings and transform them (or vice versa)"?[11] Such observations would serve to guide the study of ritual and ceremony as the means by which the body is inscribed by culture and works to create religious and philosophical systems.[12]

Michel Foucault moved the discussion of embodiment from the realm of ritual practice to that of politics, discourse, and power relations.[13] Foucault's work helped to point out that medical systems are the result of culturally specific moments in history. Foucault makes the case that all medical systems, including western biomedicine, are formulated and directly influenced by the religious, philosophical, political, and economic worldviews in which they take shape. In *Birth of the Clinic*, for instance, Foucault argues that if not for the unique historical positioning of western capitalism, Protestantism, and enlightenment philosophy, the biomedical approach to the body would not have been possible. Foucault explored biomedicine's origins in the shifts during the seventeenth and eighteenth centuries away from living patients and toward the analysis of dead bodies.

As the dissection of cadavers came to be the source of information about living bodies, western medicine was fundamentally altered. This new medicine was entirely material, focused on the body as static flesh rather than as a dynamic process of interaction with the environment.[14] What Foucault argued, convincingly, was that the modern biomedical view of the person-in-a-body was the result of a unique moment in western history, one that was informed by specific philosophical, economic, political, and religious sensibilities.[15] This view is useful when reflecting on the imposition of biomedicine on colonized peoples. Biomedicine was seen by colonial authorities as the only rational way to approach healing, a perspective entirely overlooking the fact that biomedicine itself was the product of a particular cultural moment.

Many feminist scholars have gone on to reinterpret Foucault's work (which virtually ignores gender), finding his approach useful toward the overall project of deconstructing cultural perceptions of the gendered body, revealing hierarchical power relations and the modes of coercion and constraint inherent in those relations.[16] This idea of the cultural construction of the body has been instrumental in challenging race- and gender-based biological determinism. Denise Riley, for instance, has critiqued the notion of the female body as "that obstinate core of identification, purity, and mothering which helps to underpin the appeal to 'women's experience.'"[17] The point is that if gender expectations are learned, rather than innate, they can be changed. Once cultural narratives have been thoroughly deconstructed, she argues, "both 'the body' and 'women's bodies' will have slipped away as objects, and become instead almost trace phenomena which are produced by the wheelings-about of great technologies and politics. . . . In a strong sense, the body is a concept, and so is hardly intelligible unless it is read in relation to whatever else supports it and surrounds it."[18] For Riley, the body "becomes visible *as* a body, and *as* a female body, only under some particular gaze, including that of politics."[19]

Judith Butler has carried this conversation further, arguing that any material foundation of bodies that might exist is entirely inaccessible: bodies can only be experienced or accessed through language. Hence, for Butler, there is no body that is not socially constructed. As she argues, "there is no reference to a pure body which is not at the same time a further formation of that body."[20] Butler argues that gender, sex, and embodiment are processes of performativity. When we perform our gender and ritually repeat cultural norms, Butler argues, we are bringing bodies into being. Cultural definitions of the normal and the abject define those bodies that are allowed to "matter" and those that *do not matter.* The body is a "historically contingent nexus of power/discourse," creatively determined by the unique historical positioning in which it is located.[21]

Foucault, Riley, and Butler have worked toward a deconstruction of the body and the self so as to uncover hidden power relations, the hierarchies and the inequalities that perceptions of the body quietly reinforce. Such scholars have argued that this deconstructing of the embodied self is a necessary step toward political change and personal renewal.[22] While Butler's notion of the body might be said to appear passively constrained by the power inherent in culture and society, she does disrupt assumptions about the nature of the embodied subject in a useful way. The embodied subject here is problematized, taken "outside the terms of an epistemological given."[23] In opening up such categories, one might argue, possibilities for change and resistance become available.

Perhaps most important for this project is the way in which Foucault and those who came after him have complicated the idea of "power" and pointed out the ways in which marginalized communities exert power of their own. Within Foucault's writing, power (a force or energy that is pervasive, omnipresent), ought not to be confused with domination (the expression of unequal power, used to control and constrain a person or population).[24] For Foucault, power is not simply something held by one party and used to subjugate another but rather that which exists between groups and individuals, within hidden mechanisms that both support and challenge unequal and hierarchical relationships. Power relations thus act as "matrices of transformation," which are not static, but constantly changing over time, and moving in more than one direction.[25] As Jana Sawicki has argued, populations are subjected to relations of power, but "wherever there is power, there is (always) resistance."[26] This notion is helpful when considering communities' responses to colonialism. Embodiment, health, healthcare, and Native responses to colonization take place within a complex network of power relations, wherein resistance can occur in unexpected places, and in subtle ways.[27] Given this, ahistorical statements about Native acquiescence, victimization, or accommodation to colonization are at best reductionistic and at worst simply inaccurate. Looking at history through the lens of a more nuanced notion of power, one can see that resistance to colonization can exist where least expected and that the negotiation of power is never complete. This nuanced notion of power also encourages one to consider the role the body plays within networks of power relations, acting as the very site where power relations are inscribed, resisted, and transformed. According to Foucault, the body can be seen as text, inscribed with the discourses of power, in a nuanced movement of accommodation and resistance. In similar ways, Native communities continue to engage in acts of creativity, negotiation, and resistance that center on the ways in which the body is perceived, health is understood, and healing is pursued.

These theoretical perspectives can be helpful, then, in pointing out several key ideas. First, they highlight the culturally specific nature of the body, illness, and gender. Second, they point out that such narratives are part of ongoing power relations. Euroamerican and Native illness narratives, for instance, can tell us as much about politics and identity as they do about people's experiences of illness. Finally, these more nuanced notions of power relations help to call attention to the sometimes covert and often creative ways in which Native people responded to colonial encounters.

The Marxist Materialist Critique: Bodies in the Flesh

To that end, it may also be helpful to consider a very different theoretical approach to the body, one held by scholars often informed by Marxist theory who have balked at the approach exemplified by Foucault and Butler. These authors argue that a focus on the culturally constructed nature of the body ignores material economic concerns. They contend that the deconstruction of body, self, or identity as mere cultural constructions prevents political mobilization and genuine social change. Forget symbols, language, and processes of cultural construction, they argue: focus instead on economic and political disparities that affect the self within that body. Consider for instance Terence Turner's critique of Foucault, in whose work he sees "a focus on conceptual or linguistic representations of the body and an indifference to the body as an objective physical reality." As far as Turner is concerned, "Foucault's body has no flesh."[28]

To some degree I share this critique of theoretical approaches that reduce the body purely to culture and language or that suggest the body can never be accessed directly. Anyone who has experienced childbirth, extreme hunger, thirst, or injury can attest to the fact that there are moments when we transcend language and when the material reality of our bodies imposes itself upon us. Indeed, the ability to suggest that bodies as such are purely cultural constructs of language and culture seems to me to come from a place of enormous privilege, where the material needs of the body are so far at bay that one need not pay them mind. As Turner argues, focusing *too* extensively on the symbolic nature of language and how it shapes our view of the body can lead us to miss some very pragmatic concerns.

Turner also argues that Foucault's notion of power as existing within a state of constant negotiation without end leaves no room for resistance: one can never escape these networks of power. Hierarchies can never be undone, only shifted. The result, Turner argues, is a depoliticizing move that advocates acquiescence to the status quo.[29] Feminist theorist Terese Ebert likewise critiques theories concerned with the deconstruction of discourse and identity, seeing them as inherently apolitical. As she writes, such approaches are "aimed at extending middle-class privileges—especially the free consumption of pleasures and fulfillment of desires—instead of engaging social change as the fundamental restructuring of the relations of production in order to end exploitation and provide all people with equal distribution of social resources."[30] And as Gail Weiss has argued, an overemphasis on the cultural construction of our bodies "runs the danger of disembodying them by presenting them as merely the discursive effects of historical power relations" and, in doing so, ignoring the very physical realities that continually shape the ways in which the body is experienced and understood.[31]

Further, as many scholars have pointed out, deconstructing bodies, selves, and modes of identity runs the risk of dismantling those very categories of identification that make political mobilization and meaningful living a possibility. As identities and essentialist categories have been challenged by poststructuralist theorists, many marginalized communities have reacted by claiming that such categories are in fact necessary for political action to occur. If feminists deconstruct the concept of "woman," how can women join as a political force? If terms such as "Native" or "Indigenous" are made meaningless, then on what basis can American Indian peoples stake a claim for identity, for community, for rightful ownership of their land? How can individuals craft a meaningful identity when the identifiers they rely on have become unstable? These questions are vital to the discussion at hand. I would argue that deconstructing Euroamerican inscriptions of the Native body can help make clear the hidden power relations and modes of domination within colonial history. But the same gaze may also be counterproductive when turned upon Native discourse. In what can all too easily become a recolonizing move, theorists who would seek to deconstruct Native narratives about their own identity run a risk of effectively creating a depoliticized space that reinforces colonial hierarchies.[32] As Aaron Glass has argued in his study of Kwak'waka'wakw ritual, while it is useful to challenge the racial stereotypes of the past, arguments about the cultural construction of contemporary Native identity run the risk of denying the authenticity of cultural creativity. Glass writes: "Anthropology has spent the last century helping to dismantle the notion of racial determinism, arguably in the best interests of Native people. . . . [But] now deconstructivist, academic theories of culture threaten to undermine aboriginal performance of culture."[33]

Such arguments raise the question: can scholars reflect critically upon the cultural construction of bodies and identities without losing sight of on-the-ground political concerns? Does a study analyzing Euroamerican and Coast Salish understandings of the embodied self simply work to reify inequalities by ignoring the real material concerns of Native populations? If one concludes that bodies are culturally constructed, or if they are the blank matter upon which cultural narratives are inscribed, if they have no meaning outside of language, then must one not also conclude that illness, pregnancy loss, poverty, colonialism, and *genocide* are merely linguistic constructs without material consequences? That is a conclusion I am certainly not willing to make. When turning to the study of health and the body, it seems to me imperative to remember that these stories, while shaped by cultural locations, are still the stories of living, breathing, bleeding, sometimes painful, sometimes healing bodies. I would argue that regaining a sense of embodiment, of living within a body, while simultaneously recognizing the role of culture and language in how one experiences that body, is a difficult but necessary challenge, for the body itself is the location where any resistance can occur.[34]

A Middle Way: Symbols with Consequences, Bodies with Agency

There are two important and interrelated issues here. The first concerns whether or not critical reflection upon why and how we think about the *body* as we do can be done without losing track of the body as a physical, material reality. The second is whether or not one can deconstruct the self, and its attendant personal and political identities, without stripping groups and individuals of the power to define themselves and so mobilize for change. Indeed, central to my argument is that people-in-bodies (embodied subjects) are at the same time shaped by their cultural context *and* are conscious, acting entities that challenge political structures and change their world. The embodied subject is shaped by its cultural context, but it also actively works to transform that context in turn. While Butler has argued that thinking about how the body is constructed by culture "is not opposed to agency, it is the necessary scene of agency."[35] I would agree with other scholars who insist that recognition of the material presence of the body is necessary to affirm individual and collective agency to resist domination. As Monique Deveaux has argued, deconstructivist theories can treat individuals "as cultural sponges rather than active agents."[36] Susan Bordo, in a similar move, has likewise argued that postmodern theories ignoring the material reality of bodies miss locations of resistance, of agency, and of the real embodied consequences that cultural discourse carries. The body, she argues, should be seen "as a battleground, rather than a postmodern playground."[37] For Bordo, the materiality of the body *must* be considered alongside its discursive expression, in order for politico-economic realities and possibilities for resistance to be recognized.

On this theoretical middle ground one recognizes that economic and political inequalities are reinforced, maintained, and resisted through symbolic means, and hence it is worthwhile to understand and interpret the symbol systems that are at play. At the same time, it is the body itself that has the agency and resiliency to subvert, affect, and influence the way cultural narratives become inscribed on it.[38] As Elizabeth Grosz has argued, "Far from being an inert, passive, noncultural and ahistorical term, the body may be seen as the crucial term, the site of contestation, in a series of economic, political, sexual, and intellectual struggles."[39] Camilla Griggers has also been successful at integrating the discussion of cultural sign systems with a Marxist materialist critique of the politico-economic conditions that set those signs in place. It is necessary, she argues, first to decode the sign in order to break down the inequalities that it perpetuates.[40] The lived experience and the representation of that experience are both important and can be differentiated, as Janis Jenkins and Martha Valiente have described them, as "raw" bodily experiences and "'cooked' linguistic, ethnopsychological representation."[41]

Scholarship within the relatively new field of environmental history provides a helpful example of moving toward this middle path. Since the 1970s environmental historians have wrestled with how to portray the body as both a symbol and a material reality that suffers under dangerous conditions.[42] In the 1970s historians such as Alfred Crosby, William Cronon, and Carolyn Merchant began considering bodies, and Native American bodies in particular, as metaphors for thinking about the histories of epidemic disease. Concurrently, Conevery Valencius argued that the symbolic language around bodies and illness revealed how people viewed their surrounding landscape.[43] In the 1990s the scholarly conversation took a radical shift away from this attention to symbolic language and toward a focus on the material consequences of labor conditions and environmental contamination.[44] By the beginning of the twenty-first century environmental historians had come to a middle path, concerning themselves with both the cultural significance of bodies and how those cultural constructions translate into material consequences. Linda Nash, for instance, carried on Valencius's analysis, exploring how settlers in California's Central Valley viewed their bodies in relationship to the surrounding landscape. Early settlers, she argued, saw a clear interrelatedness between the health of their bodies and the health of the landscape. However, when older understandings of well-being, based on humors, vapors, and miasmas, gave way to modern germ theory, people lost this sense of a connection between body and place. But with the increasing awareness of the impact of pesticides on both human and ecological well-being, this view of body and place as being tied together has found a rebirth.[45] The work of Gregg Mittman is also important here, demonstrating how understandings of diseases are relational and place-based and how illnesses take on meaning within particular social and economic contexts.[46] This most recent scholarship shares an engagement *both* with the locally specific culturally constructed nature of bodies and places and with how those meanings translate into the material experience of illness, labor, and leisure.

Such approaches are important to consider if the goal is a fuller and more nuanced understanding of both raw embodied experience and the way that experience is understood by Native and non-native peoples. From this perspective, discourses around the body do indeed reinforce relations of power and inequality that have concrete and material consequences.[47] The history of Native communities brings this notion into sharp relief. The stories told about illness and embodiment are not merely postmodern wordplay but translate into very tangible realities: governmental policies, missionaries' programs, tribal initiatives, and individual illness experiences.

This middle ground can be vital when considering Native and Euroamerican discourse about what it means to be a healthy self, and what the proper relationship between self, body, and community ought to be, because in between the diseases themselves and the illness narratives told to make sense of them is the space for personal and collective transformation.

Getting Local: Illness Narratives and Standpoint Theory

If one is to follow this middle way, arguing that yes, bodies materially exist, *and* it is worthwhile to think about why we experience them the way we do, what then? If we have determined that definitions of health and illness cannot be understood apart from the embodied subject, how are we to get at these elusive notions, particularly when talking across cultures? If the goal is to get at culturally distinct notions of embodied subjectivity—an endeavor that requires considering cultural location, material experience and religious worldview—it is helpful to return to Arthur Kleinman's illness narratives.

Illness narratives recognize the material reality of bodily experience, possibilities for agency and resistance within that body, and the culturally and religiously specific (and thereby potentially malleable) understandings of what it means to be a self-in-a-body. The goal of such an approach is to understand culture or personal experience as it is seen from within. Such cultural analysis enables one to gain a better understanding of the worldview and ethos that construct what it means to be a healthy self and of how that self can be reconstructed through healing techniques. It is the experiential view from within, of the body as lived, which might be said to unite symbolic discourse and material concerns: for the embodied self must live materially, but it must also live meaningfully.

Feminist standpoint theory has made the case for such local perspectives, seeking to situate the self within particular embodied experience. Emphasizing the *lived-body*, standpoint theory affirms the materiality of the body as well as its location in culture. As Susan Bordo has argued, "We are standing in concrete bodies, in a particular time and place, in the 'middle' of things, *always*. The most sophisticated theory cannot alter this limitation on our knowledge."[48] By reemphasizing this notion of positionality and location, standpoint serves as a possible middle ground between biological determinism and cultural relativism, offering methodological possibilities for getting at culturally specific views of the embodied self.[49] In many ways these perspectives serve as a direct challenge to one of the foundational voices with western philosophy: Rene Descartes.

Beginning with consciousness of his existence, Descartes (1596–1650) reasoned the existence of two separate spheres of human life: material body and intangible mind.[50] For Descartes truth was that which could be directly apprehended by the mind, and the mind became the arena of the self. This self was scarcely embodied: the conscious self was ontologically distinct from the body, which was a purely material, machinelike entity, bound by the laws of nature.[51] This disembodied subject was reflected within what would be called the master-subject of the Enlightenment: an autonomous, private self, separate from the public sphere, from society, and from the body. This subject, because of its ontological detachment from the material world, being only incidentally and temporarily housed within flesh, was capable of purely objective knowledge, capable of seeing the external world with an untainted eye, and also of critical self-reflection, of turning the eye inward. It had the ability to know everything from nowhere.[52] To put it another way, one's embodied location was irrelevant to true knowledge.

This Cartesian legacy was carried on within clinical medicine, which concentrated its efforts upon a body that was viewed as predictable, machinelike, and ruled purely by material causes.[53] While clinical medicine came to rely on radical materialism ("Is there a *real* cause of this illness, or is it *just in your head*?"), the mind was left to psychotherapy, and the soul was left to the church.[54] But this Cartesian legacy has been challenged by voices both within the Euroamerican tradition and without who have explored the interrelationship between self and body and have argued for the importance of embodied perception as a means of knowing. One of the most vocal of these is Donna Haraway.

Haraway argues that taking up these local, particular perspectives necessitates accepting that one can see only partially, that one's knowledge can never be universal. "The knowing self," she argues, "is partial in all its guises, never finished, whole, simply there and original; it is always constructed and stitched together imperfectly, and therefore able to join with another, and to see together without claiming to be another."[55] Haraway calls for such "situated knowledges," to emerge from "a doctrine of embodied objectivity."[56]

> We need to learn in our bodies . . . to name where we are and are not. . . . Objectivity turns out to be about particular and specific embodiment . . . only partial perspective promises objective vision. . . . I am arguing for politics and epistemologies of location, positioning, situating, where partiality and not universality is the condition for being heard to make rational knowledge claims. . . . I am arguing for a view from a body, always a complex, contradictory, structuring and structured body, versus the view from above, from nowhere, from simplicity.[57]

Haraway challenges universal truth claims, even those put forth by the sciences, insisting that even scientific scholarship "is a contestable text, and a power field."[58]

Attempting to gain a sense of culturally specific views of the embodied subject and to do so in ways that empower local identity making and political mobilizing requires what Chandra Mohanty describes as "historically and culturally specific" studies that involve "careful, politically focused local analysis."[59] Such studies should provide spaces for individuals to describe their embodied subject position: what they have learned from the unique standpoint that they hold as embodied subjects.[60]

While standpoint theory insists that objective universal knowledge is an impossible ideal, it does not suggest the abandonment of knowledge altogether. Rather, standpoint theorists suggest, if we do not pursue knowledge of "everything from nowhere," then we ought to pursue knowledge of "something from somewhere."[61] This sense of partial knowing, of knowledge grounded in embodiment, is an important element of this book, because it provides a means of considering the diverse, local, and particular nature of embodied subjects. It provides a means whereby culturally distinct expressions of health and wellness and unique approaches to healing can exist side by side, each with meaning, relevance, and efficacy. I do not claim to present *the* Euroamerican or *the* Native American view on health and wellness. Indeed, there is no such thing. Rather, my goal throughout is to present many different positions and standpoints, to observe common themes and trace common threads, but also to affirm the diversity of opinion, the multiplicity of perspectives.

How We Know: Perception and the Interrelational Self

Calling for a return to locally situated case studies and a focus on personal illness narratives brings us back to some of our original questions: what is this body and how do we know it? What relationship do "I" have with my body? Building on the work of Edmund Husserl (1859–1938) and Martin Heidegger (1889–1976), Maurice Merleau-Ponty (1908–61) argued that the key to understanding perception lay in the lived-body and being-in-the-world. The self exists in a body, and as such the external world is always mediated through the processes of perception. For Merleau-Ponty, perception is derived from fleshly experience as well as cultural significance. As he insists, "I am not in space and time, nor do I conceive space and time; I belong to them, my body combines with them and includes them."[62] It is the perceiving self as part of a perceiving world that lays the groundwork for all modes of thinking about the world.[63]

Merleau-Ponty has argued that at a perceptual level, our bodies are not objects to us but an integral part of ourselves as perceiving subjects. From the level of perception, it is then appropriate to ask *how* our bodies came to be objectified in the first place.[64] Merleau-Ponty suggests that it is through processes of reflection, through bringing experience into language, that the body becomes objectified.[65] For Merleau-Ponty some experience is indeed more *real* than other experience, being less obscured by culture or language (though never completely without them). The origins of perception and knowledge of this *real* lie in embodied experience.

Merleau-Ponty took this a step further, arguing that perception and embodied experience never exist in isolation but are in fact the result of dialogue and exchange between self and Other.[66] Perception of other people and of the earth itself is possible because that which is perceived is active, initiating.[67] Perception thus becomes a conversation, a relational exchange, between observer and observed. As Merleau-Ponty has put it, "every perception is a communication or a communion . . . of our body with things." The fallacy of objective thinking, he argues, is that it rejects "all phenomena which bear witness to the union of the subject and world, putting in their place the clear idea of the object as *in itself*, and of the subject as pure consciousness. It therefore severs the links which unite the thing and the embodied subject."[68] Rather, Merleau-Ponty calls for a return to perception from a body, in an embodied location, through which one can achieve a renewal of a sense of exchange, interaction, and relational perception with the world.[69]

Recognizing perception as intrinsically shaped both by embodied experience and by relationship to the world (its cultural as well as its ecological milieu) has led many writers to suggest a definition of the self that has more to do with orientation, position, and perspective than with disembodied detachment. Anthropologist Thomas Csordas, for instance, has suggested a definition of the self as an "indeterminate capacity to engage or become oriented in the world, characterized by effort and reflexivity."[70] In contrast to the Cartesian master-subject, the embodied self here is one that is not finite, bounded, or purely individual. Rather it is a location, an orientation, and dependent upon one's situation and relation to the surrounding social world. What then is the nature of the self? Csordas suggests, "Our answer might be that if it is elusive, it is because there is no such 'thing' as the self. There are only self processes, and these are orientational processes."[71] Such perspectives draw an image of the self that exists in a relationship of give and take with the social and ecological landscape in which it dwells.[72] From this perspective, the embodied subject is not so much a *thing* as a *process*.[73]

If the embodied self is not a thing, but rather a "process," then healing-as-self-making takes on new meanings as well.[74] Instead of "curing disease," healing becomes a means of orientation or direction within the ongoing experience of self-making and collective survival. Healing, as Csordas describes it, is a "self-process" located in the body, which "acts as the existential ground of the self." Simply put, *healing is the ongoing act of self-making*. It is not a finite destination but an ongoing experience.

Body and Self within Native American Healing Traditions

While all the theoretical approaches I have described seek to destabilize Cartesian dualism and the master subject, none appears to be successful. Foucauldian postmodern deconstructivist theory attempts to displace the subject and the body by examining the cultural narratives that go into constructing them. Marxist materialist scholars respond that such theoretical moves lose sight of the materiality of the body, of the economic and political structures that continue to oppress large numbers of disadvantaged communities. Feminists like Susan Bordo, Elizabeth Grosz, or Camilla Griggers have responded to this critique by seeking to embody both material bodies and their concerns with cultural analysis, while standpoint theorists have taken a similar approach, calling for situated local knowledges that are partial and perspectival. Other scholars such as Maurice Merleau-Ponty and Thomas Csordas have argued for a look at the lived-body as it is experienced from within. While these theoretical movements have gone far, they continue to struggle with the same theoretical dilemmas. No school of thought mentioned has been able to leave fully behind a distinctly western notion of the embodied subject: mind/body dualisms continue to surface in different guises. The culture/nature, body/spirit dichotomy remains: one or the other seems to be perpetually either dominant or entirely absent. One way to get beyond these dualisms, I would suggest, is to step outside western epistemologies and consider the worldviews and ways of knowing that can be found within the indigenous traditions of North America.

While scholars within Native American religious and cultural studies have not often made explicit connections with the theoretical conversations so far discussed, I would insist that they have a great deal to contribute, illustrating points of convergence and providing new perspectives on what it means to heal and to be a whole self. Indeed, one of my central goals in the present work is to bring Native perspectives into this conversation.

Within the field of Native American studies numerous scholarly works provide particular frameworks for thinking about the nature of the body and the self.[75] Discussions of Native American identities challenge notions of identity as static, arguing instead that Native identities have been multifaceted, complex, in-process, and continually in negotiation. Contemporary scholarship on Native American identities, for instance, makes clear the complex and seemingly paradoxical nature of personal identity.[76] Such studies describe many individuals working to affirm an identity that is indigenous (or Lakota, or Diné, or Coast Salish), even as they are continually reframing what that means, and how such identities can be sustained within the lived experience of contemporary America. Maureen Trudelle Schwarz, for instance, describes an *emerging self* within contemporary Diné (Navajo) healing and ceremonial traditions. As she explains, for the Diné, the self is a work-in-progress, where "personhood is developed gradually."[77]

In Therese O'Nell's work on healing traditions and understandings of mental health in the Flathead Nation, she discusses a similarly complex notion of identity. Intermarriage and varying degrees of engagement with the non-native world require individuals continually to negotiate and clarify their sense of self, for themselves and for others. As she explains:

> Thus not only do some Indian families become fragmented with the critical bifurcation of the world into Indian and white, good and bad, but ultimately *selves* are fragmented for some as well . . . being Indian is a complicated and high-stakes venture. Indian identity at the Flathead Reservation is not simply given—by formal enrollment, by birth, by degree of blood, by language, or by cultural practice. Nor is it consistent for individuals across all contexts. No set of core characteristics defines an essence of Indianness that remains valid at all times, for all people, in all places.[78]

O'Nell's work provides a rejoinder to those concerned about the depoliticizing potential within deconstructing essentialist categories of identity. In her experience, identities are not being challenged by abstract theorizing but by the people themselves. Their own lived experience is complex and multilayered. But the apparent challenge is not so much for Native people themselves, she suggests, who may experience their identity as "a seemingly paradoxical combination of several contexts," but rather for those who insist on "the supposition of a single essence of Indianness."[79]

Following her discussion of the complex and multifaceted nature of Native American identities, O'Nell goes on to point to the interrelational nature of self within Flathead culture, where individualism can be seen as a kind of pathology and interdependence as a sign that one is healthy and more closely modeling "really Indian" identities.[80] O'Nell describes a "psychology of interdependence" among this community, where depression has been construed in distinctly Flathead terms that reflect Flathead notions of the self. This is a community where depression is more commonly associated with loneliness. In a context where each person is seen as belonging to the collective, reinforced through modes of "reciprocity and social responsibility," loneliness and depression occur when that collectivity is compromised. As she writes:

> Loneliness expresses the anguish of finding oneself outside usual or expected relations of compassion and exchange. . . . [Loneliness is] the lament of the loss of "real Indians," [it is] a plaintive cry for compassion, for incorporation into networks of caring and exchange. . . . At base, this psychology of interdependence constructs the Flathead self as highly invested in making and maintaining of relationships, particularly family relationships. Within this psychology of interdependence, disruptions in or losses of relationships can be tantamount to disruption or loss of the self. . . . Loneliness, as it appears in Flathead narratives of individual and collective experience, is an idiom that seeks to reclaim the very relationships and identities it heralds as missing.[81]

The proper response to the loneliness of others is "pity," which O'Nell describes as the "local term that encapsulates the Flathead stance toward the interdependent self. Out of pity for those who are hungry, ill, grieving or simply lacking in something, mature persons are moved to generosity."[82] Loneliness and pity become the "key elements structuring interpersonal interactions at the Flathead Reservation."[83]

O'Nell's work challenges views of health and well-being that are based on Euroamerican models of individualized identity. Many other studies similarly emphasize local views of self that are based on concepts of interrelatedness, where the boundaries between self and other are porous or even nonexistent. As Judith Blackfeather argues in her analysis of Lakota culture, "The values and customs from the European perspective emphasize competition and independence, while the [Lakota] Indian community strives for interdependence, collective responsibility, and cooperation through a definitive hierarchy."[84] She argues that an emphasis on balance instead of competitive dualisms, of tribalism instead of individualism, often sets Native traditions apart from the dominant Euroamerican culture.[85] Richard Voss, Victor Douville, Alex Little Soldier, and Gayla Twiss agree, arguing that Lakota views of the self are such that "the notion of a separate, independent, individual ego is foreign to Lakota cosmology. Each person is a living testament as well as a collective legacy of his or her ancestral spirits and the spirits of creation.

. . . The boundaries between 'self' and 'non-self' are remarkably permeable and fluid, and . . . the self can cross interpersonal borders to include other people."[86] Voss and colleagues contend that the Lakota term *wicozani*, harmony and balance, fits this notion as well. Here, "balance" is not about an individual, perfectly poised, but a self that is maintaining "proper interconnections among family, tribe, and clan with moral, political, and ceremonial life."[87] This notion also calls to mind the Diné (Navajo) concept of *Sa'ah Naghai Bikeh Hozho*, a term that synthesizes the goals and ideals of Navajo spirituality. Scholars of Navajo religious traditions have offered numerous definitions, but most agree that this central phrase emphasizes a life lived in beauty, balance, and harmony with one's world.[88]

Other studies emphasize the interrelational nature of identity not only in terms of the human community but in terms of the natural landscape as well. In these texts, knowledge and personal identity are the result of embodied experience and come from being in relationship with particular places. Keith Basso, Crisca Bierwert, Richard Nelson and Robert Thornton, for instance, all discuss the way in which places (and the beings that inhabit them) participate in relationships with human beings. Places "speak" and play an active role in shaping human spiritual, social, and ethical worlds.[89] As Bierwert and Nelson emphasize in particular, these are relationships with sentient places that participate in ongoing living relationships that are continually being renegotiated and maintained.

The work of Basso, Bierwert, Nelson, and O'Nell, along with that of Voss and Blackfeather, present cultural perspectives on the self that emphasize the interrelational, processual self over the kind of static individualism seen within the classical Cartesian framework. In doing so, such case studies demonstrate that within these cultural systems, identity is something continually taking shape in the context of living, dynamic, and complex relationships. In the chapters that follow I explore these ideas within the context of Coast Salish and Chinook history and culture.

O'Nell's work also illustrates the importance of situating case studies within their particular cultural and historical contexts as she struggles to reconcile the diagnosis and definition of depression in the Diagnostic and Statistical Manual of Mental Disorders (DSM) with the way in which the ailment is understood by the Flathead themselves. Understanding the Flathead perspective, she explains, requires knowledge of the Flathead Nation's historical experience of colonialism, disease, death, place, and community. When she entered the community with the DSM definition of depression in mind, she was blinded "to the relational, historical, and moral meanings of Flathead 'depression.'"[90] As she explains, "the medicalized vision of 'depression'," which assumes a "universality," and "'givenness' of 'real depression' calls into question the primacy of cultural processes in human experiences of disorder, relegating culture to the marginal position of 'influencing' the universally recognizable disease of depression."[91] Depression means something very different for Flathead people, for whom "depression is the natural and esteemed condition of the 'real Indians,' those who have 'disciplined hearts,' those who have transformed their sadness over present and past losses into compassionate responsibility for others."[92]

Importantly, while O'Nell's work makes clear that the experience of pathology is culturally specific, she does not call for abandoning general categories, such as the diagnostic language within the DSM. Instead, she encourages scholars and clinicians to bring the DSM with them. Universalist categories are helpful, she insists, and in some ways essential for the work that needs to be done. At the same time, they should not be given a privileged place of authority, and should be continually subjected to reevaluation, in light of local interpretations and epistemologies.[93]

Studies of such "local interpretations and epistemologies" help illustrate the importance of illness narratives as tools for healing in American Indian communities. Eva Garroute (Cherokee) and Kathleen Westcott (Anishinaabe), for instance, have explained that such narratives allow a patient to "draw out the culturally located meanings of her medical situation, to contrast her own perspectives with those of her healthcare providers, and to explain the consequences of cultural knowledge for her medical decisions."[94] Other studies of personal illness narratives, such as Maureen Trudelle Schwarz's study of Diné cancer narratives, help to exemplify the way in which illness narratives both reveal the unique worldview and philosophy of the self and themselves work as tools for healing, affirming indigenous perspectives and traditions. The work of Michelle Jacob (Yakama), Garroute and Westcott, and Rodney Frey likewise illustrate the powerful way in which oral traditions and sacred stories function as means of meaning making within illness, and the (re)creation of a working identity, both for individuals and for tribal communities.[95]

Scholarship such as this makes clear that there is no simple, unitary way of thinking about the self or the embodied subject. The view of the self is culturally distinct and complex. Here are alternate modes of perceiving the embodied subject that strive to get beyond the classic Cartesian dualism and its finite, closed, or individualized self, while still allowing for a *self* to exist. The embodied self might be multiple, porous, communal, relational, interactive, reciprocally dependent, fluid, in transition, becoming, or a combination of these. But somehow, within those spaces of flux and negotiation, there remains space for political identity and collective sensibility. Native American religious and cultural studies demonstrate that understandings of illness are locally specific and culturally constructed, and that the stories and symbol systems constructed around bodily experience have had material, devastating consequences.[96]

Illness, Healing, and Cultural Genocide

By seeking to provide space for indigenous voices, perspectives, and experiences, I seek to articulate indigenous views, a "something from somewhere" that can challenge seemingly monolithic notions of the body, the self, and what it means to be healthy. And indeed, these different perceptions of the embodied subject are not merely opportunities for debate over discourse and symbol: they translate into the very material health and wellness of individuals and communities. Disease, illness, healing, spirituality, the suppression of indigenous approaches to health, and a history of federal policies that undermined the Native social structures and land base have presented persistent challenges to the spiritual and communal integrity of American Indian people. Such challenges have been manifest within and enacted through the bodies of Native people throughout Native North America, an experience sometimes referred to as "cultural genocide."[97]

The use of the term *genocide* is controversial at best and worth some discussion. The most commonly referenced legal definition of genocide comes from the United Nations Convention on the Prevention and Punishment of the Crime of Genocide, adopted in 1948. The legal definition is the "intent to destroy, in whole or in part, a national, ethnic, racial or religious group," by killing, "causing serious bodily harm . . . deliberately inflicting on the group conditions of life calculated to bring about its physical destruction . . . imposing measures intended to prevent births within the group," and "forcibly transferring children of the group to another group." The original draft of the resolution included a reference to "cultural genocide" as well, but this reference was removed from the final statement, reportedly at the behest of western nations who feared that their colonial interests might be construed as falling within this legal definition.[98]

Numerous historians have sought to make the case that the historical experience of American Indian people qualifies as a kind of genocide, citing the removal of children to boarding schools, nonconsensual sterilization of Native women, the impact of epidemic diseases, violence by the United States military, and vigilante massacres.[99] Others have opposed the use of the term, arguing that it was not the official policy of the United States government to eradicate Native people, and thereby "intent" to eliminate American Indians as a people remains to be proven.

Cultural genocide is not a legal term but one used by scholars of Native American culture and history as a way to call attention to the severity of the material consequences that result from the suppression and destruction of culture. George Tinker uses the term in his 1993 book *Missionary Conquest: The Gospel and Native American Cultural Genocide*. Tinker sets aside the question of intention. He argues that regardless of intent, cultural genocide can be defined as imposing "a new cultural model for existence on Indian people" and that the "destruction of Indian cultures and tribal social structures" resulted in "devastating impoverishment and death."[100] Tinker argues that individuals with "good intentions" can still be guilty of or complicit in cultural genocide. "Cultural genocide is more subtle than overt military extermination," he argues, "but is no less devastating to a people."[101] He goes on to define the term as

> the effective destruction of a people by systematically or systemically (intentionally or unintentionally to achieve other goals) destroying, eroding or undermining the integrity of the culture and system of values that defines a people and gives them life. . . . It involves the destruction of those cultural structures of existence that give a people a sense of holistic and communal integrity. It does this by limiting a people's freedom to practice their culture and to live out their lives in culturally appropriate patterns. It effectively destroys a people by eroding both their self-esteem and the interrelationships that bind them together as a community.

This includes an "attack on the spiritual foundations of a people's unity by denying the existing ceremonial and mythological sense of a community in relationship to the Sacred Other."[102] Tinker argues that cultural genocide is carried out in four ways: politically (through the loss of political autonomy), economically (through enslavement, exploitation, and pillaging of natural resources), religiously (by destroying "the spiritual solidarity of a people"), and socially (by profoundly disrupting the structures that create coherent communities).[103]

The term *genocide* evokes a strong emotional response, and perhaps that is why it is at times necessary. It calls our attention to the profound importance that culture, religion, and identity have for the material well-being of individuals and communities. The way we think about and approach bodies, health, wellness, and healing is not symbolic wordplay but literally a matter of life and death. My work can be situated within this larger conversation of cultural genocide because it illustrates the profound consequences of the loss of culture and identity.

At the same time, while it is important to make clear the material consequences of illness and the federal policies aimed toward the eradication of Native cultures and communities, I want to emphasize as strongly as possible that the story does not end there. While Native communities were in many ways devastated by their encounter with epidemic diseases, political and cultural suppression, the loss of land, and the loss of younger generations, they have also worked to rebuild bodies and communities. As this chapter has portrayed, power does not move in one direction. It is not simply held by a single group to be wielded over another. Rather, the relations of power between individuals and between communities are complex, continually in motion, continually being negotiated. Even federal policies have shifted and changed over time, moving from an era of overtly seeking the assimilation of Native people and the eradication of Native cultures to policies that have promoted and sought to protect Native cultural diversity.

This book contributes to a large corpus of work that complicates colonial narratives portraying Native people as victims confronted with the monolithic overpowering force of "civilization." Instead, Native people have responded creatively to political, economic, and social change, incorporating elements of colonial cultures, religions, and political systems in ways that ensured cultural, political, and physical survival. "Power" here is not unidirectional, nor is it the purview of a single group. Both Native people and non-native settlers operated and negotiated within complex networks of political, economic, social, and spiritual power. By examining the experience of the tribal communities on the lower Columbia River and around Puget Sound, we can see the central role of health, healing, and embodied ritual practice in indigenous responses to colonization. It is in the daily, lived experiences of Native communities that power relations are navigated, cultural creativity is allowed to flourish, and resistance is daily embodied.

The chapters that follow contribute to the growing scholarship on Native American healing traditions and understandings of the self. I return to this conversation in the conclusion, pointing out the ways in which Coast Salish traditions provide unique perspectives on the nature of the self, the embodied subject, and what it means to be healthy. It is my belief that for broader comparative theoretical conversations to get beyond the seemingly eternal idealist-materialist back and forth, we need to step outside Euroamerican tradition and consider indigenous understandings of the self that begin with fundamentally different ways of knowing and of being.

Two

Illness, Healing, and Missionization in Historical Context

2. "The Fact Is They Cannot Live"

Euroamerican Responses to Epidemic Disease

> So you see, Providence has made room for me, and without doing them more injury than I should if I had made room for myself, viz killing them off.
>
> —NATHANIEL WYETH, 1834

> This calamity which God sent these Indians on account of their abominable lives came to visit them every year, and always made some of them its victims.
>
> —REVEREND MODESTE DEMERS, 1845

In 1905, nearly seventy-five years after the first missionary arrived in western Oregon and Washington territories, Ezra Meeker wrote, "I have been trying for two years to find out something about missionary work at this point, but there is nothing left to find out. The fact is that religious work of the early missionaries among the Indians was a complete failure at Nisqually, Salem, the Dalles, Wailatpu, at Lapwai, and everywhere else."[1] Despite concerted efforts throughout the nineteenth century, Christian missions appeared to have had relatively little success in converting Native communities. One important reason for this failure was the impact of epidemic diseases and the different ways that Euroamericans and Native Americans made sense of and reacted to these illnesses.

This chapter offers an analysis of how nineteenth-century Euroamericans described, interpreted, and understood the epidemic diseases that struck Native Americans. It lays the groundwork for understanding the challenges contemporary communities face as a result of this historic devastation.[2] Euroamerican views of indigenous health and healing changed over time, and these changes shaped their approach to Native communities. This chapter is concerned with the early years of contact, primarily between traders and newly arrived missionaries.

At first Euroamericans described the Pacific Northwest in utopian terms, a place filled with a healthy, hardworking population who would soon be won over to the gospel. Within a few years, however, their letters and journals showed a dramatic shift. Confronted with staggering rates of disease, these early settlers were forced to modify their perspective. To a great degree Euroamericans blamed the soaring mortality rates on Native people themselves, their culture, their (im)morality, and especially their healing practices. I argue that because of a theology that left little room for ritual or embodied practice, early Protestant missionaries in particular were quick to abandon all hope, giving up their posts or turning their attention to Euroamerican settlers. Catholic missions encountered similar challenges. But while they shared a great deal with their Protestant counterparts, their sacramental theology enabled them to cope better with a sick and dying people. Because of a theology that imbued ritual practices such as baptism and last rites (also known as extreme unction) with salvific power, Catholic missionaries were able to proceed in the midst of vast suffering with some sense of success. While Protestant and Catholic missionaries agreed in many respects as to the nature and cause of epidemic diseases, their different theological views of the embodied subject shaped their different responses to those diseases.

Early Missionary History in the Pacific Northwest

The earliest Protestant missions in the Pacific Northwest arrived in the 1830s, though Christian influence had been present earlier through the unofficial—and at times unorthodox—presence of explorers and traders. Methodists Jason Lee, Cyrus Shepherd, and Philip Edwards arrived with some of the first settlers in the Willamette Valley in 1834, founding the first mission in Oregon Territory at Willamette Station in present-day Salem, Oregon. In 1836 Anglican Reverend Herbert Beaver founded a short-lived mission at Fort Vancouver, which lasted until the fall of 1838. Several missions followed east of the Cascade Mountains. In 1836 Congregationalist missions were founded among the Nez Perce by Henry and Eliza Spaulding, and among the Cayuse by Marcus and Narcissa Whitman, who would be slain in 1847. In 1837 a Spokane mission was founded at Tshimakain by Elkanah and Mary Walker, along with Cushing and Myra Eells. Protestant missions were virtually absent from the Puget Sound region until a "futile" attempt by Methodists David Leslie, William Holden Wilson, and Dr. John Richmond at Fort Nisqually, an effort that lasted only from the spring of 1839 until the fall of 1842.[3]

The earliest Catholic mission west of the Cascades was undertaken by Father Francois Blanchet and Father Modeste Demers, who established their mission on the Cowlitz River in 1838, where they worked to "regularize" métis marriages and instruct the Cowlitz and Nisqually.[4] In 1839 Blanchet created the Catholic Ladder, a graphic depiction of Biblical history that worked as a mnemonic device. The Ladder was given to twelve Lushootseed visitors who reportedly took the document with them back to Puget Sound.[5] (In 1845 Protestant missionaries Henry and Eliza Spaulding would create a "Protestant Ladder" to counter what they saw as Catholic propaganda.) In 1840, when Blanchet traveled north to Whidbey Island, he found that local leaders "had already taught their fellow villagers to make the sign of the cross and to sing verses of certain hymns" and were familiar with the Catholic Ladder.[6] But, astonished as he was to find Natives singing hymns, much remained to be done, and he was frustrated by the persistent presence of idolatry, gambling, and polygamy.[7] Catholic missions were undertaken east of the Cascades as well, organized by Pierre de Smet in 1842. Two of the most influential individuals in this region were Charles Pandosy and Eugene Casimir Chirouse, who ministered to the Yakama from 1848 to 1856.[8]

Despite this promising beginning, when Demers and Father J. B. Z. Bolduc visited the area only three years later in 1843, they found that interest in conversion had waned.[9] As Barbara Lane, Wayne Suttles, and June McCormick Collins have suggested, the initial wave of interest appears to have been politically motivated, as Salish leaders employed new rituals and rules as a temporary means of social control.[10]

History of Epidemics

The failure of early missions in this region cannot be understood without considering the impact of epidemic diseases on Native populations in the Pacific Northwest. Epidemics swept throughout the Northwest beginning as early as the 1770s, a full generation before Lewis and Clark visited the region. The devastation brought by subsequent waves of illness has been well documented in various historical sources but is worth briefly summarizing here.[11] Prior to the arrival of Europeans the most common causes of death among Native communities in western Washington appear to have been fishing and hunting accidents and complications arising from childbirth. Threats of starvation or food-borne toxins were rare, and while some contagious diseases were certainly present, morbidity as a result was less common.[12] This changed dramatically with the arrival of smallpox sometime between 1770 and 1790.[13] Robert Boyd argues that the first smallpox epidemic arrived in the 1770s, traveling down the coast from present-day British Columbia and Southeast Alaska to Oregon and moving inland as far as the interior Columbia Plateau.[14] These epidemics brought mortality rates ranging from 30 to 80 percent. The illness itself was only the beginning of the devastation, as survivors suffered from malnutrition due to the loss of subsistence providers and cultural breakdown as other social, economic, and ceremonial aspects of life were brought to a halt.[15] Smallpox epidemics recurred between 1800 and 1810; tuberculosis followed in the 1820s; measles arrived with the Hudson's Bay company in 1821; "fever and ague" (most likely malaria) decimated western Oregon and the Columbia River tribes in the 1820s and 1830s. Between 1835 and 1847 outbreaks of meningitis, smallpox, influenza, mumps, and dysentery are recorded. Measles would return in 1848 and smallpox in 1853. And throughout, syphilis and gonorrhea (likely introduced to the region by Euroamerican sailors in the late eighteenth century) spread among Native communities at devastating rates.[16] It has been estimated that Native populations in the Northwest declined by 88 percent between 1805 and 1855.[17] When the first traders, missionaries, and settlers arrived in this region, then, they encountered cultures and communities already decimated by disease and that had undergone profound social, cultural, and political change as a result.

Horatio Hale, philologist of the U.S. Exploring Expedition in the Pacific Northwest from 1828 to 1842 described the impact of one such epidemic:

> At the period of the visit of Lewis and Clark [the lower Columbia] was the most densely populated part of the whole Columbia region, and it so continued until the fatal year 1823, when the ague-fever, before unknown west of the Rocky Mountains, broke out, and carried off four-fifths of the population in a single summer. Whole villages were swept away, leaving not a single inhabitant. The living could not bury the dead, and the traders were obliged to undertake this office, to prevent a new pestilence from completing the desolation of the country. The region below the Cascades, which is as far as the influence of the tide is felt, suffered most from this scourge. The population, which before was estimated at upwards of ten thousand, does not now exceed five hundred.[18]

When the first Methodist and Catholic missionaries came to the Columbia River and the Willamette Valley in the 1830s and 1840s, they also witnessed the devastation wrought by disease. As Rev. George Gary wrote in his diary: "This day I had an interview with J. L. Parish, a local preacher from Clatsop, mouth of the Columbia River. . . . From his account of the Clatsop and Cheenooks Indians, they are passing away like the dew; there are but four children under a year old in both tribes. He thinks less than ten under six years old and over one. There are perhaps in the Clatsop tribe, 100; Cheenook, 300, including old and young."[19] Methodist missionaries Daniel Lee and Joseph Frost also reported their frustrations with the situation: "It had been reported that the Kilemooks [Tillamooks] were a numerous tribe of Indians, but they are like most of the other 'numerous tribes' in the country, very 'few and far between.'" Lee and Frost estimated their numbers at no more than two hundred in all. On February 26, 1842, Lee and Frost described the devastation around them: "But two children are now living out of ten or twelve that were born, to our knowledge, among the Indians of our neighborhood since last November, besides a number which were destroyed by their mothers in the earliest dawn of infancy. I saw several of those that died natural deaths, which were perfect masses of putrification before they expired, in consequence of disease which they inherited from their parents."[20] For missionaries, the loss of Native populations was not only tragic but a lethal blow to their own success: a successful mission required a healthy Native population to sustain it.

At the same time, for some Euroamericans advocating settlement, the devastation wrought by epidemics appeared to be a sign that God favored Euroamerican settlers rather than unbaptized Natives. As an 1844 commissioner of Pacific Northwest local government wrote: "This country has been populated by powerful Indian tribes, but it has pleased the Great Dispenser of human events to reduce them to mere shadows of their former greatness. Thus removing the chief obstruction to the entrance of civilization, and opening a way for the introduction of Christianity where ignorance and idolatry have reigned uncontrolled for many ages."[21] For advocates of Euroamerican settlement, epidemics were a tragedy but a providential one. Nathaniel Wyeth commented on the rapid demise of the inhabitants of Wappatoo Island (now Sauvie Island, on the Columbia River north of present-day Portland).[22] He wrote in September of 1834: "A mortality has carried off to a man its inhabitants and there is nothing to attest that they ever existed except their decaying houses, their graves, and their unburied bones of which there are heaps. So you see, as the righteous people of New England say, Providence has made room for me, and without doing them more injury than I should if I had made room for myself, viz killing them off."[23]

To make sense of such responses it is worthwhile to consider some of the key historical narratives at play within Euroamerican views of the body and the self. As the texts demonstrate, many of the dominant nineteenth-century Euroamerican approaches to the body emphasized control and constraint. Deborah Lupton has argued that the civilized body, as implied by early nineteenth-century observers, was one that was "controlled, rationalized, and individualized, subject to conscious restraint of impulses, bodily processes, urges, and desires."[24] Indigenous expressions of the body, on the other hand, were largely viewed as being *out* of control—and thus leading to illness and death. Such views were shaped by a series of strict dualisms common in nineteenth-century western European and Euroamerican culture: nature and culture; passion and reason; individual and society; woman and man; body and mind; savage and civilized. Within these dualisms were implied hierarchies: the body must be controlled, subjected to the mind; passion to reason; the individual to society; women to men; the savage to the civilized.[25]

It is important to keep in mind that in the images of "the native" that they constructed, Euroamericans were telling their own stories.[26] As many contemporary theorists have pointed out, the creation of self-identity depends on the definition of that which one is *not*. Hence, as Edward Said, Roy Harvey Pearce, and Robert Berkhofer have demonstrated, "civilization" gains meaning only if there is a "savage" against which it can be contrasted. The self that some Euroamerican settlers constructed was a self that was carefully controlled, a self that was placed in contrast to the unrestrained and ambiguously defined existence of "the savage." The value of constraint grew to nearly fetishistic proportions on the Northwest frontier, where many found themselves in the midst of wilderness, without congregation or community, and faced with the daily terrors of sickness and death. In the midst of such a context, their construction of "the Indian" helped to lend definition to the small Euroamerican population. Of course, as later chapters demonstrate, Euroamerican observers missed a great deal of Native culture that placed an enormous value on discipline, self-control, and individual autonomy—but these were beliefs and practices occluded from the view of most early observers.[27]

Early letters written by missionaries and traders seeking to secure financial support for their efforts had described a nearly utopian image of this region, praising indigenous skill, ingenuity, and the wealth of the land. The language in these letters draws upon what Roy Harvey Pearce and others have referred to as the Noble Savage, an image of utopian natural man. George Simpson, who chronicled an early visit to the Columbia as part of a trading expedition on behalf of the Hudson's Bay Company, had written to mission boards and financiers as early as 1824 that the Native communities were good humored, excellent traders, who enjoyed a powerful and well-organized political system. They were "honorable, manly" men, living in a bountiful countryside that provided a wealth of resources: fish, roots, berries, game, and furs. He stressed that as a whole they were healthy, except for *imported* diseases. They bathed regularly, were great swimmers, lived in settled villages, and were exceptionally eager for white men to come and bring them the Gospel. "I do not know of any part of Northwest America where Natives could be civilized and instructed in morality and Religion at such a moderate expense and with so much facility as on the Banks of the Columbia River," he wrote.[28] According to John Brown and Robert Ruby, early visitors to the region noted its abundance of food resources and thriving indigenous populations.[29] Thanks to predictable salmon runs, the populations rarely knew hunger: the Chinook salmon began their runs in March and continued until May. Runs continued until fall with sockeye, humpback, coho, steelhead and dog (chum) salmon. During the winter, communities relied on winter runs of fish as well as smoked and dried salmon, cached roots (camas, *wapato*, fern, thistle, cattail, and skunk cabbage), and dried berries that had been gathered during the summer months. Many families traveled in summer to fishing camps along the Columbia and the coast and in winter to shellfish gathering sites such as those on Willapa Bay, to the north along the coast. As early observers recorded, these communities relied relatively little on hunting. The river, Puget Sound, the ocean, and native plants amply provided the necessary materials for life. Many early recorders considered the Chinookan communities at the mouth of the Columbia to be among the wealthiest and most powerful on the coast; they controlled access to trade along the Columbia and made the most of their strategic position.

But when writers witnessed the impacts of disease firsthand, the discourse changed. The stereotype of the Noble Savage gave way to its counterpart: the wild man, living in dark depravity and in need of the saving grace of civilization. In stark contrast to earlier utopian voices, missionaries and traders wrote as early as 1835: "They live miserably on the Columbia—and children die under the operation of head flattening—and there is a great want of means of subsistence."[30]

Throughout the various extant texts, Euroamerican settlers generally failed to recognize their role in the importation of epidemic diseases devastating Native communities, obscuring how illness might have resulted from contact with Euroamerican culture. Nor do documents make reference to Euroamericans' acquired immunity to the illnesses that devastated Native communities. Rather, personal accounts from the era suggest that in the opinion of many Euroamerican settlers and missionaries, Natives died because of their "abominable lives," as Rev. Modeste Demers put it in the 1830s. Throughout, Euroamerican disease narratives of this era are consistent in blaming the vast extent of Native mortality in the Pacific Northwest on the Native people themselves.

Fur traders, who depended on a thriving indigenous population for both physical survival and economic success, mourned the devastation around them while also placing the blame on the Indian people themselves. Fur trader Peter Skene Ogden experienced one such epidemic during the 1830s. Trappers and traders had fallen ill, but had made use of their "seasonal supply of medicines," the "bark and tonics" which they kept on hand to ward off fever and infection. As a result, Euroamerican traders were relatively unscathed.

> Such was the visitation as we experienced it; but with the native populations, alas! The case was different. Who shall describe the sufferings

> of these unsophisticated children of the wilderness; or who depict the forlorn condition they exhibited while subject to such a scourge? [Ogden describes two villages of approximately sixty families each being completely wiped out within a month.] This may be easily accounted for in the trust which these poor, deluded savages reposed in the juggling mountebanks with whom the science therapeautic rests among them; and their total neglect of the precautions that were recommended by us for their adoption. Maddened by fever, they would rush headlong into the cooling stream, where, in search of relief, they found only the germs of dissolution.[31]

Similar sensibilities are expressed by John Work, post head of Fort Simpson in 1848: "There have been several deaths among the Natives, and from the almost utter impossibility of getting them to take proper care of themselves while under the disease, it is to be feared it will prove fatal to numbers more of them."[32] Regarding the practice of using a sweat lodge to cure ailments, Hudson's Bay Company clerk John Dunn argued in 1846: "The remedy generally did its intended work; and something more; it cured the disease, but killed the patient."[33] Describing an 1843 epidemic, Jesuit father Jean-Baptiste Bolduc made a similar conclusion: "White people do not die from it, but it almost always affects their health. The Indians die very frequently because they cannot resist the temptation of drinking cold water, and when the fever overcomes them they at once run and dive into the river which causes instant death."[34] Such observations, while in many ways sympathetic, nevertheless suggest a view of Native people informed by prevailing views of the day: Natives were "unsophisticated children of the wilderness," unable to resist temptation, and rushing headlong toward death.[35]

Some Euroamerican settlers also blamed the epidemics on Native morality—or rather what Euroamericans saw as *immorality*. In what is perhaps a classic case of blaming the victim, high rates of syphilis and gonorrhea were attributed to the promiscuity of Native women, not to the Euroamerican sailors and traders who brought the diseases with them. Lewis and Clark made note of the sickness among the Chinook, recognizing it as the same brought to the Natives of Baja by Spanish sailors. David Thompson recalled that "when the Americans first landed here in 1810, there was but little of it [syphilis] among the Natives; but it was soon communicated to them by the whites, who brought it not only from New York, but also from the Sandwich Islands." Despite this, they attributed its presence to the "wantonness" of the Chinook women; what they described as a lack of morals, which "within a few years can ruin them so that the entire race will perish."[36] O. Larsell reported that by 1814 venereal disease "had reached epidemic proportions among the fur traders," due to their "contact with native women," and the "spread of these diseases was facilitated among the Clatsops and Chinooks especially, by the low sexual standards of these tribes."[37] Cox likewise described venereal diseases as "wages of infamy," "the natural consequence of this state of general demoralization, and numbers of the unfortunate beings suffer dreadfully from the effects of their promiscuous intercourse."[38] The diseases had become such a dire problem that an official of the Northwest Fur Trading Company lamented, "It might seriously affect our commerce."[39] According to Dr. Romanowsky of the Russian-American Company, the source of many illnesses lay in Native propensities toward indulging "in orgies of lovemaking."[40]

Writing in the 1850s, Anson Henry, physician to the newly created Grand Ronde reservation, felt that venereal diseases would never be conquered among the Indians, as "this disease could only be conquered by a change in behavior," which he thought highly unlikely.[41] And in 1853 ethnologist George Gibbs described the Chinook and Cowlitz as "diseased beyond remedy, syphilis being with them hereditary as well as acquired."[42] He observed that venereal diseases and smallpox were both introduced by non-natives but nonetheless continued to blame illness on Native behavior and lifestyle. Illness was due to "their carelessness in regard to dress, the slight shelter from rain and exposure permitted by their wandering habits, and the dampness of the climate," the fact that "prostitution is almost universal" among them, and that "chastity is so entirely wanting in both sexes."[43] Native women were described as promiscuous, licentious, and out of control, and Native peoples were seen as reaping the consequences of their immoral lifestyles. Such narratives suggest a view wherein illnesses were attributed to the failure of Native women and men to conform to Euroamerican sexual standards, with virtually no attention given to the role Euroamerican men played in these sexual relationships or in the importation of non-native diseases.[44]

In a similar vein, Demers likewise appears to have attributed Native sickness to sin and immorality:

> Before the year 1830, they were the most numerous tribe inhabiting the banks of this river. This rendered them proud and haughty. Besides this, they were rich; but about this time came the disastrous malady known by the name of fever-and-ague, which carried a great many to their graves. In the heat of the fever they would leap into the river in the hope of relieving themselves of their suffering, but they found death as quick as it was certain. It was found necessary to burn a whole village where the dead bodies were piled upon one another; for the survivors were not capable of burying their dead. This calamity which God sent these Indians on account of their abominable lives, came to visit them every year, and always made some of them its victims. We are told they reformed their lives, except those who lived near the fort, who are wicked and demoralized on account of their communication with the whites.[45]

Demers's text is striking in its apocalyptic tone, as he attributes the mass deaths to their "abominable lives" and to being "proud and haughty." Regarding the Kalapuya, Demers is scarcely more optimistic. He finds here as well an inclination toward sin that has led to their illness and death. As he writes, "They were numerous before the fever, but are now reduced to a small number, which keeps decreasing every day. They are poor and lazy; thieving may be considered their predominant passion. They wish to keep away from the missionaries as much as the Cowlitz Indians wish to be near them. Hardly any of them were seen by the vicar general at the chapel assisting at instructions."[46]

"Juggling Mountebanks" and "Arrant Humbugs": Indigenous Healers and Disease

If some observers felt that immorality or a lack of civilized self-control was the primary cause of illness among the local Native population, they also agreed that traditional healers were the greatest obstacle to people's salvation.[47] As blame for venereal diseases, smallpox, malaria, and influenza were laid upon Native morality and cultural practices, fur traders and both Protestant and Catholic missionaries alike sought to liberate Native communities from these baleful influences. John Dunn wrote in the 1830s that he considered his primary responsibility to be to stop the "barbarous native practices like their impostures of priests, who, to show divine approbation stick daggers into flabby parts of patients without drawing blood."[48] Father Eugene Casimir Chirouse, of the Oblates of Mary Immaculate (OMI), also "recognized the 'conjurors' or shamans as his natural enemies among the natives," along with "polygamy, gambling, magic and sorcery, intemperance in the use of liquor, warfare among bands, and flattening the heads of infants."[49]

While maintaining an allegiance to their traditional healers, some Chinook and Coast Salish did selectively appropriate elements of Catholic ritual and doctrine. They did so, however, in ways that met their particular needs and meshed with their worldview and experience, while resisting a full-scale conversion. Many Native communities sought out baptism for their sick and dying, but their continued loyalty to traditional healers left Catholic missionaries concerned. As Demers wrote:

> This adhesion to burial rites and tamanawas [a generic term from Chinook *wawa*, typically referring to spirit power or Native religious rituals in general; spellings vary] will cause the missionaries to be more prudent in baptizing. We have learned not to trust the repeated promises they make to us to not have any recourse to the tamanawas if the baptized child gets sick. You may see that progress has been slow among them so far; their customs and habits are so inveterate that it will take a long time for religion and the fear and knowledge of God to unroot

> and destroy them entirely. This year the mission will lend to the Indians seed potatoes. . . . [Perhaps] the peas and potatoes may make them forget the berries and the camas.[50]

Demers posited "medicine men" as the primary opponents of Christianity among Native communities, giving voice to an ongoing concern among Catholic and Protestant missionaries alike.

Demers argued that these individuals were the "closest thing" to religion among the tribes. "Previous to the coming of the missionaries no traces of worship had ever been noticed among the Indians. They had some ill-defined notions, but no religious ceremonies or functions. . . . Each tribe had its priest, or medicine man, as he was more properly called, but he exercised his ministry, if so it may be styled, only with regard to sickness and to effect a cure. . . . The Indians had in him the greatest confidence, and willingly disposed in his favor all they possessed in order to be cured."[51] De Smet expressed a similar perspective. As he argued, "Among the aborigines of Oregon there is no trace of any religious worship. They have a belief which consists in obscure traditions; but no external forms of religion are visible among them. The juggler exercises his profession, though it is almost universally done in behalf of the sick, for the purpose of curing them. Though nearly all of these tribes, of whom we are speaking, possess no particular form of worship, they are naturally predisposed in favor of the Christian religion, especially those who live in the interior."[52] While Catholic theology has argued for the presence of "natural religion" within pre-Christian cultures, Demers and De Smet both saw little evidence of genuine worship or the "external forms" of religion, apart from healing traditions. But Demers and De Smet were unable to reconcile such healing practices with the sacramental system that defined worship as they understood it.

With Native healers as their primary competition, Protestant missionaries likewise constructed images of Native healing and healers that presented them as the dangerous Other. Within missionary rhetoric, Native healers were everything Christian missionaries hoped *not* to be: healers were dangerous, unethical, extortionists, and frauds. Methodists Daniel Lee and Joseph Frost present a secondhand account of these "blood-thirsty" curers certain to motivate missionaries working on the frontier:

> Formerly it was a prevailing custom for the "medicine men" at the dancing festivals to lacerate their flesh with sharp stones or knives, making deep cuts; and while the blood was gushing out, scoop it up in their hands, and drink it, to appease and gratify their blood thirsty tamanawas that raged within. Probably it was pretended by these deceivers that their "familiars" delighted in blood, in order to inspire the poor dupes of their black art with an abiding dread of their displeasure, who could commend the service of such malicious agents. The limbs and bodies of many exhibit scars which originated in this diabolical practice.[53]

In 1843 Father Bolduc recorded similar observations of healers near Fort Vancouver on the Columbia River, portraying them as hucksters who seemed to delight in the grotesque:

> When one hears someone is ill and goes there, it is very difficult to force a way through the Native doctors and medicine men. These are the ones who abuse the credulity of the others, making them believe that all illness is caused by material things entering the body. To cure them, or to extract these objects they suck the effected parts till the blood comes. They claim then that they have found in the blood the objects that caused the sickness. Sometimes it is a small piece of squirrel skin, sometimes a fishbone, etc. etc. Lately a celebrated medicine man extracted from his patient's throat a little knife but the imposter fell a victim to his lie, for the patient saw that it was too large to swallow. The poor doctor almost lost his life. This is the way these medicine men are exposed, the sick one dying claims that bad medicine caused his death. Later I will describe to you at length the methods of the medicine man in all their forms, but I warn you, in advance, it is quite possible you may become ill in reading about it as it is all truly disgusting.[54]

Bolduc's narrative suggests not only that traditional healers trafficked in the grotesque but also that they were con artists with no real ability to cure. As Northwest Company clerk Ross Cox complained, "Every Indian village has its quak doctor, or, as they call him, 'strong man of medicine.'"[55] And fur trader John Dunn lamented in 1846 "the frauds still practiced by their crafty conjurers on the credulity of the natives."[56] For Demers, aboriginal healers were not merely con men but bullies who exerted control over their communities through threats of violence.

> Everywhere we meet the same obstacles which always retard the conversion of the Indians, namely: polygamy, their adherence to the customs of their ancestors and, still more, to tamanawas, the name given to the medicines they prepare for the sick. This tamanawas is generally transmitted in families, and even women can pretend to the honor of making it. If anyone is sick they call in the medicine-man [*sic*]. No danger of their asking him what he wants for his trouble; they would be afraid of insulting him. Whatever he asks is given him without the least objection; otherwise they may fear everything from that doctor, who will not fail to take his revenge for a refusal by sending some misfortune, or some sickness, or even death through his medicines to the one who refused him, be he fifty leagues off. If anyone is dead, such a one killed him.[57]

With such an opinion of traditional healers, Demers could find ample motivation for opposing such dangerous figures. Surely, the people would be thankful to be liberated from such scoundrels?

Indeed, Protestant and Catholic missionaries alike expressed a strong desire to liberate Native people from these deceptions, to show them that such "crafty conjurers" were merely delusional. But they struggled to do so. As George Gary, Methodist missionary at Willamette Station, wrote on December 18, 1844:

> About sunset I visited the Indian lodge; here is a sick woman, the wailing for two nights past are for her recovery, directed by the medicine man or conjurer. I believe little or no medicine in such cases is given; the cure is to be effected by wailing, they lie by and sleep during the day; the most of them are now asleep. About eight o'clock the Indians have begun their night work; they howl and wail most dreadfully. Oh,

> if I could enlighten them, how gladly would I do it; two important and insurmountable impediments in the way, one is, I have not their confidence, so as to have any influence over them or access to them; the other, I cannot say a word to them they can understand. My sympathies are deeply enlisted yet I cannot do them a particle of good.[58]

Father Bolduc also experienced difficulties when confronting traditional healers. Since few would attend church services, Bolduc visited Native people in their own homes, where he occasionally witnessed the efforts of healers and lamented his inability to challenge them effectively:

> Every day I had to visit lodges. That task imposed on me by the indifference of a large number whom I was obliged to hunt up, in order to bring them to the instruction. Fever afflicted the tribe and I lacked remedies. The sick had recourse to an old woman who was reputed to be skillful in healing. The old woman would rub her hands, apply them to the sick, then bring her mouth close to them and utter strange sounds and whistles. The pus issuing from her mouth was expelled with the same ceremony; which was, she claimed, the patient's malady. She earned her living by this trade which she exercised quietly; but they tell me that these charlatans ordinarily make a frightful uproar for entire days and nights, accompanied by a thousand gestures and contortions which are to serve in the healing of the sick one. It will be difficult to put an end to this disorder; for the natives have faith in the words of these charlatans, but woe to the doctor if the sick one dies, for he is accused of having killed him, and his life is in danger.[59]

Bolduc's account highlights the way in which Euroamerican observers encountered Native healing. Such traditions appeared bizarre, irrational, and yet persisted in maintaining a hold within Native belief systems. Given Bolduc's own understanding of health and wellness, it would be difficult for him to see indigenous healers as anything other than hucksters.

While representations such as these tell us relatively little about the genuine practice of traditional healers of the time, they do tell us something about how missionaries wanted to perceive themselves. If indigenous healers were deceitful, wild, unrestrained charlatans with malicious intent, motivated by profit and power, then Christian missionaries could affirm a view of themselves, by contrast, as rational, restrained, selfless, and truthful. Such narratives also provide a truly striking illustration of the ways in which healing and illness are culturally specific. Confronted with traditions, practices, and disease etiologies so foreign to their own, early traders, missionaries, and settlers could only see them as the work of charlatans, deceiving the naïve. And indeed, given how ineffectual traditional healers were when faced with imported diseases, Euroamericans had little reason to take them seriously.

"This Phial of Wrath": Disease, Power and Coercion

While non-native settlers and missionaries strongly opposed indigenous healers, Euroamerican medical care was slow in arriving to these communities, if it arrived at all. As Bolduc mentioned, missionaries rarely had any kind of material remedies to offer. The first recorded instance of western medical care being offered to a Native person in this region was in 1796 when the ship's surgeon aboard the *Ruby* offered some form of medicine to Shelathwell, a Chinook chief. In 1803–5 Lewis and Clark carried kine-pox with them along their journey to the Pacific and reportedly instructed the Natives with whom they met to make use of it.[60] Most noteworthy was the work of Dr. William Fraser Tolmie, who joined Hudson's Bay Company in South Puget Sound in 1833.[61] Tolmie was the first doctor to live in Puget Sound, and he "enlisted help of local Indians to search for herbal cures to problematic diseases," such as malaria. He immunized local Indians against smallpox and offered such medical care as he was able to give.[62] With his help, in 1837 the Hudson's Bay Company made a concerted effort to stop the spread of a smallpox epidemic. Dr. Tolmie reportedly vaccinated Native people at Fort Vancouver in June, and on July 10 at Fort Nisqually he reported that "all the women and Children of the place" had been vaccinated against the disease."[63]

Such efforts reveal a deep concern on the part of traders and missionaries alike to protect and preserve indigenous populations as much as they could, both for humanitarian purposes and because such populations were vital for effective trade. However, their efforts are noteworthy in part because they were so unusual. For the most part, Euroamericans had little to offer, and when they did they often justified withholding medications out of fear of recrimination: should their attempts fail, they did not want to be blamed for the death of the individual.[64]

At the same time, offering medical assistance was one way that Euroamerican traders and missionaries were able to encourage a cooperative indigenous population. Some early settlers even made direct use of the threat of illness and death to score political and economic advantage. While early Euroamerican settlers to the region never fully understood Native disease etiologies, they knew enough to employ these for their own ends. One of the most striking examples of this is attributed to Duncan McDougal, official at Fort Astor in 1811. Ross Cox reported the incident in his 1831 journal, and Washington Irving of the Pacific Fur Company likewise recorded the event in 1836. That the account was popular enough to be recorded in several places and become part of Euroamerican folklore of the region suggests that such tactics retained a certain charm for future settlers. I quote the story at length there:

> Mr. McDougal, we are told, had recourse to a stratagem by which to avail himself of the ignorance and credulity of the savages, and which does credit to his ingenuity. The natives of the coast, and, indeed, of all the regions west of the mountains, had an extreme dread of smallpox; that terrific scourge having, a few years previously, appeared among them, and almost swept off entire tribes. Its origin and nature were wrapped in mystery, and they conceived it an evil inflicted upon them by the Great Spirit, or brought among them by the white man. The last idea was seized upon by Mr. McDougal. He assembled several of the chieftains whom he believed to be in the conspiracy. When they were all seated around, he informed them that he had heard of the treach-

ery of some of their northern brethren towards the Tonquin [a ship reportedly destroyed by the Nuu'chah'nulth or the Quinault] and was determined on vengeance. "The white men among you," said he, "are few in numbers, it is true, but they are mighty in medicine. See here," continued he, drawing forth a small bottle and holding it before their eyes, "in this bottle I hold the smallpox, safely corked up; I have but to draw the cork and let loose the pestilence, to sweep man, woman and child from the face of the earth." The chiefs were struck with horror and alarm. They implored him not to uncork the bottle, since they and all their people were firm friends of the white men, and would always remain so; but, should the smallpox be once let out, it would run like wildfire throughout the country, sweeping off good as well as the bad; and surely he would not be so unjust as to punish his friends for crimes committed by his enemies. Mr. McDougal pretended to be convinced by their reasoning, and assured them that, so long as the white people should be unmolested, and the conduct of their Indian neighbors friendly and hospitable, the phial of wrath should remain sealed up; but, on the least hostility, the fatal cork should be drawn.[65]

Other traders and settlers reported using similar tactics. Captain Dominis, angry that the Chinook had not brought him the largest and best beaver skins, "told them that they would all soon die." In some versions of the story, he "hung an evil sail in a tree," while in others he held up a vial, much like McDougal.[66] Subsequent outbreaks of smallpox and the "cold sick" [perhaps malaria] were blamed on Dominis.[67] Another example of the use of illness narratives to constrain Native communities comes from the writings of James Swan. While living at Shoalwater Bay in the 1850s Swan presented himself to the local Chinook and Chehalis as a physician, though he had no medical training.[68] Because of the fear and respect that Native people had for healers, Swan was able to exert control over local Native communities, procuring free labor and maintaining a strict hierarchy of influence. He described one particular instance of this:

I turned their belief in my medical knowledge to good account on several occasions, and was able, by a very simple experiment, to save all of our cabbages, of which the Indians were very fond. We had been annoyed, while packing our salmon, by thousands of crows, who would light down in flocks on our salmon, and eat them up before our eyes. . . . At length one day, while overhauling my trunk, I found a paper of strychnine. I immediately put some on three or four salmon, which I laid out for the crows. Down they came and gobbled up the fish, and then, with a squawk, would roll over on their backs and die. In this manner I slew a great number, and it had the effect of frightening the rest so bad that they did not trouble us any more. The Indians saw the whole affair, and at first were very much pleased to see me kill those "bad birds," as they call the crows; but old Suis told them she was afraid, if I got vexed, that I might put some of that white medicine where they themselves would be poisoned. I assured her such would not be the case except with the cabbages, for I had found some of her people had been helping themselves. . . . I sprinkled every cabbage-head with flour, which I had previously put into a blue paper similar to that the strychnine was in. The effect was excellent, we never lost another cabbage.[69]

By engaging such tactics, some Euroamerican traders and explorers attempted to use their limited understanding of Native disease etiologies to elicit a cooperative population. Men such as McDougal, Dominis, and Swan helped to craft a discourse of the body in which Euroamerican men held the power of life and death in their hands, Native compliance and acquiescence resulted in continued health, and any challenges to Euroamerican authority put Native communities at risk of death and disease: a powerful threat to communities already ravaged by smallpox, malaria, and syphilis.

Early missionaries in the region did not make use of overt threats like those of McDougall, Dominis, and Swan. And yet they did make strategic use of illness in order to encourage cooperation and conversion. For instance, when Father Chirouse established his mission at Tulalip in 1858, he had Stlabebtikud, an Upper Skagit religious leader, tell the gathered crowd: "'If you are sick, you are going to die. If you are not baptized, you will not reach the good country.'" An observer later recalled that as a result, "all the old people got baptized so when they die, they would go to good places."[70] According to Native disease etiologies, if these illnesses were truly brought by white settlers and their spirit powers, then only those same spirit powers (in this case the Christian God) could successfully cure them.[71] Alexandra Harmon has noted, "Because the King George men's spirit allies were reportedly capable of causing or curing the new illness, some natives deemed it prudent to propitiate the Christians' deity . . . some appealed to the King George men to treat their illness or accepted smallpox vaccinations."[72] Indeed, "the pestilence itself was reason to suspect the presence of powers greater than natives' own spirit powers."[73] Furthermore, as Harmon has argued, aboriginal cultures had a precedent for seeking outside aid, as it was traditional to "consult doctors outside their communities," particularly when confronting an unknown ailment.[74]

This, combined with the devastating cultural and spiritual losses caused by the epidemics, led many Native communities to be at least temporarily more receptive to conversion. An example of this can be seen in a report in the *Christian Advocate and Journal* by Henry Perkins, head of the Methodist Wascopam mission at the Dalles on the Columbia River from 1838 to 1844:

> The great plague or sickness, eight or nine years previous, had greatly lessened their numbers, and in a manner dispirited them. At the same time they were led to believe that this dreadful mortality was through the influence of white traders: they therefore stood in awe of all white men, and looked upon them as yielding a secret power which was to them incomprehensible; while a few looked upon it as rather a punishment sent from Heaven on account of their former atrocities. But, from whatever cause, there had been peace among them for several years, and they were in a state, therefore, to give attention to the message of salvation.[75]

Chirouse likewise reported that the Tulalip seemed "much more humble and more fearful of God" since the most recent smallpox epidemic.[76]

If illness prepared Native people for the gospel, missionaries also saw conversion, at least at first, as a path toward wellness. Implicit was the promise that being "Christian" and "civilized" meant a healthier approach to life. On March 3, 1839, Demers described those good and godly Indians with whom he had met during his travels. They were those who eagerly sought out priests such as himself, demonstrating a "zeal and eagerness to know God." In his list, he included the [Great] Lake Indians, the Colville, the Okanogan, the Cowlitz, and the Walla Walla. And he also described the ungodly, recalcitrant Indians, those who refused the call of God and treated priests, and himself, with contempt. Of these, he referred in particular to the Chinook and the Kalapooia of the Columbia River, who, he observed, were wracked with illness. Markedly, Demers omits any mention of illness among his "good" Indians. In Demers's writings, health is implicitly correlated with Christian conversion, while those who refuse the holy call are described as languishing in the worst of illnesses. A "good Indian" appears to be a healthy one. Bad Indians, on the other hand, were more likely to encounter illness, death, and destruction.

And indeed, in cases where vaccinations were available, there was often a direct correlation between conversion and physical health. It was simply the case that those living in proximity to missions were most likely to have access to vaccinations. Dr. Tolmie wrote in 1837 of his regret that supplies required that vaccination efforts were primarily "limited to local natives, trading partners, and prominent men."[77] As Chief Factor James Douglas wrote to the Hudson's Bay Company on December 5, 1844, "food, medicine, and advice were liberally dispensed to the Indians living about the establishment, but these formed a small part of the suffering thousands who were crowded into distant villages beyond the reach of our aid."[78] During the 1862 smallpox epidemic, Father Chirouse reported that he oversaw the vaccination of thousands of Native people throughout Puget Sound. As a result, as he wrote, the baptized survived, while the unbaptized were "ravaged."[79] As noted by George Guilmet and colleagues, "purposeful or not, there was a selective process involved in this differential treatment. The most acculturated segment of the native population was given an edge in survival and future increase that was not shared with the unacculturated majority."[80] The greater survival rates of those living close to missions and trading forts helped to reinforce the view among Euroamericans and Native people alike that conversion ensured better health.[81]

Within traditional Coast Salish and Chinook disease etiologies, white settlers, missionaries, and physicians were very likely not seen merely as passive carriers of germs but were instead viewed as the intentional bearers of illness and death. The fact that new diseases arrived more or less concurrently with these new people would have been proof enough that these were powerful people who had brought disease with them. That some Euroamericans actually *claimed* to have done this (so as to procure Native compliance) certainly would have validated these initial fears. And when they claimed to have abilities to cure such illnesses (through offers of vaccination or conversion), from a Native perspective they confirmed their guilt, for within local belief systems only those intimately familiar with a disease-causing object or spirit power could heal the ailment it caused.

Native communities were not naïve. They were clearly aware of the political implications and the shifts in power inherent in such epidemics and the fact that non-native communities generally survived, while Native communities were far more often ravaged by disease. For nineteenth-century Chinook and Coast Salish peoples, there was little doubt that these new illnesses came from white settlers. As Cox observed, "It is believed in the north-west that this disease [smallpox] was willfully introduced by the American traders among the Indians of the Missouri, as a short and easy method of reducing their numbers, and thereby destroying in a great measure their hostility to the whites."[82] As early as 1804 Lewis and Clark recorded that the Chinook with whom they visited along the Columbia River blamed the arrival of smallpox on the first ship that entered the Columbia. The ship had fired cannon shots, which "they believed, had sent clouds of lethal smoke upriver and into tributary streams, contaminating them with death."[83] And Dr. Tolmie noted on September 28, 1833: "A Sinnamish [*sic*] hunter tells a long story of the arrival of two American ships at Cape Flattery, and that the Chiefs threatened to send disease amongst them if they did not trade beaver. It appears that an American Captain who lay for sometime in the Columbia, the season the intermittent fever first appeared, is considered by the Indians to have left the malady in revenge for not receiving skins."[84]

Indigenous disease etiologies, which saw a relationship between disease and the spirit-power that caused disease (in this case the Christian God) placed missionaries in a position to profoundly influence Coast Salish and Chinook practices and worldviews.[85] Despite that advantage, however, success remained slow going. Epidemic diseases ultimately proved too much for traders and missionaries alike, depriving them of the indigenous population they depended upon to build their missions. Early nineteenth-century observers came to see Native people as suffering from deceitful traditional healers, while their cultural practices and moral standards further increased their susceptibility to disease. With this pervasive perspective, it was not long before Euroamerican observers came to see Native people as innately ill. As Gibbs had argued, to be born Indian was to be born ill: illnesses were "hereditary as well as acquired." For nineteenth-century Euroamerican settlers, Native mortality rates were not the result of dramatic demographic, social, and political changes, or the importation of non-native diseases, but rather the result of Native characters and cultures that seemed to doom them to extinction.

"The Fact Is, They Cannot Live": The Decline of Early Protestant Missions in the Northwest

Despite efforts at material assistance and rhetorical coercion, early Protestant missionary efforts in the Pacific Northwest floundered. Native people refused conversion even as they were dying at alarming rates. Despite the expectations of early settlers who predicted that the region would be an ideal mission field because of its peaceful villages and abundant resources, Protestant missionaries in particular found their efforts frustrated at every turn.[86] Whether Chinook, Clatsop, Tillamook, Kalapuya, Nisqually, or Chehalis, communities stubbornly refused conversion and saw little appeal in joining a congregation. Methodist missionaries Frost and Lee recorded their frustrations in journals and letters. "The Indian," Joseph Frost wrote, had "no god," no religion, and looked "no further into futurity than the canoe in which his body may be deposited."[87] Lee and Frost recollected that while they devoted time to "relieving the sick among the Indians," not knowing the language stopped them from doing any good. As a result "the Indian doctors resumed their practices, and a large proportion returned to their former vices. . . . Three quarters and more appeared careless and indifferent about the teachings of the gospel, and many of these were even against hearing it preached, that they might go on in their heathenish practices and in direct opposition to its commands, unrestrained."[88] Lee went on, "These Indians are the most degraded human beings that we have met with in all our journeyings, taking them as a whole. There is not one among them that can be considered virtuous. And, in consequence of disease, which cleaves to them from their birth, and the many murders committed among them, they are rapidly wasting away, and the time is not far distant when the last death wail will proclaim their universal extermination. It is truly heart-rending to see, as we have, how the 'last enemy' chases them 'from the cradle to the grave.'"[89]

As early as 1834 Frost, disheartened by high rates of mortality and low rates of conversions, despaired of any hope for his Methodist mission. "They are very few in number, and their number is continually decreasing. But two children are now living out of a number that have been born among them since we have been here. The fact is, they cannot live, for the most disgusting disease is entailed upon them from the womb. And this is the case universally, at least, in the lower country. I am quite confident, from the observations which I have been enabled to make, that there never will be any thing like a permanent Christian Church raised up among them."[90] Frost concluded that his efforts and those of other missionaries had been in vain, and their funding would be better spent elsewhere. The Indians, he was certain, were destined to disappear.

Other Protestant missionaries came to share Frost's view of the hopelessness of the case. As former Indian Agent T. W. Davenport recalled, "looking at the humiliating results of missionary work in the Willamette Valley by devoted men and women who preceded the pioneers with no other purpose than that of civilizing and Christianizing its aboriginal inhabitants, we should not wonder at the incredulity of the Oregon people as to the practicality of any further attempts in that direction." In 1851 Davenport argued that "only a few wandering, diseased, and degenerate remnants were left of the once powerful tribes that reveled in the veritable Garden of Eden."[91] And indeed, only four years after the malaria outbreak that he described, Frost had abandoned the Native population completely:

> Indeed I do not think the present adults will ever be benefited by missionary effort, and the children are so much diseased from their birth that but very few of them live to manhood. The Christian cannot but feel for them and pray for them, as he sees them fading away. . . . These are the mere dregs of former tribes, so much dispersed, and so migratory in their habits, and so much diseased and withal having so many different languages, which are so very imperfect as a medium of communication, that nothing encouraging can be expected. . . . Their circumstances are such that I fear they never will be much benefited by the Gospel. . . . Although it is exceedingly painful to reflect that we have laboured and toiled in vain, yet it is my sincere conviction that the money that is being expended in sustaining several of us in this field under present circumstances and in view of future prospects, might and ought to be expended to better purpose elsewhere.[92]

Reverend H. K. Hines, Methodist missionary at Willamette Station, expressed a similar sentiment. Frustrated by indigenous resistance to Christianity, and disheartened by the rising death toll, Hines considered abandoning the field. The cost and effort involved in maintaining the mission were too great, and logistics of communicating with a sparsely populated and linguistically diverse region were simply overwhelming. Finally, in 1843, discouraged by the persistent indifference demonstrated by Native peoples of the Willamette Valley toward Christianity, Hines wrote to his superiors, recommending that the mission redirect its efforts toward white parishioners. Linguistic diversity was again presented as an obstacle to effective missionary work. Of the estimated fifteen hundred Indians remaining in the valley, there were seven distinct "clans," each with a unique language.

> A man might spend ten years in the acquirement of Indian languages and then not be able to communicate the truths of the gospel to but a few hundreds of these perishing heathen. . . . They are a broken and dispirited race of men. No motive can be presented before them that will have the least tendency to induce them to engage in any enterprise from which they are not fully satisfied that they will reap present benefit. Exhort them to build houses, cultivate lands, etc., and they will meet you with the reply, "It will do no good, we are all dying off, but a little while ago our people were numerous and powerful. The Elk and Deer were plentiful and we had enough to eat, and the cold sick was not among us, we were rich, and we were happy, but the Boston and the King George people came among us, and brought the cold sick with them, since then we have been dying very fast. It will not be long before we shall all be dead." And indeed there is no life nor spirit nor energy among them, they are a stupid and melancholy and a doomed race of men. . . . So far as extending missionary operations among the different clans of this lower country is concerned, there is but little probability that it ever will, or ever can be affected to any extent.[93]

In a letter filled with resignation, Hines insisted that there was "nothing to warrant the Board in making or being at the immense expense necessary to support the Mission" to the Indians.[94] If it should remain at all, he went on to argue, the mission should direct its efforts solely toward Euroamerican settlers. In his *Mission History* Hines chronicled what he perceived as the heroic careers of Oregon's missionaries, and he argued that their failure was due to no fault of their own. Guided by a belief that the Indian people as a race were incapable of survival and that Euroamerican communities were destined to inherit the territory, Hines concluded his mission history:

> We do believe that, as a race, the Indians furnished the least hopeful field for permanent religious culture the church has ever experienced. . . .

> In the history of this world there have been few peoples so destitute of those ideas that make for power and organizing progress. How unlike our Aryan forefathers. They were vivid, resourceful, prolific. They outgrew the boundaries of their primitive home. They pushed into Western Europe and the British Isles. Thus that race spread itself. It founded cities and built commonwealths. It ordained worship. It caused the wilderness to blossom and deserts to rejoice. Our American Indian race did none of these things. . . . They lacked the revolt of genius against stupidity, of ambition against the gross imitation of sensualism. No stranger ethnic anomaly ever dropped into the flow of human history. We note the fact as, in one aspect, explaining the strange outcome of one of the most romantically conceived and vigorously and self-denyingly prosecuted missionary movements of modern times, a movement that seemed to leave the people for whom it was designed in ruins, but left a splendid residuum of civilization and Christian life for the sturdier race that so speedily came after them.[95]

Informed by ınineteenth-century notions of racial determinism, disillusioned missionaries concluded that Native peoples were simply incapable of rising to the challenges of the modern era. Hines and his peers were frustrated by their lack of success among Native tribes, shocked at their rapid demise, and unwilling to claim any responsibility for the crisis. As a result, Protestant missionaries concluded that Native inhabitants were destined to perish, and should be abandoned to their fate.

"To Baptize the Children, the Sick, and the Agonizing": Catholic Missions and Disease

Though they shared many basic assumptions with their Protestant counterparts, early Catholic missions differed in important ways as they continued to try to bring their would-be parishioners within the fold. Catholic missions outlasted most of their Protestant colleagues. There were several reasons for this. First, Catholic notions of "natural religion" allowed for a sense that God spoke to Native people in some form but that they lacked the fulfillment of revealed religion. This gave them a foundation upon which to build. A second reason, perhaps more important for our discussion here, is that Catholic sacramental worship gave them a means of ministering to a dying population that Protestants lacked.

To understand this distinction better, it helps to consider the view of the body guiding each tradition. In many ways, these perspectives have their origins in Plato's notion of the body-as-prison-of-the-soul. As Thomas Kasulis has argued, this notion was further developed within early modern Catholic and Protestant theology: within Catholicism's notion of the embodied spirit, and Protestantism's insistence on justification by intellectual or spiritual faith and not by embodied works. These two traditions, while affirming the essential distinction between body and soul, constructed it in different ways. The prevailing view within early modern Protestant theology perceived physical actions as virtually unimportant: it was the expression of faith within the disembodied mind that saved the soul.[96] By contrast, the prevailing view for many Catholic missionaries was that the body acted as a necessary vessel for the spirit, and embodied action and ritual had a direct impact on the state of the immortal soul.

These perspectives on the body would influence how Protestant and Catholic missionaries dealt with the Northwest epidemics of the nineteenth century. While Catholics shared Protestants' notions of the division between body and soul, a dominant Catholic view of the embodied subject allowed for a soul *within* the body. Because of this, the embodied practice of sacramental worship could have a very real effect toward salvation. Most important, the administration of baptism and last rites required little actual religious instruction, did not necessarily rest on the faith of the believer, and could nonetheless be spiritually transformative.[97] As Father Adrien Croquet, missionary to the Grand Ronde, recalled in September 1864, "There we began our work of our sacred ministry among the savages who sojourned on the margins of the Bay, and began to baptize the children and others of the adults who were on the verge of death. The office of baptism as you may well judge among the savages was yet with short religious instructions, a necessary precedent on the existence of God, the creation and the fall of man."[98]

While Catholic missionaries were also faced with a recalcitrant population that was dying at an alarming rate, they did not despair and abandon their work as Protestants did but instead modified their goals. They found hope in their ability to offer the sacraments of baptism and last rites for a dying people. This "mission-as-last-rites" narrative gave Catholic missionaries a way to create meaning within a desperate situation: they could not save Native lives, but they could save their souls.[99] And indeed, while Native peoples on the whole ignored priests' calls to conversion, they did welcome baptism and extreme unction at death. Missionaries such as Demers, Bolduc, and Chirouse made the most of these opportunities. Between July and November of 1857, Chirouse added five hundred people to the baptismal registry. On another occasion, during a visit to Vancouver Island, he reported baptizing four hundred children on a single occasion. Chirouse himself performed the last rites for Chief Seattle on the Suquamish reservation at Port Madison in 1866. By 1868 the Oblate Fathers in the Puget Sound region were reported to have baptized 3,811 people. Large-scale baptisms were an important feature of reports from the missionary frontier. As Bolduc wrote:

> I baptized 132 children. . . . This child, aged about seven years, had hurt himself dangerously. His relatives told me that he had not been baptized, and I made them understand that I would baptize him presently. However, after some moments given to instruction, I heard outcries and chanting, which made me presume, that those unfortunates were devoting themselves to their superstitious medicine in order to cure the sick little fellow. I hurried toward them, and . . . I expressed my sorrow and indignation that they had begun the medicine without warning me. In spite of what I was able to say to prove the impiety and absurdity of it, the medicine continued, and I was obliged to go away. The next day, as I was going to see the child, I learned that he was dead. My poor heart was about crushed and mangled beneath an enormous weight. My God, how fearful are Your judgments! I was returning plunged into

> bitter sorrow, when an inward voice seems to say to me that all was not beyond hope. I retraced my steps, and in fact the child was still in agony! Then I manifested my indignation without reserve. I spoke out in masterly fashion, and without waiting for the relatives' consent I poured the regenerating water upon the head of the dying one, and a few minutes later he was in the arms of the Saviour. . . . [100]
>
> At the end of the same day (May 20th) about six hundred Natives of the Klallam tribe arrived with their chief, come to ask one of us missionaries to baptize one of the children who had just arrived dangerously ill from the other side of the bay. I went there, examined the child, baptized it, and some moments after it tasted the happiness of the elect. How much my fatigue is rewarded by this consoling memory that I came to open the door of heaven to this poor child! . . . The natives here are still indifferent in matters relating to works of salvation. I must admit, however, that they are becoming tractable little by little; they cause little trouble now in letting themselves be baptized at the time of death; some even show eagerness. . . . The Natives inhabiting the country from the mouth of the Columbia up to Ft. Vancouver were visited this year by a dysentery that has more than decimated them. Those at Cowlitz also suffered the same fate. Of thirty of the latter who became its victims, only four refused to become Christians. . . . In spite of these fatigues I experienced great comforts, and hope that the good God has been pleased to bless my feeble efforts for the salvation of the dying.[101]

As these powerful examples show, rather than abandon their work, Catholic missionaries responded to high mortality rates by shifting their focus: if they sadly resigned Native communities to death, they still took comfort in deathbed conversions and administering the last rites, sometimes en masse, offering suffering people eternal salvation, if not temporal healing.

There is no way of knowing for certain how Native people understood baptism and extreme unction, but the fact that such "conversions" did not tend to be lasting indicates they certainly interpreted them differently than the Catholic fathers might have hoped. In

1844 Bolduc expressed his frustration on this point. "They are essentially lazy, apathetic, inconstant, and insensible to all that one can tell them about religion. They are attached to their superstitions to a point that one doubts whether they will ever be converted. Out of the large number of those near us, I see only three or four adult Christians. . . . Most of the adults agree to be baptized at the moment of death, but it is very seldom they come to the mission for that purpose."[102] At times, however, Native people sought him out, seeking baptism. In one letter to his superiors he happily recorded one instance in which "several Indians from the mainland" arrived to find him: "On seeing me, they threw themselves on their knees around me and expressed themselves thus: 'Priest, we have walked for four days to come to see you, we have walked day as well as night with nothing to eat . . . we implore you, have pity on us, as we know there is a Master in Heaven but now know how to please him. Come, baptize our children as you have baptized these here.'"[103] Elsewhere he mentions that the children in question were deathly ill: the parents appear to have made the trip under great duress rather than out of eagerness for conversion. On February 15, 1844, Bolduc recorded the words of an elderly Cowlitz woman, who said to him: "Your words are good, but they tell us that all the children who have been baptized at Fraser River are dead or die immediately. However, since you say that it is a good thing we will believe you, so that these will see the Master on High after their death, baptize all that are in our camp; show them your kindness for they are pitiful, they nearly all are dying."[104]

Early Catholic missions to the Northwest thus came to see their role as providing people with eternal salvation as they stood at death's door. Father Louis J. D'Herbomez, who joined the Oregon missions in the 1850s, agreed that "experience has proved all too clearly that all the good we can hope to do among the Indians of the Oregon and Washington territories can be reduced to this—to care for the Indians who are still benevolent toward us (and their number decreases every day), to baptize the children, the sick, and the agonizing."[105] The work of such missionaries thus soon became that of offering baptism and last rites, transforming the soul through embodied ritual.

A better understanding of indigenous disease etiologies helps to shed light upon the decision of large numbers of Native people to receive last rites from early Catholic missionaries.[106] Within traditional Coast Salish and Chinook beliefs, medicine men and women had both the power to cause illness and the power to cure it. If Native people saw priests as fulfilling a similar role, they may have seen the Catholic fathers as holders of the disease-causing spirit power that was killing them. As such, these priests would be the only ones able to offer a cure. This can be seen, for instance, in a conversation with a Cowlitz elder, recorded by Bolduc in 1843. He related that the Cowlitz, ravaged by disease, had recognized that its arrival coincided with that of Father Demers, and what they saw as his disease-causing spirit power. "He told us that Father Demers had visited their camp several times and that they were actually now afflicted with trembling fever."[107] The fathers' claim that baptism was a solution to Native illness would have been, to Native ears, an admission of culpability. Bolduc made clear that illnesses were divine punishment from the Christian God, and in claiming to have the solution, he essentially announced his own involvement with the cause, and hence the cure, of the epidemic. With this in mind, participation in baptism could be seen as a strategic accommodation, quite in keeping with indigenous healing practices.

In Bolduc's later letters he suggested that the Cowlitz attributed such spirit power to him as well. Bolduc described the fear with which people responded to a small mechanical device he had brought along: "Many people opened their eyes with fright when they saw for the first time the phenomenon. . . . The Indians are convinced that I have *tamanawas* (shaman's spirit of the medicine man), a very protecting spirit, and even that I have very strong medicine."[108] He also described the fear with which Native men and women of high rank regarded Demers, fear that would be unfounded, given his poverty and lack of physical prowess, except for his potential strength as a spiritual person who might have the ability to cause sickness. As Bolduc joked, "That young Yougletat Chief who saw Father Demers, approached the missionary crawling on his knees and trembling in his whole body. I would be very satisfied to be taken as a slave by a party of the warriors of that nation; I would be certain to subdue them in a short time."[109] If Demers was held responsible for the sickness, as the evidence would suggest, and the illness persisted even after his departure, it is not surprising that the Native communities regarded him with great caution. Given traditional disease etiologies, these communities responded as they would to one with extremely dangerous spirit powers.

It can be argued then, that the decision of many Native people to be baptized coincided with traditional practice as a ritual act mandated by Demers's spirit power and fitting within indigenous modes of perceiving illness and curing. If Demers's spirit power was at fault for the crisis, and Bolduc shared this same spirit power, than the only hope was to affirm a relationship with Bolduc's spirit power, through its requested ritual action of baptism. Acquiescing to such a ritual act, however, did not necessarily imply conversion. For instance, while Blanchet is said to have baptized 122 children in a single Upper Skagit village on a single visit, local oral histories recall that while many were content to have their children baptized, parents did not necessarily adopt the Catholic faith. Many "rejected it after hearing it," while others did not hear it at all.[110]

People cannot simply live; they must live meaningfully. When confronted with the unthinkable, we shape our experience into a meaningful narrative; we must make sense of what we see. When early settlers and missionaries first arrived in the Pacific Northwest in the nineteenth century, they were struck by Native peoples' wealth, their complex social networks and strong communities. But when faced with Native deaths on a massive scale, they were forced to confront a profound question: why did we live, when they could not? Early generations of missionaries, settlers, and explorers made sense of their experience by drawing upon existent sacred stories and worldviews within their own cultures. Some concluded that Native people died because their practices were so different, so out of control, so unhealthy. Others argued that they died because their own healers deceived them and led them astray. Such illnesses were surely sent by God, most Euroamericans concluded, to subdue the Native people, so that they might be controlled or moved aside.

These early years of settlement and missionization in the Pacific Northwest were thus years in which Native communities were ravaged by disease, their communities and cultures experiencing enormous upheaval, at best, and complete destruction, at worst. Missionaries who attempted to reach indigenous communities, primarily on the Columbia River, in the Willamette Valley, and in southwest Washington, found their efforts stymied by high mortality rates as well as Coast Salish and Chinook loyalties to their traditional healers. Within a few short years Protestant missions had abandoned the field altogether, and Catholic missions had turned their attention almost exclusively to the offering of baptism and last rites. For the most part, missionary activity in the region was all but abandoned by the mid-nineteenth century and did not begin again in earnest until the establishment of the reservation system decades later.

3. "Civilization Is Poison to the Indian"

Missionization, Authenticity, and the Myth of the Vanishing Indian

> The world's people will credit [the missionaries] with hastening the red brother towards the vanishing point. The belief is common that civilization is poison to the Indian, and Christianity is reckoned as part of civilization.
>
> —T. W. DAVENPORT, 1851

In the latter half of the nineteenth century the nature of illness and the ways Euroamericans interpreted and responded to Native health changed in pivotal ways. This was due in large part to dramatic demographic and political shifts that occurred at this time, alongside the creation of a reservation system and the relocation or consolidation of a majority of indigenous people within Oregon and Washington onto those reserved plots of land. Two central concerns inspiring the creation of reservations were the removal of Native people so as to free up land for settlement by Euroamerican immigrants, and the protection of an indigenous population that was felt to be at risk from contact with the corrupting influences of white society. The reservation system allowed for increased control on the part of missionaries and government-appointed Indian agents, better enabling them to curtail indigenous practices and traditional healers directly. Rapid industrialization and a non-native population boom transformed the region and the ways in which non-natives viewed the original inhabitants of the region.

This chapter looks at how a second wave of missionary efforts developed in the late nineteenth century, taking place within this different setting of reservation communities and residential schools.[1] While earlier generations of missionaries had concluded that epidemic diseases were divine justice visited upon a sinful people, this later era was marked by a discourse assuming that civilization was lethal to "the Indian." Since indigenous people were equated with a romanticized past, these "children of nature" could not survive within the industrialized world. Their only chance was to be quarantined on reservations, away from the corrupting influence of whites, until they passed away into history or, with the aid of missionaries and boarding schools, successfully assimilated, leaving their Indian identity completely behind them.

Such efforts were strongly guided by nineteenth-century views of cultural evolution. Prevailing ideas among Euroamerican scholars and within popular thought were that human cultures existed on a linear evolutionary continuum. Scholars such as E. B. Tylor, Lewis Henry Morgan, Herbert Spencer, and Auguste Comte borrowed from biological theories of evolution to argue that human societies progress through set stages of development, from savagery to barbarism to civilization. Such thinkers often incorporated a kind of social Darwinism, arguing that "survival of the fittest" (a term coined by Spencer) could be seen at work among human communities and societies.[2] These authors expressed a firm faith in progress, arguing that human societies were on an evolutionary path, growing from the simple to the complex, flexible to ordered, general to specialized, crude to technological. In this perspective, "primitive" societies that had survived into the modern age, like those of Native American communities, were simply less evolved: they were located farther down the linear evolutionary scale of human progress and development. While their evolution had been slower than that of western Europeans, given the inevitable march of progress one could rest assured that these cultures would eventually grow into the light of civilization, leaving their "primitive" beliefs and practices behind. This was a philosophy built upon an assumption of the inherent superiority of western European and Euroamerican cultures and the inherent inferiority of indigenous cultures and practices.[3] While such ideas would be largely rejected among late twentieth-century scholars, they were enormously influential in the late nineteenth and early twentieth centuries.

At the same time Native people were becoming increasingly hidden from the view of most Euroamericans, either because they had been removed to reservations or residential schools or because they had outwardly assimilated to contemporary modes of dress, employment, and lifestyle and so were simply not recognized as "Indian" by the non-native population. As Native people became less visible (as well as declining demographically), Euroamerican society became increasingly nostalgic for the "children of the wilderness," who they felt were "passing away like dew." Popular thought dictated that just as the natural world must give way to "progress," so traditional cultures must fade away in order for industrialization and urbanization to proceed. And within this idea, the image of Native people became relegated to the past, a figment of historical nostalgia, while living Native communities vanished from people's consciousness, being virtually unseen except in moments when they appeared to fulfill white expectations of what "an Indian" should look like. Within this narrative, Native people would either assimilate to dominant culture and live or remain mired in the past and perish. In either event, the end result was the same: the "true Indians" would vanish.

The Reservation Era in the Pacific Northwest

Reservations played an important part in this moment of history and were influenced by various and contradictory narratives of the age. Some policy makers hoped reservations would isolate Native people from the broader American experience, either to protect non-native settlers from dangerous savages or to protect Native people from corrupting white influence. Other policy makers saw reservations as only a temporary stopover on the way to assimilation: reservation agents, missionaries, and schools would provide Native people with the tools they needed to enter the larger Christian, capitalist society. At that point reservations would no longer be necessary and would be opened up for settlement. The paradoxical result was that reservations removed American Indians from the immediate experience of most non-native people, even as they strove to facilitate the assimilation of Native people into the broader American context.

The creation of reservations across the Northwest differed dramatically by region. In British Columbia, for instance, no treaties were made, but small reserves were gradually created to accommodate individual villages. In most instances indigenous communities were not removed but were able to live on their ancestral village site while (theoretically, if not actually) maintaining access rights to traditional fishing, hunting, and gathering sites in the region. As a result "every village site in use and nearly every fishing camp became a 'reserve' and nearly every village became a 'band.'" Such an approach allowed each village to maintain its own territory, rather than being removed and thrown together with those from other villages, as more often happened in the United States.[4] The hope of the British Columbian provincial government was that creating small reserves such as these would encourage assimilation, in part because Native communities would be forced to seek work in nearby non-native communities.[5] The result was that 140 Indian reserves were created in British Columbia between 1850 and 1871 alone, in comparison to eighteen in Washington State and ten in Alberta.[6] By the 1930s British Columbia was home to more than fifteen hundred small reserves, dispersed throughout the province.[7]

The situation in what would become Washington and Oregon was dramatically different. Rather than creating small local reserves, Washington territorial governor Isaac Stevens intended to gather all indigenous peoples together onto a single consolidated reservation. When he encountered the strong resistance of indigenous communities, who refused to move far from home territories and live with many whom they historically counted as enemies, he was forced to give up his initial plan.[8] Instead, between 1854 and 1855, he created ten reservations for the entirety of western Washington. These treaties included more than 17,000 Native Americans, and released 64 million acres of land for settlement by Euroamericans, retaining 6 million acres for Native people.[9] In December 1854 the Treaty of Medicine Creek was signed, which concerned the southern Puget Sound and established reservations at Puyallup, Nisqually, and Squaxin Island. Within the terms of the treaty, Native inhabitants agreed to "accept authority of an Indian agent, to forbid the sale or use of alcoholic beverages within the reservations, to free their slaves, and not to trade with 'foreign' Indians or allow them to live on their reservations without the consent of the agent.[10] In return, the government agreed to establish a general district agency, to maintain a school for the children, to provide a smithy and carpenter's shop, to employ a smith, a carpenter, and a farmer to instruct the Indians in these occupations, and to provide the Indians with a physician."[11] The treaty also ensured the important "right of taking fish at usual and accustomed places."[12] January 22, 1855, saw the signing of the Point Elliott Treaty with the Duwamish, Suquamish, Snoqualmie, Snohomish, Stillaguamish, Swinomish, Skagit, and Lummi, which created the Tulalip, Swinomish, Lummi and Port Madison reservations. On January 26, 1855, the Point No Point Treaty with the Klallam, Twana, and Chemakum created the Skokomish reservation. On January 31, 1855, the Neah Bay Treaty established the Makah reservation, while also recognizing their hunting, fishing, whaling, and sealing rights. And on July 1, 1855, Quinault, Queets, Hoh and Quileute signed the Quinault River Treaty, creating the Quinault reservation. Reservations continued to be formed in the following years, including the Muckleshoot reservation in 1857, created to accommodate bands excluded from 1855 treaties, and in 1864 and 1866 non-treaty Chehalis and Chinook were granted the Chehalis and Shoalwater Bay reservations. Some of these families chose to join kin on the Quinault or Quileute reservation, while others stayed on family land as individual homesteaders.[13] In 1889 and 1893 the Quileute and Hoh were both granted their own reservations. Three small Klallam communities were also later granted reservations: Lower Elwha, Jamestown, and Port Gamble. The reservation system in western Washington was made largely without regard to kinship patterns, intervillage relations, or other precolonial systems of social organization. And those left out of treaty-signing processes "were expected to join their neighbors with reservations; generally, however, they refused to move."[14]

Oregon reservations were even more centralized. The Oregon Donation Land Act of 1850 provided 320 acres to settlers—without first securing release of land from Indians. Treaties were not negotiated with Willamette Valley tribes until 1851–53, and Euroamericans moved onto the lands well before the treaties were ratified.[15] The Grand Ronde reservation was created to accommodate the Native population who had survived the massive depopulation of Native western Oregon by the epidemic diseases of the first half of the nineteenth century. Between 1854 and 1857 survivors from the Willamette Valley were relocated to the reservation and were gradually joined by Native people from southern Oregon, driven from their homes by gold-rush-inspired massacres and forced relocation.[16] In all, many of the survivors of the Shasta, Kalapuya, Molala, Rogue River, Kilicktat, Chinook and Tillamook nations moved to the Grand Ronde reservation. Since most did not speak English, this multiethnic and multilingual community was forced to rely upon Chinook *wawa* in order to communicate.[17] Religious and cultural life at Grand Ronde thus involved enormous cultural diversity, particularly in religious ceremonies and healing traditions, which were carried on well into the early twentieth century.[18] Grand Ronde was terminated in 1956, reorganized as Confederated Tribes of Grand Ronde in 1974, and re-recognized in 1983. Some Chinook refused to move to Grand Ronde and remained in their ancestral homes along the Columbia River. This community organized into the Chinook Indian Nation and petitioned for federal recognition in the late twentieth century. By 2010 the tribe had more than two thousand members but remained unrecognized by the federal government.[19]

As my work is primarily concerned with the Puget Sound region, it is worth taking a closer look at historical and demographic changes that took place there during the latter half of the nineteenth century. Before the first American settlers arrived in Puget Sound in 1845, the only non-natives in the region were a few nomadic trappers. By the end of 1850 there were five hundred Euroamericans in Puget Sound. By 1852 there were several thousand.[20] By the 1860s, less than twenty years after the first settlers arrived in the region, Tacoma and Seattle had become thriving port communities, drawing Native people from throughout the Pacific Northwest to trade, work, and be part of the new settler society.[21] High rates of intermarriage marked these early years, despite a series of laws intended to outlaw mixed marriage and delegitimize children of such unions. However, as Coll Thrush notes, such laws were difficult to enforce as "it was difficult to find jurors and attorneys who did not have Indian family members" themselves.[22]

Between 1880 and 1920 Seattle and Tacoma grew at an explosive rate, impacting local Native populations enormously and resulting in the loss of traditional camping, fishing, and hunting locales. Increasing pollution and overharvesting decimated populations of local fish and wildlife.[23] One Native Seattleite complained that he had been told they "had to stop fishing, 'or they will be arrested.'"[24]

Native demographics changed dramatically during this time as well. After 1855, when settlement of the region began in earnest and Native Americans were quickly outnumbered by Euroamericans, illnesses changed. Venereal diseases, tuberculosis, and measles had displaced smallpox and "fever and ague" as the main killers of Native people.[25] By 1872, for instance, "a large proportion" of the Skokomish tribe was reported to be ill with syphilis, though many of these individuals may have been misdiagnosed.[26] In 1877 another smallpox epidemic struck the Seattle-Tacoma region, disproportionately affecting Native people.[27] Between 1850 and 1870 Native populations dwindled from 7,000 or 8,000 to 3,000. At the same time Euroamerican populations in the region were rapidly expanding. In 1860 Native Americans made up half the population of the Puget Sound region, but by 1890 they were outnumbered 20 to 1. Between 1870 and 1890 Tacoma grew from 1,107 to 42,837, and Seattle, which was only founded in 1868, had 36,000 people by 1890.[28] By 1900 Seattle had become a regular stop for Native people seeking seasonal labor from all over the Pacific Northwest, from southern Oregon to Southeast Alaska to the Columbia Plateau. The population of Native Seattle grew, becoming increasingly diverse.[29] This era is remarkable then for the major changes it brought to indigenous lives: the move to reservations, dislocation from traditional village sites, the growing impact of Euroamerican influences, and creation of diverse, cosmopolitan urban Indian communities in Seattle and Tacoma.[30]

Missionization in the Reservation Era

By the mid-1840s missionary efforts were on the decline in the Pacific Northwest. While they had certainly had an impact on the shape of indigenous religious and cultural life (discussed at length in chapter 4), they had failed to make the kinds of inroads for which their founders and funders had initially hoped. Protestant missions in particular either were closed or turned their attention to the growing numbers of Euroamerican settlers, while the few Catholic missions that remained concentrated their efforts in fewer locales. For the most part Native communities returned to their own ceremonial traditions, integrating some elements of Christian ritual and mythology and retaining what they could of their own cultural and religious practices.

While most Native communities in Washington and Oregon were confined to reservations by the late 1850s, even there they received relatively little attention from Euroamerican missionaries. A Clackamas Chinook oral narrative recorded by Jacobs recalled the days of a Catholic mission at Grand Ronde. The piece presents the priests in a comical light and illustrates to some degree how ineffective missions had been in this community. As one woman told him, "When the person-who-continually-prayed (a Catholic priest) first came to this place, he told them, 'you should pray all the time, the above chief (God) will see you then. But if you do not believe it, then you will have tails (and you will remain just like the animals you are), like the various animals that run about in the forests.' Now, my husband's mother would say, "Dear oh dear! Probably it would be something different (and really funny) when we play (women's) shinny. We would whip each other with our tails!"[31]

The ability of missionaries to influence Native communities did not gain ground until the 1870s with the implementation of President Grant's Peace Policy, which sought to reform the corrupt Bureau of Indian Affairs and reduce conflict between religious denominations by appointing Christian missionaries to oversee reservations. This began a second era in missionary work among these communities, as the federal government divided reservations up among various religious denominations. Some of these assignments were made regardless of which religious group had first established a presence on the reservation: Catholic missions might be displaced by Protestants. Among the Tlingit in Southeast Alaska, for instance, people familiar with Russian Orthodoxy were suddenly presented with Presbyterian missions.[32] The Neah Bay reservation, including the Makah and Quileute, were assigned first to Christian Union and later to Methodists.[33] The Skokomish-Twanas, Squaxins, and Klallams were assigned to Congregationalists, while the Puyallup, Nisqually, and Upper Chehalis were placed in the care of Presbyterians.[34] The Presbyterian minister Reverend M. G. Mann, for instance, arrived to minister to the Puyallup in 1876, and he also visited the Nisqually and Chehalis regularly, building churches there in 1880 and 1881, respectively. The Swinomish, Tulalip, Port Madison, Lummi, Suquamish, and Muckleshoot reservations were assigned to Catholic clergy, under the supervision of Eugene Casimir Chirouse, OMI. After working with the Yakama from 1848 to 1856, Chirouse had been reassigned to Tulalip, where he remained from 1857 to 1878. Chirouse authored a grammar and catechism in Coast Salish and the first English-Salish dictionary. He appears to have been relatively well received at Tulalip, with a loyal following of parishioners.[35] Reverend Myron Eells claimed in 1887 that in addition to the Cowlitz, Nisqually, and Tulalip, "the Snohomish, Port Madison, Muckleshoot, Lummi, and Swinomish reservations [had] been under the teachings of the Catholics" since the 1850s.[36] Michael Kew has likewise concluded that conversion to Christianity, Catholicism in particular, was nearly universal among the Central Coast Salish by 1900, largely as a result of Chirouse's efforts.[37]

However, reasons for conversion were complex and stemmed from a multitude of different motivations. Some experienced a genuine faith conversion. Others found elements of the new faith appealing and participated in a selective manner. Others recognized the pragmatic necessity of working with one's Indian agent, in order to ensure that one's family had access to resources, education, and material support, and adapted to changing contexts to meet their own pressing needs. Consider for instance that when a group of Nooksacks moved from Tulalip to the Lummi reservation in 1876, their Catholic status put them at risk of being dispossessed of their homes by settlers. In response, the Nooksacks became Methodists.[38]

If Chirouse was the most influential missionary figure in central Puget Sound during this era, one can argue that in the south the greatest impact was made by two brothers: Edwin and Myron Eells. In 1871 Edwin Eells, son of Cushing and Myra Eells, was appointed to govern the Puyallup-Nisqually agency, which also included the Skokomish-Twanas and the Squaxins. He remained there until 1895. In 1874 his Congregationalist brother Reverend Myron Eells arrived and took over ministerial duties in the region. He continued in this work until his death in 1907. Myron Eells would go on to publish a hymnal in Chinook *wawa* in 1878, and became an avid scholar of Coast Salish culture, keeping detailed journals of his observations that offer a wealth of information about the state of Coast Salish practices, beliefs, and material culture of the time.

The Suppression of Indigenous Medicine and Culture

Despite the fact that Myron Eells made a careful study of southern Coast Salish religious and cultural life, he was also firmly committed to the eradication of that culture. For him, the survival of the indigenous population of the region was absolutely dependent upon their conversion to Christianity and their assimilation into Euroamerican culture. Eells was particularly concerned with the elimination of Coast Salish religious and healing traditions. He associated such indigenous healers with greed and deception when he wrote that they demanded "large fees, and sometimes in advance, for healing the sick."[39] This claim is not borne out by ethnographic evidence from the early twentieth century, which tells us that while healers were greatly respected and often feared, they rarely demanded payment (though they might accept gifts), and some refused any kind of payment at all.[40]

By contrast, Eells saw Coast Salish healers as professional hucksters, deceiving their communities. As he described it: "Sometimes a person who has much intercourse with the other world persuades one who is in the best of health that he has visited the spirit land and seen the spirit of his dupe there, and the latter is thus frightened into having a tamanous. Again, when some credulous individual has been ailing a little for a long time, but not sufficiently to feel that he needs to employ a medicine man, one of these arrant humbugs takes a fancied journey of which he soon announces, and once more there must be a tamanous."[41]

Myron Eells observed that healing practices, which he called "tamahnous over the sick," continued to be the primary obstacle to Christian influence and Native conversion. As he wrote, "This kind of tamahnous has more power over the Indian mind than any other. The others have reference in a general way to religion, and are partly practices to wile away the time in the winter, or to call people together for a social time; but this has reference to their lives. It is material, intensely practical."[42] While Eells's theology offered promises of otherworldly salvation, it was hard-pressed to compete with religious practices that met the "material, intensely practical" needs of the lived-body in community.

Nineteenth-century observers (such as Eells) noted high rates of somatic complaints among their wards but were rarely able to offer adequate medical care.[43] While reservation officials often included an agency physician, he was generally extremely limited in training, funding, and pharmacopoeia and did not often venture out into the communities he served. When care was available, it often did more harm than good. In 1903, for instance, it was reported that among the fifty-six families living on the Skokomish reservation, in twenty families there were no children—due either to sterility or to the death of all the children. While it is extremely difficult to be certain about determining the origins and diagnoses of historical ailments, George Guilmet and colleagues concluded that these high rates of infertility and early mortality were caused at least in part by misdiagnosis: physicians assumed most were infected with syphilis (though Guilmet challenges this), and the common treatment for syphilis at the time was heavy doses of mercury iodide.[44] Mercury poisoning can cause sterility or death.

Even when biomedical care was available, most Native people avoided it. As Reverend Eells recalled, "They are slow to use the white man's medicine (although on the reservation they are furnished free of charge), often preferring their old remedies in slight cases of illness, and in severe cases their tamanous. If a medicine cures quickly they like it; but if after a few days they are not well, they abandon it. Those who live off reservation seldom have any treatment except in the old style."[45]

While missionaries and the American government were relatively unequipped to provide adequate medical care to American Indian communities, they simultaneously worked to outlaw and eliminate indigenous medical and religious practices.[46] During their time working with indigenous communities in south Puget Sound, the Eells brothers continued to struggle against traditional healers and were forced to call upon the threat of physical force to curtail healers' practices. Their efforts were backed by the superintendent of Indian affairs for Washington Territory, who in 1871 had banned "Indian doctoring" altogether.[47] As Myron Eells wrote: "About 1871 or 1872 the Agent E. Eells had orders [to prevent traditional healers from practicing] from the Superintendent of Indian Affairs for Washington Territory, but it was simply impossible. The Indians would hide away, or leave the reservation, or doctor at night to cure the sick in their way, and not an Indian would dare to testify to the fact." In 1885, for instance, Edwin Eells tried to stop well-known medicine man Tenas Charley from curing the sick, attempting to have him arrested. However, tribal police were fearful of his possible anger and refused to do more than politely request that he pay the agent a visit. Agent Eells then threatened to call upon the army to enforce the law, and Tenas Charley surrendered. As Myron Eells recalled, "So after dinner he came down and delivered himself up. He was put in jail for ten days, and fined forty dollars. It did him good, for he learned not to oppose the government, and became in many ways a better Indian."[48]

The active suppression by reservation officials alongside the loss of elders to disease, hunger, and poverty meant that many communities were soon without the care of traditional healers, a loss that struck a devastating blow to indigenous cultures and communities. As George Guilmet and David Whited have argued, healing was "but one part of a larger philosophical system" that included "religion, economics, politics, and medicine." When one part of that system was damaged, the whole web unwound.[49] The devastation of epidemics, the loss of traditional healing systems, and the impact of the reservation on extended kinship communities and local economies inspired many younger people to try to assimilate into the dominant Euroamerican culture, leading to further disruption of joint family households and traditional knowledge.[50]

Educating for Assimilation

As described in the previous chapter, an earlier generation of missionaries to the Northwest had attributed epidemics and staggering mortality rates both to Native peoples' "abominable lives" and to divine Providence. By the 1880s a new generation of missionaries had arrived, with a new narrative. With the backing of the federal government and the military, missionaries and agents such as the Eells brothers were able to exert a degree of influence and control over their reservation communities in a way their predecessors could not. And they were operating from a different discourse regarding indigenous mortality. Like their predecessors, missionaries of the late nineteenth century believed that the indigenous population was fading away. However, this later generation was inspired by nineteenth-century notions of cultural evolution to see their demise as a necessary part of the path toward progress, civilization, and industrialization. Euroamerican popular imagery of indigenous people located them squarely in the past, as part of nature that must be tamed, of a precivilized barbarism that must necessarily give way to progress. Only two options remained for indigenous people: assimilate into Euroamerican culture, leaving one's indigenous culture and identity completely behind, or die. Many missionaries of the time saw it as their primary task to assist those who were able to assimilate into a Christian, Euroamerican culture, abandoning their indigenous identity to the mists of history.

Ideas of cultural evolution would be highly influential within the creation of residential schools for Native children. Those who advocated the removal of Native children from their home communities shared the view that Native cultures were less evolved and that children would benefit from access to the civilized accomplishments of Euroamerican culture. Such perspectives differed from many race-based theories of evolution in regarding Native people as *capable* of being civilized. It was argued that Indian children had the best chances of success and survival if they were removed from their home communities, instructed in English, converted to Christianity, and taught vocational trades.[51] Local mission schools were established as early as the first reservations, and many more were founded following Grant's Peace Policy of 1869, which placed reservations under the governance of Christian denominations.[52]

Three types of residential schools existed in the Pacific Northwest: off-reservation federal boarding schools, reservation boarding schools, and mission schools that were generally located on or near a reservation. The Carlisle Indian School in Carlisle, Pennsylvania, was the first centralized, federally funded off-reservation boarding school, founded in 1879 by Captain Richard Henry Pratt. The school focused on cultural transformation. Dramatic photographs depicted "before and after" images of Native students, arriving with long hair and traditional dress and later coiffed and dressed in Victorian style, seated in classrooms.[53] The second such federally sponsored institution was the Chemewa Indian School in Oregon, founded in 1880 in Forest Grove and relocated to Salem in 1885, in part to have access to better agricultural lands. Initially all of Chemewa's students came from Washington State, from the Puyallup and Nisqually reservations in particular. By 1920 the school enrolled 903 students from ninety tribes. Some traveled from as far away as Alaska. Such schools concentrated their efforts on preparing students for manual vocations, and Chemewa placed strong emphasis on agriculture, dairy farming, and animal husbandry. An early pamphlet promoting the Chemewa Indian School presents images of young Native men being trained at "blacksmithing," "wagon making," and "shoe making."[54]

The federal government also established on-reservation boarding schools, though school officials worked diligently to curtail contact between students and their families, limiting visitation to proscribed times and often maintaining on-campus residence for nine months out of the year. Administrators of both off-reservation and on-reservation boarding schools tried to eliminate all signs of Native language and culture, strictly enforcing "English-only" policies.[55] Small reservation schools were founded on the Chehalis, Skokomish, and Makah reservations, though all were closed by 1896. In Tacoma, Cushman Indian School boarded Puyallup students beginning in 1873. By 1901 the school housed 350 students from throughout the Northwest and Alaska. The school closed in 1920.[56]

The most prominent mission school in this region was the Tulalip Mission School, founded in 1857 by Father Eugene Casimir Chirouse and located at Priest's Point near the Tulalip reservation. By 1868 the boys' school was joined by a girls' school, under the direction of the Sisters of Providence. The school was the first federal contract Indian school, receiving federal funds to maintain its buildings, while the Church provided other necessary materials and resources. Under its founder, the school had a complex relationship with Salish culture. As a scholar of the Lushootseed language, Chirouse preached his sermons in both English and Snohomish as well as translating prayers and Bible stories into the local language.[57] At the same time, Chirouse felt called to educate young Indian children in English, in the Christian tradition, and in vocations such as farming and animal husbandry. Girls were trained in domestic skills such as sewing, baking, and housekeeping. He also endeavored to eradicate drinking, gambling, polygamy, and intertribal violence among the local communities. It does not, however, appear that Chirouse sought to eradicate local indigenous languages, nor the culture as a whole.[58]

However, when the school became a federal facility in 1901 (now known as the Tulalip Indian School) the transfer to federal control brought with it an era of severe cultural repression. Speaking Native languages or engaging with traditional cultural activities were thereafter forbidden. The federal institution welcomed students from throughout the Northwest and offered education through the eighth grade. Many students would then transfer to Chemewa to complete their secondary education. The Tulalip school would close in 1923, leaving Chemewa Indian School as the only remaining federal boarding school in the region.

School attendance was made mandatory by federal law in 1893. Strictly speaking, Native students were not required to attend boarding schools. However, it was also policy that local Indian agents would pressure families into sending their children away to school. Agents were given the authority to withhold rations and annuities or threaten parents with jail time if they did not surrender their children, some as young as six years old.[59] Understandably, many parents resisted.

From the 1880s to the 1930s schools worked hard to stamp out Native language, culture, and religion. Discipline was harsh, including being locked in isolation, physical beatings, and withholding of food. Schools typically followed a military model, with carefully regulated daily schedules. Students were marched from one activity to another, and discipline was strictly enforced. Students typically spent the first half of the day in classes, studying English, geography, U.S. history, reading, and writing. The second half of the day would be spent working ("vocational training") in the kitchens, fields, barns, or workshops.

Students experienced fear, loneliness, and confusion as they were removed from their homes, families, and communities. Many did not speak English and had no way of communicating with those not from their home communities. Young people were generally housed and schooled by age, so siblings and cousins were not necessarily able to seek each other out for comfort.[60] Most schools were underfunded: food and medical care were inadequate, and schools were often found to be unsanitary and poorly insulated. Disease could run rampant. Tuberculosis was a great threat to students at the Tulalip Indian School, for instance. Larger schools had their own cemeteries for those students whose bodies were not sent home. Chemewa Indian School's cemetery contains the bodies of 189 students.

Despite all this, some people have reflected on the school experience positively, thankful for the opportunity to learn, enjoying the social exchange and the fun of participating in school sports, theater, and music. The dominant narrative within American Indian and Canadian First Nations people's recollections on the residential school era, however, is extremely negative. High rates of physical and sexual abuse, neglect, and homesickness, coupled with the sometimes violent suppression of Native cultures and religions, traumatized many students. Some institutions had shockingly high rates of physical and sexual abuse, while others were more humane, better funded, and better able to provide a safe and healthy environment.

The student's experience also appears to have depended on age at the time of arrival at the school. Christine Quintasket (Okanogan), also known as Mourning Dove, provides a good example.[61] When she first attended school she was far too young and was traumatized as a result. When she returned at an older age, she welcomed the experience and would later go on to become an author who chronicled the history and culture of her people. Proximity to home appears to have been another factor that influenced a student's experience. Students who were able to attend schools closer to home (and hence able to return home for regular visits) tended to do better than those forced to travel far from home and unable to see family for months and sometimes years at a time.[62]

The Meriam Report, commissioned by the federal government in 1928 in part to investigate the conditions of Indian schools throughout the country, found that conditions at most residential schools were unacceptable. The report detailed poor diet, poor sanitation, high rates of disease, poor medical care, excessive physical labor demanded of students, crumbling infrastructure, unacceptable teaching, and outdated curriculum content.[63] For all their faults and their good intentions, residential schools were a product of their moment in history and of the prevailing views toward American Indian people at the time. With a strong belief in progress and the necessity that "primitive" and "barbaric" cultures give way to civilization, many Euroamericans felt that only two possibilities stood before Native people: assimilate or perish. In either event, Native people were assumed to be vanishing into history.

"Civilization Is Poison to the Indian"

Contemporary commentators agreed that missions worked very effectively to remove "the Indian problem."[64] As Indian Agent T. W. Davenport wrote as early as 1851, "The world's people will credit [the missionaries] with hastening the red brother towards the vanishing point. The belief is common that civilization is poison to the Indian, and Christianity is reckoned as part of civilization."[65] According to Davenport, missionaries were both savior and executioner. As Methodist Episcopal Bishop J. W. Bashford wrote on September 5, 1878, the Catholic missions and "the slower pace at which they led their wards toward the white man's civilization at least kept the Indians alive longer than did the Protestants, with their more rapid rate of progress." But both efforts arrived at the same end: "all contributed, if not to the speedy, at least to the orderly settlement" of the Northwest and removal of its Native inhabitants.[66] It was not merely the lack of civilization that threatened Native survival—but the actual presence of civilization as well. Civilization was considered lethal to indigenous people.

Missionaries working in the early reservation era often shared these sentiments, hoping that the reservation boundaries would protect their wards from the unwholesome influence of Euroamerican society. Reverend Myron Eells held this view and strongly opposed efforts to grant citizenship and land allotments to south Puget Sound Natives, which would end their tribal status, open up the reservation to white settlement, and further expose the Coast Salish under his care to the more debased elements of white society. In such a context, he argued, vices were certain to arise, as were illnesses in general. Eells noted that contact with civilization had had a weakening effect on the Skokomish and Squaxin under his care. In the 1880s he argued that "many have died from diseases caused by the transition from a savage to a civilized life. . . . Colds and rheumatism are far more common and fatal than when they were uncivilized."[67] He also noted that contact with Euroamerican civilization had increased the difficulty of childbirth for Native women, resulting in higher mortality rates for mothers and infants.[68]

In the minds of some Euroamericans, demographic decline, coupled with notions of the inevitable demise of Native peoples in the face of progress and civilization, worked to justify the devastating impact that settlement and introduced diseases had on the indigenous population. As Thomas Nelson Strong wrote in 1906, "The white man had no need of war or violence in his dealings with these Indians, nor did he employ them, for the Sahalee Tyee, the Indian God had struck before him," clearing the land.[69] By constructing such narratives drawn from the myth of the vanishing Indian, some nineteenth-century Euroamerican settlers crafted an image of American Indians as passively, almost benignly making way for progress and industrialization, at the behest of God almighty.[70] Euroamericans simply could not conceive of a surviving Native population that remained culturally Coast Salish or Chinook. They must utterly assimilate (and thereby cease to be), or they must die.

Consider, for example, Davenport's recollections, an important testimony to this view. He first mentions that "when I arrived in the Oregon Territory in the year 1851, the Chinook had become extinct."[71] This is obviously an erroneous statement, given the presence of Chinook communities at the time and their survival today. The point is that to Davenport, they were already gone. Their actual presence was irrelevant because they had ceased to exist as the "genuine Indians" of his imagination. Later, however, Davenport notes the death of one of his Chinook interpreters, evidence that they were not "extinct." Though the man was shot, an investigation was never carried out: "He was a half-breed Indian," Davenport explained, "and as a rule, inquiry as to the cause of death in the whole or half breed Indian stops at the bullet hole."[72] Death of Native people, according to the dominant discourse of white society, was simply to be expected.[73]

This perspective appeared to be confirmed by the demographic changes that hit Puget Sound between 1880 and 1930. The rapid industrialization of the region was disastrous for indigenous people trying to maintain their traditions within their ancestral locations. Those who remained did so because they were able to adapt to life in the new urban environment, becoming, as Coll Thrush argues, "almost invisible."[74] While numerous Native Americans made the cities of Olympia, Tacoma, and Seattle their home, within the narrative of the vanishing Indian, these apparently assimilated individuals were no longer "real Indians." Real Indians could not be well adapted to a modern economy. They could not be integrated into an urban society, speak English, or drive trucks.[75] As far as local Euroamericans were concerned, there were no more "real Indians" to be found. Or if they existed, they lived on reservations and were rapidly fading away. Thrush notes a poignant example of this. When the city of Seattle needed to replace the Chief-of-All-Women totem pole, an iconic image in Pioneer Square, they hired carvers from Alaska rather than consider local artists. Southeast Alaskan Natives such as the Tlingit and Haida were considered still to be "real Indians," both because they came from a "totem pole culture" and because they were farther removed from urban life.[76] Whether because they had been removed out of sight onto reservations, or assimilated into white society, or because local communities did not live up to romanticized images of what a Native person should look like, Coast Salish people had vanished from view.

Thrush further argues that because of being perceived as a vanishing race, the indigenous population was no longer seen as a threat. Instead, the image of the Indian or the Noble Savage came to serve an "allegorical purpose." As "actual Native people" became "overshadowed by symbolic Indians in Seattle's urban imagination," Euroamerican popular culture appropriated indigenous terminology and symbolism for its own, using these as means for expressing a nostalgia for the wilderness, for the pioneer spirit, and for the loss of natural places and the frontier lifestyle to urban development.[77] As non-natives built their suburban homes, they borrowed names from Chinook *wawa*, selecting words that were "picturesque" and "quaint."[78] Consider, for example, that between 1911 and 1914 Seattle's main public festival was the "Potlatch," an awkward appropriation of Native imagery and stereotype, employed to boost the standing of local business leaders and investors. As Thrush points out, Seattle's name itself honors the "seemingly noblest of savages," but in order to do so relies "on two premises: a notion of a vanishing race and a belief in inevitable Anglo-Saxon supremacy."[79]

This fascination with indigenous culture and the myth of the vanishing Indian were both driven by Euroamerican notions of "authenticity." For much of colonial history, Euroamericans have privileged what they defined as "authentic" Indian culture and have sought it out for museum collections, private curios, and other forms of cultural tourism. But of course this begs the question: what makes for "authentic" indigenous culture, and who gets to determine what is authentic? Since the late nineteenth century, Euroamerican popular culture had constructed a narrative of what made for authentic Indian culture. Within this schema authenticity required a kind of racial purity: only "full-bloods" could be considered truly authentic. To be of mixed ancestry was suspect. Further, as Paige Raibmon puts it, the authentic was "traditional, uncivilized, cultural, impoverished, feminine, static, part of nature and the past." Authentic Indians, then, were part of "a noble and tragic past but had no role in the future." To be authentic one could not be "modern, civilized, political, prosperous, masculine, dynamic, or part of society and the future." And so, by this logic, assimilated Indians could not be Indians at all. To survive modernity intrinsically disqualified one from any claim to authentic Indian identity.[80] As Raibmon concludes, "according to prevailing notions of authenticity, Aboriginal people could not be 'Aboriginal' and 'modern' at the same time."[81]

Yet ironically, since the late nineteenth century many non-native people have been inspired by a romantic primitivism and have sought escape from modernity through the appropriation of indigenous imagery and mythology. The boy scouts and fee-for-service vision quests are immediate examples that may come to mind.[82] And to some degree, Native communities have cooperated with these narratives of authenticity, whether it be a nineteenth-century woman posing for photos for a fee, or a twenty-first-century casino making use of indigenous imagery to market a rollout of new slot machines. Raibmon's analysis of indigenous cultural performance in the nineteenth century illustrates the ways in which Natives gained access to national and international stages by "playing Indian" and conforming to colonial expectations of what they should look and sound like—even as they often simultaneously subverted those expectations. By directly engaging with colonial expectations, and at times upsetting them, Native communities were able to challenge directly the notion that authentic Indian culture could not coexist with modernity. Performing an unsettling traditional dance at the Chicago World's Fair, for instance, simultaneously "proclaimed their cultural survival and political defiance."[83] Indigenous communities could thus collaborate in the creation of their public image and identity, even as they subtly challenged or undermined those images.

But as Raibmon argues, the catch-22 of engaging with Euroamerican stereotypes of indigenous authenticity is that Native cultures may be empowered to survive only "in a cultural formaldehyde."[84] When Native people collaborated with late nineteenth- and early twentieth-century Euroamerican appropriation of "authentic" Indian imagery, they benefited in material and symbolic ways. By selling baskets, or posing for photographs, they were able to earn a living while simultaneously demonstrating their continuing presence and vitality to a growing Euroamerican populace. But on the other hand, "their roles as photographic subjects and curio vendors fed the ideological underpinnings of political and economic systems that threatened their ability to remain self-supporting. The 'Indian Hop Picker' became a poster child for the industrial development of the region. She attracted the sources of her own disenfranchisement."[85]

Such stereotypes have had profound consequences for Native health and wellness, influencing missionaries and government officials who designed policies based on the assumption that Native communities were passing away. Federal policies actively sought to suppress traditional healers, forcing those who maintained their traditions to do so underground. At the same time the federal government failed to provide anything close to adequate healthcare in response. During the first half of the twentieth century American Indian communities struggled with poverty, unemployment, and the cultural devastation brought by forced removal of Native children to boarding schools and the suppression of indigenous languages and religious practices.[86] And healthcare would remain an enormous challenge. Despite the fact that healthcare had been promised within treaty negotiations, most Native people did not have access to adequate care.[87] As Harmon has pointed out, the federal government had failed utterly to provide promised care to the Native populations of Puget Sound. "For people whose elders had judged someone's powers in part by his or her health, it was humiliating that disease felled so many friends and relatives. It was doubly galling that the government provided only one doctor—a doctor who allegedly swore and pointed guns at his patients—for more than thirty-four hundred Indians in an area one hundred miles square."[88]

Many indigenous communities in western Oregon and Washington maintained a long-standing distrust of federally provided medicine, a distrust that continued well into the twentieth century.[89] Ethnographers recorded numerous stories that portrayed historical biomedical interventions as part of a federal plot to destroy the Indian population. One Clackamas Chinook story told to Melville Jacobs in the 1950s is indicative of this tradition.

> Now one (Indian) became sick. They (whites) went to get him, they took him with them, they brought him (to their hospital). They cut his beautiful long and thick hair, they shaved it off. One person (an Indian or part Indian) I do not know where he was from was the one who took

care of the sick people. He (probably he was a hospital orderly) said to him, "Be on your guard!" He (the orderly) gave him a handkerchief. He said to him, "He (the doctor) will give you medicine. Do not swallow it. Spit it out. Here is a handkerchief. Wipe (inside) your mouth. He will try to give you water. Do not drink it." "Yes," he replied to him. And soon afterward the shaman (the white doctor) came, he brought him medicine. He told him, "Drink the medicine now!" He gave it to him, he held his handkerchief, he poured it into his mouth, he hurried and wiped it (out from inside his mouth), he spit out the medicine. He said to him, "Here is water, drink it!" He replied to him, "No." Where the medicine ran out (from his lips), his mouth (lips) was all burned. They (his relatives) went to see him, he said to them, "Come get me quickly!" They went to get him, they took him to their house. He told them about it. He said to them, "Had not that other person (the orderly) seen me I should now be long since dead. The shaman (the white doctor) is giving bad medicine to people (to Indian patients), they are dying (because of that). . . . He must have come to live here just in order to kill the (Indian) people." So she used to say. "The myth (white) people just fixed up the disease for us. They wanted this country of ours."[90]

Stories such as this reveal a cultural narrative alive in Native communities, a narrative that saw biomedicine and colonialism as being intricately intertwined and that portrayed Euroamerican physicians as having potently diabolical intentions. At the same time, such stories also encouraged individuals to seek traditional healers and abide by traditional values and ethics, rather than seeking aid from Euroamerican physicians.

Jacobs's interviews with reservation communities during the 1930s attest to a continued respect for and faith in Native healing traditions. Consider this Coos narrative: "A strong shaman [*ilxqa'in* is the Coos term for such a healer], when a person was constantly spitting (from consumption), this is what they said, when he looked at the sick person, 'It is just this that has made him ill. It is like a *gu'me'* worm that is eating him there inside him. That is what is making him cough, that thing like a *gu'me'* worm.' Then indeed he worked on the person who had that sickness, and when he took it out, they all saw it (the worm). Indeed then the sick person got well."[91] Given indigenous disease etiologies, such stories of successful cures were not without political implications. While Euroamerican healers were accused of poisoning their patients and Euroamerican hospitals were seen as places where people went to die (perhaps an accurate analysis when considering the history of Native American tuberculosis sanitariums, particularly in the first half of the twentieth century), Native healers were credited with seeing the true cause of illness and removing its source. Tales of successful cures attested to the strength of Native culture. Told at a time when white hospitals provided little hope for Native communities, these narratives of genuine cures reaffirmed the value and efficacy of traditional healers.

One oral history is worth considering at some length, because it stands in direct contrast to historical notions of the vanishing Indian unable to accommodate modernity or embody non-native expectations of "authenticity." In 1959 Melville Jacobs spoke with Mrs. Howard, a Clackamas Chinook woman living on the Grande Ronde reservation, who recalled her community's health history as described to her by her mother-in-law. Before the reservation days, she recalls, "coughing sickness" had hit the community. This coughing sickness spread rapidly, killing large numbers of people.

> Children would be running about, they would start to cough, they would run, and soon after while they were still running they would drop right there, they would die. She said, many of them died (like that, or more slowly). The cough killed them.
>
> I do not know how long a time after then, and then again they were announcing, they said, "The ague (fever and shivering) is on its way here. Dear oh dear! Now another thing!" Soon but I do not know how long after, then some one person got the ague. He lay with his back to the fire, he only got colder. They threw covers over him, but the ague got worse. His whole body shook. So long a time and then it stopped. Now he got feverish, he got thirsty for water. They gave it to him, he drank it. So many days, then he died. Then some other person too, and

also I do not know how many others got the ague. Soon then a great many of them, I do not know how many. Their village was a large one, but they all got the ague. In each and every house so many of the people were ill now. . . . The Clackamas people died (from the introduced sicknesses), I do not know how many. Only a few did not die. It (the epidemic of ague) quit even before they gathered them (the corpses that were lying around), they buried them. They were at last through with (burying) them all, and then they (the survivors) lived there.

I do not know how long afterward, then again they now got measles. Now they were again like that, they died. They drank quantities of water in the same manner again, they died quickly. They were like that (one of the people after another catching measles) for a considerable time. It (the rash) would come out on a child, he would get cold, it (the disease) would (because he had not been kept sufficiently warm), go in (into his heart or stomach), and presently he would die. Some of them went to sweat (in their sweathouse). It would come out all over them, the measles would come out on their eyes. Some of them would come out (of the sweathouse), they would pour cold water on (themselves), they would die soon after that. Some came out, they lay down, they put covers over them, they would recover. After a long time then they did not die much more from that. But it was quite a while before the disease left.

I do not know how long after, and then a pain (like heart trouble) got them. One shaman got it (learned about it) quickly, it bit him. ʔa.' ʔa.' ʔa.' it did to him. He died. They got some one shaman, he doctored them. He said, "I shall take it (the disease-power) out (from some sick person), I shall throw the disease to a dog." He took out the disease, he threw it to a dog. Presently the dogs got the disease. . . . Then after some short time now the (surviving) people became well, not many more died of it. Only their dogs all died. That is what she (my mother-in-law) said.

Mrs. Howard went on to describe a final scourge of illness that hit the community, when "right here at this place (at Oregon City) they again got fever."[92] Importantly she did not stop there but continued her narrative to describe the way in which Indian communities were shortly thereafter gathered together on the Grand Ronde reservation. The remnants of most tribes in western Oregon, including the Chinooks, Klamath, Upper Umpquas, Shastas, Rogue River Indians, Kalapuyas, and Yonkallas, were painfully separated from their homelands and brought together on this new reservation. The transition, as she described it, was not an easy one, but she went on to conclude her story by pointing out that the community was now settled and growing.

The story is an important one, placed alongside Euroamerican narratives of the vanishing Indian. It does not shirk from recalling the tragedies and dire impact of illness upon Native people. But it includes the story of the survivors. After enduring five epidemics (five is an important ritual number in oral traditions of the Northwest), the community had been gathered together at Grand Ronde. A difficult transitional period followed, when the tribes were given commodity issue foods and tents, goods to which they were unaccustomed. Mrs. Howard recalled with pride that because of an acquaintance with a white woman, she knew how to prepare the strange food they were given as rations, such as pork and white flour. They had suffered greatly, but they had survived. The story is striking today, during an era when Native people are decidedly *not* vanishing demographically or culturally. And this story is particularly poignant given that the Confederated Tribes of Grand Ronde today constitute one of the most economically successful tribal communities in the region. From the success of its Spirit Mountain Casino, opened during the 1990s, the tribe has been able to donate large sums of money to various organizations: it has built its own health clinic; provided assistance to the Oregon Health Plan (health insurance for people falling below the poverty line); sponsored a wing of the Multnomah County Library, where I researched part of this chapter; and funded the creation of an art museum featuring American Indian cultural materials at Willamette University, the university founded by Jason Lee at the Willamette mission.

By the late nineteenth and early twentieth centuries, federal Indian agents and missionaries such as Myron Eells approached their work with renewed purpose, but they remained extremely skeptical of the ability of Native people to survive *as Native people* in the modern world. By the late nineteenth century the prevailing Euroamerican narrative was that "primitive cultures" like those of the Coast Salish and Chinook were simply incompatible with the onward march of civilization. Buoyed by scholarly and popular notions of cultural evolution, policy makers argued that Native people, like all peoples, were destined to progress toward civilization or be left behind: only the fittest would survive. Some missionaries, such as Eells, felt Natives' only hope was to be isolated on reservations, removed from Euroamericans' corrupting influence. But faced with continued high mortality and skyrocketing rates of tuberculosis, venereal diseases, and a host of other ailments, few missionaries managed to sustain any hope that Native people would survive for long. Federal officials, social reformers, and missionaries turned to boarding schools in the hope that Native children could be assimilated into the broader American culture.

Turning our attention to questions of illness and healing, this chapter challenges us to ask: if we define illness as an inability to be one's true self, what does that mean in this context? From a Euroamerican perspective, Native people failed to realize the self that they should attain: a Christian, civilized self, abandoning the constraints of their primitive culture and stepping into a new modern Euroamerican identity.[93] As late nineteenth-century authors described the demise of Native populations, dwelling painstakingly upon the gruesome details, dissecting both flesh and experience, their printed observations acted as proof of the dominant cultural myth: *the Indians were vanishing*. And given beliefs of cultural evolution common at the time, this was no surprise. If natural laws dictated that all cultural groups were destined to achieve the final evolutionary stage of civilization, then Native people must leave their primitive cultures behind. In the eyes of many, failing to achieve a working identity that would meet the needs of Euroamerican society doomed Native people and cultures to death.

This history illustrates the very material consequences that emerge from cultural understandings of the embodied subject and the symbol systems with which people make meaning of their lives. Symbols and discourse guided and inspired missionaries' efforts and decisions. Informed by their sense of the embodied subject and what a working identity comprised, Euroamerican settlers and missionaries read the landscape of illness and turned toward the myth of the vanishing Indian for meaning. What should be clear is that such discursive narratives are not merely symbolic language at play: they have material results. These narratives constructed around illness—whether they were used to justify the taking of land, removal of a population, and failure to provide adequate healthcare or to celebrate collective survival—are all indicative of the political and economic implications within religious and philosophical ideas of the self. In light of these disease narratives told by nineteenth-century Native and non-native voices alike, it becomes apparent how politically potent such narratives can be.[94]

Three

Restoring the Spirit, Renewing Tradition

4. "A Good Christian Is a Good Medicine Man"

Changing Religious Landscapes from 1804 to 2005

When John Slocum was preaching, I heard that if I prayed I would have power to be a medicine man, and could cure the sick.

—MUD BAY SAM YOWALUCH, Squaxin, 1896

The distinction between the 'Native' belief system and Christianity may not be as clear and simple as most ethnographers have implicitly assumed; contemporary Coast Salish religion must be seen as the result of not one but a series of compromises and reinterpretations.

—WAYNE SUTTLES, 1987

This chapter examines the ways in which religious movements and approaches to healing among Chinook and Coast Salish communities have changed over the past two centuries, incorporating strategic elements of Euroamerican culture as they did so.[1] The preceding discussion leaves us with a question: if Euroamerican religious and medical worldviews directly challenged indigenous notions of the self and community, how could future generations integrate elements of Christianity or western biomedicine into their religious lives and healing traditions without doing violence to those very Native identities and worldviews? This in turn brings us back to a question raised in chapter 2: can we talk about identity in a way that recognizes its fluid, multiple, positional, and hybrid nature, without deconstructing it out of existence?

As I argue in this chapter, "tradition" in the Pacific Northwest has always been an evolving notion. To put it another way, change *is* traditional—when it occurs in ways that maintain core values, worldviews, and a consistent sense of what it means to be a healthy self.

Through this brief survey of the ways in which Chinook and Coast Salish religious and healing traditions have changed under colonialism, we see that approaches to health and wellness have adapted alongside changing needs, at the same time maintaining many core beliefs and values.

I begin with a discussion of the prophetic traditions that arose among indigenous populations of the nineteenth century, largely in response to social and epidemiological change. In particular, I discuss what anthropologist Leslie Spier has labeled the "Prophet Dance Movement." I go on to address how these traditions contributed to the rise of the Indian Shaker Church in the late nineteenth and early twentieth centuries, one of the predominant Native religious movements in this region. And finally, I explore the revival of Coast Salish spirit dancing in the late twentieth century. While Coast Salish religious practices have changed dramatically over the past two centuries, I aim to show here that certain foundational elements have been retained. In particular, throughout these changing traditions, the healthy self maintains a clear sense of individual identity within a complex network of relationships: relationships with fellow community members, with ancestral spirits, and with the indigenous land base. For such an embodied self to be healthy, it requires the continual navigation and restoration of these relationships as well as a clear sense of one's individual role and purpose within that community. The cultural events of the past two centuries have worked to turn the apparent tension of being both Native and modern into a space for creative possibility.

In this chapter I provide a wide-ranging survey of religious change among Coast Salish and Chinook communities as it occurred between 1800 and 2000. Such a discussion is necessarily a simplified overview of a much more complicated history. This is a synthesis of religious traditions as they occurred throughout the region. It is important to note that many of the traditions discussed differ from area to area, from community to community, and even from family to family; this should be kept in mind even as I try to paint the historical narrative in broad strokes.

Spirit Powers and Traditional Northwest Healing Practices

Precolonial religious practice in the Northwest centered on the veneration of spirit powers, or what anthropologists have labeled the guardian spirit complex (discussed in greater detail in part 4). To put it briefly, at their coming of age young people ventured out into isolated areas to procure spirit powers, *tamanowas* in the Chinook *wawa*. Martin Sampson, Coast Salish Skagit, described it this way: "Each person had one or more spirit guides or guardians, called Tamanowas; these were inherited or acquired by fasting and bathing in clean and secluded places. The Indians believed in the hereafter: that death was not the end, but the beginning of a new life, that the spirit of [people] advanced from one world to another and that the wicked lingered in this earth for a long time before advancing to the next spirit world."[2] Likewise, Wayne Suttles has described the Coast Salish *s'elya* (or spirit power encounter). According to Suttles the vision was sought, "especially during adolescence, by fasting and bathing in remote forest lakes or along lonely shores. During the vision the seeker encountered some animal, real or mythical, which conferred upon him a particular skill or became in anthropological language, his 'guardian spirit.' The seeker also received a *syowen*, or 'spirit song', which came to him some winter later in life and made him sick."[3]

Pamela Amoss, Crisca Bierwert, and Wayne Suttles have ably discussed the honoring of such spirit powers in formal spirit dancing.[4] I address this later but highlight several themes in this chapter. First, spirit dancing is characterized by relationship between an individual and that person's spirit power. Spirit powers often provided individuals with particular strengths and abilities, thus enabling them to fulfill unique roles within the community. Failure to honor one's spirit power (and thereby maintain one's personal relationship with it) impaired one's ability to fulfill responsibilities and obligations as well as potentially resulting in spirit-sickness.[5] One signifier of health was an ongoing relationship with one's spirit power that enabled one to live well within the community. Illness resulted when that relationship (and subsequently one's identity and sense of self) was compromised. Healing was secured through the restoration of these spiritual relationships, often through spirit dancing in the smokehouse (also referred to as spirit-house or longhouse) or other healing ceremonies.[6]

Broken relationships and the improper embodiment of one's identity within a community could also account for disease. Within traditional disease etiology, "conjurers" could cause illness by "shooting" disease-causing objects or powers into an enemy. In order to remove such diseases, healers coaxed the disease object out of the body through massage, song, sucking, brushing, or blowing upon the body. The spirit object was then thrown away, sent back to the person who originally sent it, placed in cold water to cool it ("when it gets cold it loses its power"), or placed in a container, sealed, and buried.[7] Such understandings of illness make clear that breaks in human relationships became embodied as illness. Relationships *mattered*. And relationships could potentially be healed through the process of removing the disease-causing object. The efficacy of such rituals required the aid of powerful spiritual entities, but it was also the power of the ritual itself, which involved the full participation of patient, healer, family, and community. A transformation occurred in the patient and in the person's lived-identity in the community when broken relationships were healed, or literally thrown away, brushed off, or buried. The ritual enactment made the spiritual and relational transformation tangible.

This notion of health and illness as dependent upon the proper fulfillment of one's identity and relationships within community is also illustrated through the notion of soul loss. When confronted with excessive trauma, contact with dangerous things, inappropriate actions or lifestyle, or the animosity of another person or spirit, part of one's soul could leave one's body. While individuals remained alive, patients were fundamentally compromised: they were literally not themselves. As a result, they were physically, spiritually, and/or mentally compromised. Until the soul was retrieved through ritual and ceremony, patients would remain impaired. If the soul was not returned through a soul retrieval ceremony, the person might die.

The significance is striking: the embodied subject here was one that was multilayered, defined by relationships with spirit powers and others in community. Illness was caused by the loss of one's soul, the loss of one's identity-within-community. And that identity was an intrinsically relational one: the patient was not restored to be an isolated individual but to fulfill a place within community. For this reason the embodied self was restored through communal effort, involving a large number of people, all dependent upon their relationships with their individual spirit powers, such as a collective gathering of people spirit dancing in the longhouse or offering support at a soul recovery ceremony. In short, the embodied self existed simultaneously at multiple levels and locations; it could be lost, recovered, or sent out to others and was dependent upon the maintenance of a complex web of reciprocal relationships.

A final key theme I would like to note within Coast Salish and Chinook healing traditions is that of restoration and renewal. Such narratives and ritual performances reenacted a journey to and return from the land of the dead. As Spier points out, "one of the most striking features of Northwest Coast myth is the occurrence of numerous tales concerning visits of the living with the dead."[8] One of the most common narratives to accompany the receiving of spirit power during an adolescent spirit quest was that individuals who lost consciousness traveled to the spirit world, established a relationship with the powerful being in question, and returned home, bringing with them new spiritual wisdom, songs, dances, rituals, and symbols. Some of these individuals went on to become religious specialists and healers. Indeed, such death and rebirth experiences appear to have been particular prerequisites for the calling of healer.[9] Healers were those who had lost themselves on dangerous spiritual journeys and found themselves again, whose relationships and levels of self identity were stretched, broken, and re-created. The knowledge and the skills gained through this process enabled these individuals to become healers themselves.[10]

This idea of a relational self potentially renewed through spiritual journeys would be maintained within the changing religious landscape of the nineteenth and twentieth centuries. Because Coast Salish religious practices were not characterized by liturgy or fixed tradition, but were highly personalized practices based on individual relationships with spirit powers, they had the potential for creative and individualized responses to unique situations. As such, they were able to adapt to changing contexts and conditions. What is most important to note here is that within such change, perspectives on the embodied subject and definitions of health and wellness maintained a remarkable degree of consistency, even within the significant diversity of Northwest religious expression. Health was determined by one's participation within a network of reciprocal relationships and the degree to which one was able to embody fully one's identity-within-community. Breaks in these relationships had material results (soul loss and illness) and could only be healed through the restoration of one's proper identity. Stories of healers who had returned from the dead provided a source of hope for renewal and restoration—that one could be made whole and find a place once again within community.

The Prophet Dance: Adaptation and Cultural Continuity

With the arrival of Euroamericans and the epidemic diseases that accompanied them, indigenous traditions of death and rebirth became increasingly important as Native communities sought out ways to respond to these crises. During the nineteenth century prophetic leaders emerged throughout the Northwest, bringing religious instruction and ritual practices that served to facilitate the restoration of a clear sense of personal identity within community by maintaining continuity with the past. Prophetic leaders drew heavily upon traditional narratives of sacred journeys between the lands of the living and the dead. Nearly all the prophets who arose during this time shared a common narrative of a near-death experience: having traveled to the land of the dead and visited with the spirits, they now returned to offer wisdom and guidance to their communities. Such a narrative meshed well with Pacific Northwest oral traditions and marked these individuals as spiritual leaders and healers. As early as the 1770s, when the first epidemic diseases reached the Northwest, prophets began calling people together, encouraging them to maintain traditional identities and ways of life.

Historian Elizabeth Vibert has taken issue with those scholars who view Northwest prophetic movements simply as responses to white invasion. As she argues, such traditions had deep roots within indigenous belief systems, and prophetic responses drew upon a bedrock of Native traditions in their response to the epidemic crises. While David Aberle, Deward Walker, and Christopher Miller have tended to downplay the relevance of precolonial religious foundations for the movements, emphasizing deprivation, stresses from contact, and socioeconomic changes, Vibert, Wayne Suttles, and Leslie Spier have argued for the importance of seeing such movements as extensions of earlier religious beliefs and practices.[11]

I would agree that while prophetic movements of the era appeared different from earlier spirit power traditions, they shared key elements in common. First, they shared elements of style and structure: people were familiar with the notion of spiritual leaders who visited the land of the dead and returned with new songs, prayers, ceremonies, and sacred stories. As Vibert has argued, "Prophets took their place within the system as Indians who had acquired the extraordinary ability to dream their souls to the land of the dead and back, and to communicate with the spirits. Similar to initiates in the spirit quest, they returned with songs, dreams and supernaturally inspired instructions."[12] Second, by emphasizing the internal logic of these prophetic movements, we can see that they also reflected traditional disease etiologies. Such movements shared a common sense of the embodied self and what it meant to be well. Within indigenous theories of disease causation, illness was often caused by spiritual disorder, such as "the intrusion of a malevolent spirit, or the injury or loss of one's own guardian spirit through wandering or desertion."[13] Prophets, those with the ability to communicate with spirits and gifted with extraordinary vision, were able to discern the causes of such imbalances, and they called their communities to ritual performances designed to restore balance and hasten the renewal of the earth. Further, by reinforcing an indigenous understanding of wellness as rooted in interpersonal relationships, prophetic voices tended to emphasize *collective* wellness rather than individual healing. The focus on restoring balanced and proper relationships remained their primary concern.

Central to their role as healers, prophets brought to their communities new songs, dances, symbols, ritual procedures, and admonitions, all designed to facilitate the community's survival through an apocalyptic era. The earliest written reports by non-natives of such prophets came around 1800, describing prophets with apocalyptic messages that responded to new epidemics and volcanic eruptions, all of which appeared to be threatening life along the Columbia River.[14] For instance, explorer Alexander Ross reported that Native people on the lower Columbia believed "that this world will have an end, as it had a beginning; and their reason is this, that the rivers and lakes must eventually undermine the earth and set the land afloat again like the island of their forefathers, and then all must perish. Frequently they have asked us when it would take place, the *its'owl'eigh* or end of the world."[15] Spier reports an Upper Chinookan prophet, reportedly living at the Cascades "long before the arrival of the whites," who predicted the coming destruction of the world with the arrival of white settlers, and its eventual renewal.[16]

Given the near apocalypse facing communities during the nineteenth century with onslaughts of disease, loss of land to white settlers, and resultant cultural disruption, prophets provided a necessary transition from local, individualized spirit power traditions to a more regional, community-based response to identity loss. The result was an in-gathering of people, who pooled their collective memories of previous traditions and crafted innovative ways to maintain traditional identity within a changing world. At the heart of these movements was a sense of health and wellness that required more than physiological balance—it required the restoration of tradition and reciprocal relationships with the human, spiritual, and natural worlds.

One way in which people achieved this was through a skillful negotiation and incorporation of new symbolic language. At a time when traditional religious leaders were lost to disease, were ineffectual against new diseases, or were being suppressed by Euroamerican agents and missionaries, prophets were inspired to incorporate modes of Christian expression. They began meeting on Sundays, in structures sometimes resembling churches; they held prayer meetings and called upon a high God. In adapting these Christian elements, Native religion was able to offer an attractive alternative to Christian missions, an alternative that was distinctly indigenous. By gathering for prayer every seventh day, for instance, Native people were presented with an alternative to Sunday church services. Such adaptations were incorporated as they were deemed useful to meet communities' needs for a secure identity, cultural continuity, and restored relationships.

Sampson provides specific examples of this when he describes prophets who emerged among the Skagit Valley tribes. The prophet La'hail'by addressed his people during the smallpox epidemics of the 1780s and 1800, and a later prophet Johnny Stick (Ha'hei'bath) came to his community in 1866, both saying that "God had commanded him to teach them a new way of life." Ha'hei'bath prophesied a new growth of huckleberries on nearby Mount Sauk, and when it occurred, the community gathered around him "to be taught the new way of life, the songs, the chants, and the prayers with which each activity was accomplished."[17] Likewise, June McCormick Collins describes another Upper Skagit prophet in the 1840s or 1850s who made use of Christian teachings as a means to exert political control over his local communities. This particular prophet built a longhouse for "'church' during summer months," but "in the winter the traditional guardian spirit dances were held in it."[18]

Various observers reported a similar event among the Plateau communities along the upper Columbia River: "A man died. They kept his body three days and then he came to. He told the people what he saw in heaven, what was right to do. . . . The Creator told him to have this Indian Religion every seven days and to sing. They counted seven days and every seventh day danced. This was the first Religion. This was a long time back when people were dying like flies. This was how the Washani Religion began."[19] The Washani, or Wáášhat, went on to become one of the most important religious movements on the Columbia Plateau, thriving into the twenty-first century.[20]

As may already be clear from these brief descriptions, one key element that enabled indigenous communities in the region to converse with Euroamericans was the incorporation of a Creator, yet even this newer notion drew upon long-held beliefs. Scholars have argued whether, prior to the nineteenth century, notions of a supreme deity like that of the Christian God existed among Northwest tribes. If it did, many argue that it is not likely that such an entity was actively revered, worshipped, prayed to, or served as the focus of extensive ceremonial activity. Indigenous ideas of a Creator appear to have been tied to earlier oral traditions of Transformer, a being (or several beings) found in oral traditions throughout the Pacific Northwest and thought responsible for transforming the earth from its condition in the mythic past to its present state. Transformer brought salmon and created a means for catching, cooking, and preserving them; Transformer assigned animals and humans to their proper places in the world; and Transformer created major landforms, human communities, and food sources.[21] For the Tillamook, Transformer was referred to as South Wind, Everlasting Man, Tk'a (Our Grandfather), or Sunnutchul. Among the Alsea, Transformer was Shi'ok, and among the Coos, Arrow Young Man, or Parents of the People; for the Kalapuyans, and for many Plateau communities, Transformer was Coyote.[22] And among the Coast Salish of Puget Sound Transformer was known as *xa'ls* in the Halkomelem and Straits region, and *du'kʷibətl* among southern Puget Sound and Twana tribes. Transformer was recognized, but not necessarily an object of reverence, Suttles suggests, until the first arrival of Christian missions.[23] According to Suttles, the Klallam have a tradition of Seqwa'ta, a female deity, associated with the earth, the sky, dawn, and the feminine.[24] Suttles also argues that among the coastal Salish the term Si'satl si'Em, literally translated from the Salish as "Chief Above," was used during the nineteenth century, accompanied by Christian symbols such as the Sabbath and the sign of the cross.[25] Among Sahaptin speakers on the Plateau and upper Columbia, notions of the Creator are expressed as Saghalee Tyee (Our Father); Honyawat (Creator), or Nami Piap (Elder Brother).[26]

My point is not that the idea of a high God may be new but rather that this idea was integrated into Native cultures in a way that maintained key elements of indigenous worldviews: Creator was often described as a relative (elder brother, grandfather), reflecting a sense of the world as shaped and held in place by kinship and reciprocity. Like Coast Salish oral traditions of Transformer, Creator's main task was to set the world in order, assigning all people and things to their proper role and responsibility. These fundamentally underlying notions of kinship and personal responsibility appear to have informed discourse about the Creator within prophetic traditions of the nineteenth century as well.

A fascinating example of the way the high god concept was integrated within Coast Salish worldview comes from a Lushootseed translation of the Lord's Prayer, composed in the mid-nineteenth century by Father Eugene Casimir Chirouse during his time on the Tulalip reservation. A 1992 analysis of the prayer by Christopher Vecsey and Lushootseed elder Taqʷšəblu (Vi Hilbert) reveals a great deal about the way in which Christian ideas were made relevant to the Coast Salish cultural context. The initial phrase "our father," Hilbert noted, was translated into Lushootseed in such a way that it suggested "a bond of kinship rather than holiness," reflecting the vast importance of kinship within Coast Salish culture. Chirouse avoided the use of the Salish word *Xaʔxaʔ*, which means more than "good," but rather suggests that which is also dangerous, holy, and supernaturally powerful, opting for kin-based "father" instead. In doing so, Vecsey argues, "the prayer's opening provides a proper meeting ground of human dimension for Christianity and Lushootseed spirituality," by reflecting the Coast Salish value of kinship.[27] The next phrase translates roughly to "Good that it be made first, good that which is your name," referring "to a name that is first among names, a name that has the highest social status." In doing so, the prayer references the value that Coast Salish cultures placed on class and rank, particularly as it was socially validated and recognized within the giving of certain names. "The second half of the phrase indicates that it is a good name, both morally and pragmatically: an ethically good, usefully good name." Rather than emphasizing holiness or otherworldliness, then, the translation chose to call people's attention to a Father who is both high-class and "usefully" good, which in the Coast Salish context would imply the support of one's kin.[28] The prayer goes on not to reference heaven but rather "the good it would be" if our Father's thoughts and intentions were followed "on this land, our territory, this earth," just as it is "there up high." The Lushootseed words here do not speak in abstractions of location but locate the good in this physical geography.

Likewise, the Lushootseed phrase for "give us this day our daily bread," is literally translated as "establish the nobility of Our Father" because He gives us "that which is our food each day," affirming the high class status of this "father," because within Coast Salish communities high-class noble persons provided food for others. Interestingly Hilbert "was surprised that Chirouse had chosen not to use a word for salmon, which might carry for the Lushootseed all the sacramental qualities of bread as food for the early Christians." Nor did he simply say "bread" but "instead used a Skagit word for food in general."[29] Finally, the prayer concludes with "let us be winners toward all of our sins, and remove from us all that is bad." The Lushootseed phrase does not equate sin with evil (or the Greek term that implies missing the mark) but rather that which is "useless." Rather than a message evocative of Christian ethics, the Lushootseed phrase is intrinsically practical: give us that which works, and keep away from us that which is useless.[30] The prayer is a powerful example of the ways in which Father Chirouse, and the Lushootseed people with whom he worked, incorporated Christianity into previously existing Coast Salish frameworks. It shows an emphasis on kinship, status, the value of providing for others, and the pragmatism of addressing material needs such as food within the lived context of this world in the here-and-now.

The inclusion of Christianity within regional religious practice also meant maintaining a highly embodied form of worship. From

Coast Salish and Chinook perspectives religious practice was first and foremost embodied religious experience: song and dance. It was never a purely cerebral affair. Just as breaks in relationships (human and spiritual) were reflected physiologically in illness, healing also required embodied expression in dance and in ritual. Father Blanchet, for instance, noted that his Native parishioners insisted on physical expressions of religion. As he wrote: "In fact I did my best to make them understand Good and Evil, they on their part promised fair, and had their devotional Dance, for without it they would think very little of what we say to them."[31]

This commitment to embodied practice can be seen within the new practices instituted by nineteenth-century prophets as well. The story of prophet and Upper Chinookan Chief Tilki provides one excellent example. Following his own death and return to life, Tilki established Sunday dances at The Dalles around 1830. Here he brought elements of Christian worship together with indigenous practice and ethos. These dances followed the traditional styles, but as he was directed in his vision, he incorporated certain Christian features, such as prayer to a high god and meeting every seventh day, on the Sabbath. As Boyd put it, "New Christian practices were being accreted to an older base that centered on ceremonial dancing."[32] The movement flourished in the Dalles for a number of years, until Christian missionaries exerted their influence to ban dancing at the meetings. Weekly prayer meetings should be sufficient, they argued. Dancing was stopped shortly thereafter (by 1840), and attendance immediately dropped off as a result. The movement itself was soon abandoned. The decline of Tilki's movement illustrates an important point: this Chinookan community on the Columbian River was not simply looking for Christianity in their own language, but for a space of expression that allowed the continuity of previous indigenous traditions and identity, expressions that were essentially *embodied* practices. It also illustrates the different perspectives on the embodied subject existing between missionaries and the Native communities of the region. While Protestant missionaries in particular emphasized a mental (and cultural) conversion, which intentionally downplayed physical expressions of worship, Chinook and Coast Salish insisted upon a faith that was embodied and physiologically experienced.

William Fraser Tolmie recorded two observations of such embodied healing traditions at Fort Vancouver and Fort Nisqually:

> Heard a howling and approaching a party of from 30 to 40 Indians, men, women and children performing their devotions. They formed a circle two deep and went around and round, moving their hands, as is done in sculling, exerting themselves violently and simultaneously repeating a monotonous chant loudly. Two men were within the circle and kept moving rapidly from side to side making the same motion of arms, and were I am told the directors or managers of the ceremony. Having continued this exercise for several minutes, after we beheld them becoming more and more vehement and excited, they suddenly dropped on their knees and uttered a short prayer, and having rested a short time resumed the circular motion. During the ceremony so intent were they that not an eye was once turned towards us, although we stood within a few yards. . . . Felt sensation of awe come over me when they knelt and prayed. . . . They have imitated the Europeans in observing the seventh day as a day of rest.[33]

While most missionaries were less than successful in their efforts among Coast Salish and Chinook communities, Native prophetic movements offered a means of reinterpreting Euroamerican assimilation, providing an alternative model that restored individuals to their place within community and the network of relationships that defined it.[34] Prophets built on earlier traditions, such as spirit journeys to the land of the dead and oral traditions of Transformer or Creator, to craft new traditions that incorporated elements of Euroamerican religions, such as kneeling in prayer and worship on the Sabbath, all the while remaining distinctly indigenous. Through their apocalyptic message, and their call to retain traditional beliefs, practices, and modes of religious experience, such cultural foundations were not entirely lost, and much survived what Eugene Hunn has called the "spiritual apocalypse" of the nineteenth century.[35]

"A Good Christian Is a Good Medicine Man": The Indian Shaker Church

In 1881 Squaxin Island tribal member Squi-sacht-uhn (John Slocum) died, visited heaven, and three days later returned to earth with a message of repentance and faith. He had been instructed by God to direct his fellow Indians in the construction of a new church, an Indian church that God intended uniquely for them. Soon, he promised, God was going to send a special medicine to the Indian people, one that would empower them to survive in these trying times. One year later Squi-sacht-uhn became ill and was again near death. His wife Mary (Thompson) Slocum left the house, overwhelmed with grief, and went to a nearby creek. As Chehalis church elder Silas Heck later recalled: "There she felt something come down from above, and flow over her body. It felt hot, and she began to tremble all over." When she came back into the house, according to some accounts, her brother began to shake and tremble as well. Mary stood over her husband, shaking and praying. By the next day, Squi-sacht-uhn was fully recovered.[36] It was decided that this "Shake" was the medicine that God had promised Squi-sacht-uhn a year before, and at a large gathering on the Skokomish reservation in August of 1883, many others experienced this same shaking power.

Indeed, after the arrival of the "new medicine" promised by God, healing quickly became the defining feature of the movement. Mud Bay Sam Yowaluch, quoted at the outset of this chapter, became one of the most prominent voices in the new church, traveling widely (often accompanied by Squi-sacht-uhn) to heal those who were sick and spread the power of the Shake. As Squi-sacht-uhn himself explained: "It is ten years now, since we began, and we have good things. We all love these things and will follow them all time. We learn to help ourselves when sick. When our friend is sick, we kneel and ask for help to cure him. We learn something once in a while to cure him. Then we do as we know to help him and cure him. If we don't learn to help him, we generally lose him."[37]

The Shaker Church's emphasis on healing took center stage during both of the major waves of evangelism that the church underwent in the late nineteenth and early twentieth centuries. Shakers set forth with the aim of healing a friend or relative on a neighboring reservation. As they traveled to Native communities and demonstrated the healing power of the Shake, they in turn garnered new converts.[38] In addition to the Squaxin and Skokomish, the Chehalis, Nisqually, Quinault, and Queets received the church as early as 1883. In 1890 a Cowlitz, having witnessed a miraculous cure among the Chehalis, took word of the movement east to the Yakama. Yakama congregations quickly became extremely active, passing the message to the Umatilla in Oregon. The movement spread north to British Columbia and west to the Makah through the Klallam at Jamestown in the 1890s. A second wave of evangelism during and immediately following World War I brought the movement to the Warm Springs and Siletz in Oregon. In the 1930s it reached as far as the Yurok, Tolowa, and Hupa in northern California. Because most congregations met informally, it is virtually impossible to gauge how many church communities were founded between 1885 and 1930. However, it is certain that the great majority of Native communities throughout the Pacific Northwest, from northern California to British Columbia, had at least a small contingent of Shakers at some point in their history.[39]

The appeal of the Indian Shaker Church may be better understood when considered within the context of the late nineteenth and early twentieth century. By the 1880s Native communities had been relocated onto reservations and found their traditional subsistence activities dramatically curtailed; access to traditional vision questing, hunting, fishing, and gathering sites had been severely disrupted, and economic changes had driven many people into wage labor activities, such as logging, the industry in which Squi-sacht-uhn was employed. Such shifts contributed to and accompanied changes in family life and political leadership and severely strained traditional kinship networks and modes of collective support. Those who had survived the epidemic diseases of the nineteenth century now struggled under new epidemics of alcoholism, malnutrition, gambling, and poverty, as well as tuberculosis, measles, influenza, syphilis, recurring smallpox epidemics, and high rates of infant mortality. Squi-sacht-uhn himself had thirteen children, only two of whom survived to raise children of their own.[40] Shakers were able to offer "God's power to heal Indians at a time when physical and psychological distress afflicted many people they knew," and when epidemics were ravaging Indian communities.[41]

Indigenous religious traditions were also hard-pressed at this time, largely because of the heavy-handed leadership of reservation agents. Beginning as early as 1871, Indian agents such as Edwin Eells worked diligently to suppress traditional religious practices and traditional healers in particular.[42] His brother, Reverend Myron Eells, lamented that traditional healers proved to be a persistent obstacle to conversion. As Indian Agent Donald M. Carr, overseeing the Yakama reservation, wrote in 1917, "It is my belief that the Indian doctors do a great deal of harm. . . . Some of the Indians keep on calling them [Indian doctors] every time someone gets sick, all of which is wrong."[43]

Traditional healers were at first opposed to the Shakers, finding in the church a new source of competition. But as agency officials clamped down on traditional healers, their attitude changed: the Shaker Church provided a means of continuing their healing practices with less risk of persecution. As Eells noted: "About this time, an order came from the Indian department to stop all medicine men from practicing their incantations over the sick. . . . And then the medicine men almost entirely joined the Shakers, as their style was more nearly in accordance with the old style than with the religion of the Bible."[44] Squi-sacht-uhn welcomed traditional healers into the church, providing that they promised to repent of any sinful habits and to cure without charging anyone for the service.[45] Hence, confronted by stern opposition from the Eells brothers and faced with arrest, imprisonment, or heavy fines, South Puget traditional healers joined the newly formed Shaker Church in large numbers.[46]

Like earlier prophetic movements, the Indian Shaker Church incorporated Christian elements and organization into its worship and in so doing enabled the survival of an approach to healing and the embodied self that reflected regional indigenous worldviews and traditions. Shakers shared a view of illness in which broken relationships or the loss of a clear sense of personal identity could result in soul loss, spiritual sickness, and physiological illness. The Shaker Church likewise shared an approach to healing that involved physically enacted rituals affirming spiritual relationships and the possibility of personal rebirth and renewal. And like indigenous prophets, the Shaker Church affirmed that one could pass through deathlike journeys and be reborn. Through its incorporation of Christian imagery and symbolism alongside these indigenous traditions, Shakers actively took hold of their moment in history, conceptualizing it and conceiving it within their own worldview.

Shaker Healing and Indigenous Approaches to Health and Wellness

The Shaker Church maintained indigenous approaches to health and well-being, albeit in a modified form. June Collins has argued that Euroamerican missions, on the whole, were rejected because they failed to provide an adequate substitute for the spirit power religion and because they did not honor indigenous kin-based ethical values.[47] By contrast, the Shaker religion was successful in recruiting adherents because it corresponded so closely to the guardian spirit religion.

Perhaps most important, the Shaker Church succeeded because it offered healing for physical and spiritual illnesses.[48] As Homer Barnett argued, "The principal virtue of (Shaker) power is its curative and restorative properties. Its acquisition brings mental and physical relief. Also, even though a person has not experienced its healing effects by possessing the power himself he can be relieved or cured of an illness by the manipulations of one who has."[49] And as Pamela Amoss observed, the Shaker movement offered spiritual power, "power to heal, power to diagnose the cause of difficulties others are suffering, and power to throw off the bondage of some addiction, usually drinking."[50] Just as spirit powers had brought with them physical health and well-being, "general well-being" likewise became a sign of one's identity as a Shaker. As Collins noted among the Upper Skagit, "Shakers and their families maintain health and live to old age because they have Shaker power to cure sickness."[51]

Spier has argued that healing practices of the early Shaker Church were "an exact parallel point for point with shamanistic curing: the operators invoke their spirit power to cure [here the Holy Spirit]; sickness is something intrusive which can be removed from the body, they brush and catch disease above the patient's head in precisely the same manner of the ancient shamans, and like them drown it in water; the operator who catches it is yanked about by the disease, although he is restrained by those who hold him about the waist, precisely as in the old manner."[52] Likewise, Barnett's description of Shaker curing practices parallels healing within the guardian spirit tradition, drawing upon similar techniques, notions of disease causation, and the ability of healers to restore a patient suffering from soul loss.[53] In a manner also strikingly similar to traditional practice, Shaker healers shake over the patient, singing the song provided by their shake, while supported by other church members, who join in song. "While waiting for the service to commence, people sit clapping their hands together quietly, rubbing their faces, or brushing evil off themselves. All these actions are similar to those of persons about to be possessed by a guardian spirit at a winter dance."[54]

The Shaker Church also maintained a traditional emphasis on ritual purity. As one church member explained it, "You got to confess your sins, be clean, in order to get the full spirit from heaven. Then the spirit can grow in your body."[55] Church members have compared the purifying process of prayers and confessions to the bathing and fasting necessary to acquire guardian spirits. As one individual noted, "'it's the same with this religion. You got to confess your sins, be clean in order to get the full spirit from heaven.'"[56] The church shares with Coast Salish and Chinook traditions a sense of the gravity associated with ritual purity and proper behavior. As Collins notes, "the guardian spirit religion and the Shaker Church share the belief that spirit retaliation in the form of illness and death will overtake the adherents who deviate from the path. Disobedience of the Shaker spirit and refusal to live in accordance with Shaker precepts brings sickness and ultimately death."[57]

The Shaker Church also shares with the guardian spirit tradition a strong emphasis on a personal, individualized relationship with one's source of spiritual power. While all church members share in the same spirit power, the Holy Spirit, each person has his or her own distinct and unique power, which is an expression unique to every woman and man. Just as Squi-sacht-uhn "received direct revelation from God," so each individual's "shake" directs the person in the proper way to worship or to heal an individual, revealing to the believer the cause or source of illness, and how best to remove it from the person's body.[58] Writing in the first half of the twentieth century, Barnett noted that Shaker practice "has become individualized, with the result that each person is believed to have his own distinct personalized guiding force. Very often individuals speak of *their* shakes."[59] Each person's "Shake" expressed itself to and through the individual in particular ways. Like one's first encounter with a spirit power, an initiate into the Shaker movement receives a vision of God or Jesus, who "sets certain restrictions upon his behavior for a designated period, [and] presents him with a costume and a song. The Shaker spirit confers some ability upon him, and if he is to use candles and bells, he receives those techniques at the same time."[60] Shakers are each given their particular "powers of God," and recognize that "certain 'helps' are specific for certain purposes. 'When people join the Shaker Church, they get different helps, one for curing, one for joiners, one for bell ringers, one for preaching, one for singing.'"[61] As in the guardian spirit tradition, Shakers have a personal relationship with the spirit that manifests in unique ways. Because of the highly individualized nature of one's relationship with God, beliefs and doctrine in the Shaker Church are not entirely formalized, allowing for personal interpretation and development.[62]

The Shaker Church inherited Coast Salish and Chinook beliefs about the origins of disease as well. For instance, Shakers shared the belief that illness could be caused by soul loss. Such a condition would necessitate that a Shaker retrieve the soul from where it had strayed. Mooney recorded examples of soul recovery in Shaker services similar to those within earlier spirit power traditions: "For a long time before a person is taken sick, they foretell that his spirit is gone to heaven and (Shakers) profess to be able to bring it back and restore it to him, so that he will not die as soon as he otherwise would."[63] As one early church member explained: "I think that the power of the old doctors turned into the new religion and was used for good."[64] Like traditional healers, then, Shakers could be gifted with a heightened discernment that enabled them to detect the location of lost souls.[65]

Like earlier Coast Salish and Chinook traditions, the Shaker Church affirmed a healthy self that existed within a network of kinship and reciprocity. Broken relationships, whether caused by offense to God or other persons, could result in physical and spiritual illness. Conflict with other people could result in illness—for a malevolent person possessing dangerous disease-powers might cause you to become ill. Or relationships could have been broken due to improper actions (sins) that placed the self in jeopardy. Importantly, in the early Shaker Church "sins" were often those actions most likely to impair one's ability to fulfill one's role within community. Hence the sins that Squi-sacht-uhn identified as the greatest offenses were drinking alcohol, smoking, and gambling: activities that threatened the health and social stability of nineteenth-century Native communities.[66]

Like guardian spirit traditions, Shaker services provided individuals with a place to nurture their own relationship with their spirit power (in this case Jesus and the Holy Spirit) within a communal setting. Hence, by providing a new mode of worship the Shaker Church reinforced Coast Salish values of individual autonomy and personal responsibility within a community. The church provided an alternative identity, along with personal status and respect.[67] It also combined common Northwest Native beliefs that individuals could acquire power from spiritual sources, and simultaneously "define their relations with other humans by displaying their new powers, thus inviting respect both for what they shared with those humans and for their unique traits and practices."[68] By providing a sense of personal value, worth, and purpose, the Shaker Church affirmed "an individual's place in an estimable group."[69]

But the Shaker Church also departed from precolonial Coast Salish and Chinook practices and beliefs in important ways. Shakers emphasized Coast Salish values of community, kinship, and individual responsibility within collective survival, but they did so in a way that expanded the notion of kinship to include the broader Indian community. During the early years of the reservation system, social cohesion was breaking down, suspicions were high, and charges and countercharges of sorcery threatened to disrupt fragile social cohesion. Alexandra Harmon has argued that some shamans had a "pernicious effect" on social relations at this time, employing their powers for malicious ends. Some profited from fears and old grudges existing between different families as previously independent villages were forced together into crowded reservations or off-reservation camps. The situation made many "more anxious and suspicious . . . to the point of paranoia. . . . Shamans were a favorite target for displaced rage," and many blamed illnesses and deaths upon shamans and strangers.[70] At a time when traditional kinship networks and community support systems were greatly at risk, the Shaker Church offered a balm to these interpersonal tensions, reinforcing and in some ways redefining the web of relationships that held together Native identity and community. Shakers functioned as "part of a struggle for a new consensus on the norms of social relations and the best means to enforce those norms."[71]

The Shaker Church took precolonial notions of kinship and community, and transformed them, presenting Church members with a tradition that encompassed Native people throughout the Northwest. Regardless of where one was from, a fellow Shaker was a brother or sister. Put another way, the movement reinforced a traditional ethic of collective survival (for spiritual efficacy was seen as depending upon a strong community) but expanded the notion of kinship to include a broader Indian community. This was a different way of seeing identity, one in which village or tribal identities coexisted within a broader sense of "Indian" identity and the sense that survival in the colonial context demanded intertribal cooperation.[72] The movement was very quickly not a Coast Salish or a Chinook tradition but an "Indian" one. As such, it played an important part in an emerging regional indigenous identity.[73]

The Shaker Church differed from Coast Salish and Chinook guardian spirit healing traditions by its more democratic nature, wherein "all pious people" had access to "a prestigious power that had formerly come to a very few—the power to cure."[74] The ability to heal was no longer restricted to those with the ability or luck to inherit or acquire powerful spirit powers. All people, young and old, can cure sickness if they are Shakers. "Every Shaker potentially had the ability to heal and cure, because every Shaker had access to the Holy Spirit."[75] Mary (Thompson) Slocum's initial gift of the Shake to the Shaker Church was a significant break from traditional practice: healing was no longer restricted to a uniquely gifted few. Now, in an era when healers were desperately needed, every devout Shaker could step forward. And they could do so at any time: the spiritual power of Shakers did not come and leave with the seasons or with particular times of one's life, as spirit powers often did.[76] This new *universal* guardian spirit power, or Holy Spirit power, was available and effective for everyone. Further, Shaker healers often worked together in pairs or groups, in contrast to Coast Salish and Chinook healers, who nearly always worked alone.[77] The newly forming church expressed this more democratic theology through such means as providing food, taking collections for those in need, and providing memorial services for the dead. It was believed that "a failure of charity within the congregation or the family (would) spoil the harmony that mobilizes the Spirit to cure the sick."[78] But while approaches to treatment have changed, "from prestige-shamanic cures to democratic-Shaker cures," Shaker traditions continued to emphasize that power came from spiritual relationships and that managing that power depended on demonstration of respect and care for spiritual relationships.[79]

Shakers took pains to distinguish themselves from an earlier generation of indigenous healers. As Mud Bay Sam Yowaluch makes clear:

When John Slocum was preaching, I heard that if I prayed I would have power to be a medicine man, and could cure the sick. . . . There is lots of difference between this power and old Indian doctoring. This is not old power. I can cure people now. I have cured some white men and women, but they are ashamed to tell it. I cure without money. God will pay us when we die. This is our religion. When we die, we get our pay from God. No, we do not believe the Bible. We believe God, and in Jesus Christ, as the Son of God, and we believe in a hell. . . . A good Christian man is a good medicine man. A good Christian man in the dark sees a light toward God. God makes a fog. A good Christian man goes straight through it to the end, like good medicine. I believe this religion. It helps poor people. . . . We were sent to jail for this religion, but we will never give up. We all believe that John Slocum died and went to heaven, and was sent back to preach to the people. We all talk about that and believe it.[80]

Yowaluch makes clear distinctions here, pointing to Shaker healers' refusal to accept payment, the ability of nonspecialists to cure, and their belief in the Creator and Jesus Christ as a source of spiritual power. Seventy-five years after Squi-sacht-uhn's prophetic experience, George Sanders, Chehalis, affirmed this distinction, arguing that spiritual power originated from the Creator. "This shaking was a substitute for the old shaman's power which was used to kill people. Shaking is God's power, and it is used only to cure the sick."[81] By 1935 a consensus seemed to have been formed that this new power was preferable to the old. As one man reflected, "Powers aren't any good anymore. Everyone wants Shaker doctors."[82]

Significantly, Shakers did not often discount the legitimacy of previous practices, even as they claimed that their healing ability came from a more powerful source. Rather than preaching that earlier traditions were false, Shakers demonstrated their ability to best malevolent shamans, curing illnesses such as spirit intrusion, or retrieving souls that had been captured by spirit powers or ghosts.[83] Big Bill, an early leader in the Shaker Church, argued that illness came from God, and so healing likewise required the ability to invoke

God's aid. Traditional healers were not malicious, he argued, but sought power from the wrong source. "It is not because they want to kill you that they [traditional healers] tamahnous over you, but they like you, and they want to cure you. One thing only God does not like. Where do you think you got this disease? In this world? No. God gave it to you, and no Indian doctor has a right to say he can cure you. If an Indian doctor goes to a sick man, the first thing he ought to do is to pray to God, and ask God's help in curing him."[84]

Of course, the main distinction between the Shaker Church and indigenous Coast Salish traditions was its incorporation of key Christian symbols and beliefs. Spier has described the Indian Shaker Church as a blend of "shamanistic performances with Catholic ritual and Protestant doctrine."[85] Christian symbols such as candles, the sign of the cross, and a belief in heaven, hell, the Trinity, and angels and devils were brought together with indigenous elements such as songs and prayers in Native languages, a distinctive notion of sin, and in particular, a healing tradition strikingly similar to Coast Salish and Chinook healing practices or *tamanawas*.[86] Shakers did not opt to adopt the Eucharist or baptism but did incorporate the censure of gambling, whiskey, and tobacco conveyed by many of the missionaries working in the Puget Sound region. In the early years of the church, Myron Eells wrote that "they held church services, prayed to God, believed in Christ as Savior, said much about his death, and used the cross, their services being a combination of Protestant and Catholic services, though at first they almost totally rejected the Bible, for they said they had direct revelations from Christ, and were more fortunate than whites, who had an old, antiquated book."[87] Shakers incorporated elements of Euroamerican religious practice that made sense within their new cultural context. In the new reservation economy, work was discouraged on Sundays and church attendance was expected. The Shaker Church gave people a Native alternative to Eells's Congregationalist services. The story of Christ, particularly his death and resurrection and his role as a voice of dissent among a people colonized by foreigners, resonated with Coast Salish oral traditions of prophets visiting the land of the dead as well as with their current political situation. The notion of direct revelation, of communicating personally with a powerful spirit, also made sense, as did the incorporation of concrete symbols (like the cross) representing that revelation.

But at the same time the Shaker Church maintained a clear distinction from Euroamerican Christianity and a strong sense of Native identity. As a non-native observer wrote to Mooney in 1882, Shakers believe:

> . . . not in the Bible particularly. They do believe in it as a history, but they do not value it as a book of revelation. They do not need it, for John Slocum personally came back from a conference with the angels at the gates of heaven, and has imparted to them the actual facts and the angelic words of the means of salvation. . . . This testimony is even better than the words of Christ contained in the Bible, for Slocum comes 1800 years nearer; he is an Indian, and personally appears to them and in Indian language reports the facts.[88]

Since the death and resurrection stories of Squi-sacht-uhn and Jesus Christ fit within well-established prophet traditions, the Bible was also not necessarily a uniquely sacred text.[89] Individuals were capable of having direct spiritual communication with the divine themselves.[90]

"You Have to Convert a Person by Shaking"

Despite members' Christian sensibilities, the movement's success became a source of concern for reservation agents and missionaries, who sought to suppress the Indian Shaker Church along with the indigenous healers that the Shakers had displaced. For the Eells brothers the Shakers seemed a particular threat, simultaneously embodying the challenges posed by "aboriginal superstition" and by the "vestiges of Catholic missionary influence."[91] In 1871 a general ban had been issued against traditional religious practice on reservations, and in April 1883 that ban was extended to include Shaker Church practitioners.[92] During this time agents ordered the arrest, trial, and imprisonment of traditional healers, Wáashat leaders, and members of the Indian Shaker Church.[93] Shakers were forced to hold services covertly, or off reservation lands. Reverend Eells reflected on the difficulty of enforcing a law among thousands of Native people, with only a handful of Euroamerican authority figures at hand. "So the agent ordered this work of the medicine men to be stopped. He lives eighty miles away on the Puyallup reservation, but there was a school teacher at Skokomish when this order was promulgated, who was chief of police; also, a farmer, physician, and two Indian policemen." Native Presbyterians on the Puyallup reservation were instructed to stand guard over the homes of the sick, in order to prevent Shakers from attempting to cure them.[94]

When a Nisqually woman sought a cure for an ailment, Squi-sacht-uhn went to see her, along with Mud Bay Louis, Mud Bay Sam, and Charlie Walker, a Chehalis Shaker who was also a practicing traditional healer.[95] Agent Edwin Eells had them arrested and put in prison for seven weeks. During the day, "bearing balls and chains," the men "were required to cut wood along the road where the other Indians were encouraged to ridicule them." Eells brought the men to the Congregationalist Church on Sunday, in irons, where his brother Reverend Myron Eells was preaching. They were seated in the front row "to humiliate them." Ridicule and intimidation continued, until Walker cursed some of those who mocked them, and one individual subsequently died. The imprisoned group garnered more community support, and Eells released the prisoners shortly thereafter.[96]

In part, the Shaker Church came into conflict with Protestant neighbors because of the direct, embodied, and experiential relationship with spiritual power that the movement afforded. In contrast to the rather dry intellectual nature of the Congregationalism that Reverend Eells offered his parishioners, ceremonialism within the Shaker Church was profoundly physical as well as spiritual. When one received one's shake, one's body shook, one's spirit was lifted, one's very self was ontologically transformed through an embodied experience. This embodied spirituality was one that called for active participation. This was not a tradition of preacher and passive audience but one in which every member of the congregation actively ministered to others, becoming a vehicle for spiritual power.[97] Spiritual illness manifested in the body, and when healing occurred it was *felt*, and *expressed*, through the body. The two identifying features of the movement are both intrinsically physical: that one's body shakes when one is caught up in worship, and that shaking provides an opportunity to provide healing from physical ailments. Adherents to the movement have been careful to point out that "the Shake" was not brought by any Christian missionaries, and that it was not present in any of the forms of Christianity in the area at the time. Rather, ritualized trembling was part of shamanic healing.[98] Indeed, much like a spirit power, "the Shake" was first given to a woman in prayer by a creek. It descended upon her as a power to cure, much like a healing spirit power would have done in a similar location.

Just as the Shaker traditions maintained a focus on embodied experience, Shaker notions of sin, illness, and healing also emphasized the importance of this life, rather than the hereafter. Barnett explains that "all Shakers are anxious about their souls, but their interest is in keeping them in their bodies, rather than in providing for them after death."[99] This emphasis on healing in the here-and-now was also reflected in Squi-sacht-uhn's first prayer, given after his death and resurrection: "Our God is in heaven. If we died He will take our life to heaven. Help us so that we shall not die. Wherever we are, help us not to die. Our Father, who is always there, always have a good mind on us."[100]

But this notion of an embodied religious practice, one that is experienced physically and that translates into physiological well-being, appeared dangerous to the Congregationalist reservation administrators. As Reverend Myron Eells complained, "Like the old system, it has much noise."[101] Arguing that the frequent and long meetings were the cause of lost work time and property, and suspecting that the shaking at prayer meetings posed a health risk to those participating (it was thought such "uncontrolled" shaking might damage the brain), agency physician J. T. Martin advised that meetings be suppressed, and "the authority of the agent was brought to bear, and to a great extent the Shaking was stopped, though they were encouraged to keep on in the practice of some good habits which they had begun, ceasing gambling, intemperance . . . and the like."[102]

One can witness the application of this administrative policy within the minutes of a special session of the Indian Police Court, held on April 14, 1884. Superintendent Chalcraft, Puyallup-Nisqually Agent Edwin Eells, Reverend Mann, and schoolteacher George Mills interviewed members of the church, along with Associate Judge Jim Walker and church members Pike Ben, Charlie Walker, and George Heck.

Church members sought to convey to those present that the church was a healing force in the community: "Charlie Walker began the discussion by saying that Mr. Mann was doing good teaching white people how to live, and John Slocum was doing good in teaching Indians. Both believed in God, and should walk together like brothers, teaching the people." But the court replied, "That which you suggest is impossible, besides, Mr. Mann and the Church have nothing to do with the question we have to decide. It is doctoring the sick, we have to talk about." Like their predecessors in the early part of the nineteenth century, the reverend, agent, and superintendent sought to make a clear distinction between "doctoring" and religion, a distinction that did not exist for Coast Salish and Chinook people. In an ironic decision, they reached what they saw as a compromise and issued an official order:

> The giving of "Shakes" to sick people in treating them for sickness is in violation of Rule 6, in "Rules Governing Courts of Indian Offences" and is prohibited, but if an Indian begins to shake and cannot stop doing so, he must not have any other person present, unless it be his wife, or husband as the case may be. Children shall not be present. . . . No one shall offer to give another Indian the "shakes" but if an Indian requests it be given him, it may be done, providing they apply to the Head Chief, Jim Walker, or the Superintendent in advance, so that both may be present to see that no Government Rule is violated.[103]

Such an order reveals the degree to which communication between Shaker Church leaders and Euroamerican officials was complicated by differing views of the embodied subject. For reservation agents and Presbyterian officials, "the shakes" and their attendant healing rites were extraneous to real spirituality, an unnecessary and dangerous addition to religious practice. The thought that such spiritual practice might first be subjected to petitions and permits, so that a healing ceremony could be conducted without breaking "Rule 6" is remarkable. Such an order suggests a definition of "religion" as something that is cerebral and personal, rather than embodied and collective.

It also suggests that, less than theology, it was the collective embodied practice that comprised a meaningful spirituality for Shaker Church members.[104] As one Shaker said: "I am a preacher, but I never had anybody tell me that I converted him by preaching. You have to convert a person by shaking."[105] Much like the missionaries who wanted Chief Tilki's prayer meetings at The Dalles to continue but wanted the dancing to stop, Indian agents wanted Shakers to continue their temperance but stop the shaking. In both instances, missionaries failed to recognize that it was the very embodied practice of dance, of physically merging with the Spirit, that made these other things possible.

And indeed, while Euroamerican missionizing failed to gain traction in these communities, the Shaker Church thrived. In 1894, for instance, Eells wrote of declining numbers in his own church but noted that the Shakers "have taken the larger share of the uneducated Indians in the Church with them."[106] Eells later noted that after twenty years in the mission field he had garnered only sixty-five church members, not all of whom were Native, while since its 1882 founding the Shaker Church had grown to perhaps eight hundred members.[107]

The ability of agents to suppress the tradition further waned with the 1887 passage of the Dawes Severalty Act, which granted citizenship to those Native people who accepted allotments of land. In 1892, encouraged by Euroamerican Judge James Wickersham (who had his own agenda of "freeing" Native land for white settlement through the allotment act), many church leaders became citizens and the church became a legally protected entity. The church was incorporated within the state of Washington in 1910, when it adopted formal church structures with bishops, elders, ministers, and regular conventions.[108] Accommodating Euroamerican political structures by becoming citizens and incorporating the church thus had a paradoxical result. The move provided Shakers with the legal protection to practice their religion and define it as they saw fit. At the same time, accepting allotments of individual parcels of land also opened up tribal land to Euroamerican settlement, furthering federal goals of assimilating Native people into the dominant culture. Debatable as the move may have been, even Myron Eells could not deny that it granted them the liberty to practice their faith. As he wrote: "Since the Indians have become citizens . . . a good share of those on the Puyallup reservations have returned to tamahnous over their sick."[109]

The Shaker Church: Tantamount to Survival

The inclusion of Christian cosmology and symbolism in the Indian Shaker Church should not be seen as acquiescence to a more powerful colonizing force but rather as a sophisticated turning of the colonial tables. The Shaker Church crafted a new symbolic system that drew from both the indigenous traditions of the Pacific Northwest and the sacred symbols of Christianity, shaping them to meet the colonial present. By infusing Christian symbols with Coast Salish values such as kinship, personal responsibility, and collective survival, the Shaker Church provided Native communities with a means of negotiating cultural transition and sustaining tribal identities.

This movement reflects Charles Long's analysis of postcolonial ritualizing in the South Pacific, wherein he argues: "On the one hand, the members of the indigenous cultures must positively undergo their domination on a historical level, but on the other hand they actively participate in and think through the meaning of this historical domination in mythical modes. . . . [They] now undertake the creation of a new cultural myth that will enable them to make sense of the mythic past and the historical present in mythic terms."[110] The Indian Shaker Church remains a powerful part of Native American life in the Pacific Northwest in part because of its ability to think through their experience in mythic terms. As Pamela Amoss put it, the Shaker Church enabled people "to tap into the power of the alien God without rejecting the native concepts of what humanity is and how it relates to the supernatural."[111]

The Indian Shaker Church is a dramatic illustration of the ways in which a new cultural narrative can unite what Long calls the "mythic past and historical present." When the Shaker Church emerged, some of the greatest threats to community well-being were alcoholism, poverty, gambling, despair, and a sense of powerlessness in the face of colonial control. Shaker healers were able to subvert colonial control, reclaiming authority from the colonial Christian God, and to secure a means for healing the ailments of the colonial historical moment. The church provided a sacred narrative in which one's suffering worked toward a greater good, where sobriety and hard work were to be rewarded, and where the community could join together in a collective spirit to support and nurture one another through crisis and cultural transition. It affirmed the power of the older traditions and was a means by which distinctly "Indian" views on the world could be seen as vitally relevant. By 1909 even H. H. Johnson, Indian agent for the Puyallup-Nisqually district, was forced to admit: "The Shaker religion has done much to better the Indians."[112]

The Shaker Church reshaped Christian symbols and ideas, giving them meanings that meshed with and reinforced indigenous values and beliefs. The cross, bells, church, and Holy Spirit became a means of affirming the centrality of kinship and community, of healing as a fundamentally embodied spiritual endeavor, and of the importance of maintaining a distinct indigenous identity. As an expression of the multicultural experience of Native communities of the last 150 years, the Shaker Church reflects the potential for hybridity and adaptation within indigenous traditions. As Thomas Buckley has argued: "The notion that the Shaker Church is a 'continuation' of an authentic Indian spirituality, an 'evolution' of it, as a Church member said to me in 1978, rings false only as long as we view modern Native American history in terms of polarities: Indian/Christian, traditionalist/Shaker, this faction/that faction."[113]

All this speaks powerfully to the view that indigenous communities in the Northwest were not passive victims of colonization, epidemic diseases, and the powerful coercion of reservation agents and Euroamerican missionaries. As Long has written, people found "it necessary to create . . . a possibility of freeing themselves symbolically from what they must passively endure. In responding to the experience of western domination, [such movements] create on a symbolic level so that their own creativity will possess a value freed from Westerners' categories. On this sacred level they can manipulate the symbols, even become them and act them out when possessed, and thus understand and dominate them, although they may consider themselves to be controlled by them."[114] The Shaker Church illustrates this ability of people who have confronted colonialism to create on a symbolic level, to appropriate, reinvent, and *become* the symbols of Euroamerican Christianity, and in doing so to transform them.

Michael McNally has asserted that indigenous reinventions of Christianity "contained social change, enough to respond to changing circumstances of survival without compromising basic (indigenous) values." He argues that such an effort is "a resourceful attempt to forge a new kind of community around the more fundamental" indigenous values, where "symbolic accommodation" is indeed "tantamount to survival."[115] Members of the wider Shaker Church were able to craft elements of Christianity into new symbols with new meanings and new powers that reinforced traditional ways of viewing the world, giving their values, community structures, spirituality, and healing traditions an arena in which they could survive, even within a radically transformed historical context. The Shaker Church carried core indigenous values that were shared by the diverse array of Native communities from Vancouver to northern California and, in so doing, facilitated a wider network of support, communication, and spirituality essential to Native survival at the turn of the twentieth century.

In his history of the Coast Salish, Elmendorf summarized the mid-twentieth century as an era of "disintegration, death of older culture participants, waning survival of Shakerism, apathy."[116] Indeed, Coast Salish communities were severely challenged during the first half of the twentieth century. As Suttles notes, this era "saw a decline in economic opportunities for Indians made worse by the Depression, a decline in the use of Native languages, due especially to their suppression in residential schools, and a decline in influence of mission-founded churches."[117]

The Shaker Church took on the dominant role of religious life among Coast Salish and Chinook communities during this time, in part because of these very economic and cultural stressors, and because of the severe restrictions placed upon spirit dancing associated with the guardian spirit tradition. From 1884 to 1951 potlatches and Indian dances were illegal in Canada (and actively suppressed beginning in 1910), and they were severely restricted in the United States by the Bureau of Indian Affairs.[118] Because of such suppression, spirit dancing and potlatching went underground, being practiced only "in the privacy of modern homes" or in reoccupied "old smokehouses in winter." Funerals, for instance, provided an opportunity for potlatches, preserving indigenous beliefs regarding death and the afterlife.[119] Spirit dancing in Canada reached its lowest point around 1900, nearly dying out, and was carried on by only a few more traditionally minded families. In the 1930s public performances of spirit dances became briefly popular, and some dances, such as the Sxweywey, were performed by paid dancers during summer festivals. Some performers purportedly rationalized that it was safe to do so because if the spirit powers referenced in the dance existed at all, they were present in the human world only during the winter months.[120]

Elmendorf's historical narrative (published in 1960) ends on a pessimistic note. But he was not witness to the renaissance of political activism and pride in Native culture that accompanied the movements for fishing rights and tribal sovereignty and the revival of Native religious practices that came into force in the 1970s. A revival of winter spirit dancing began in Canada as early as the 1950s, providing a means for widely scattered reserves to forge social and spiritual ties. But it was during the 1960s and 1970s that spirit dancing began to see a real renewal.[121] Between 1967 and 1972, for instance, thirty-four people were initiated into spirit dancing longhouses in the Fraser River Valley. By the 1990s more than that number were initiated in the Fraser Valley every year, and sometimes nearly that many might be initiated into a single longhouse. As interest in spirit dancing began to be taken more seriously, public performances came to an end, and the dancing has become increasingly concealed from public view. By the 1980s spirit dancing had become a major force within Coast Salish religious life in British Columbia and was entirely closed to the public. Ceremonies are now private, invitation-only affairs.[122]

The history of spirit dancing differed somewhat among the off-reservation Upper Skagit in Washington State, who did not experience the kind of religious oppression faced by tribes on Canadian reserves and United States reservations. According to Collins, as late as 1942 nearly everyone over twenty-five still had a guardian spirit and participated in guardian spirit dancing. Most were also members of the Shaker Church and had been baptized Catholic. Everyone fifty years old or older had been on a spirit quest as a child, nearly everyone spoke Skagit, and at least four shamans had active practices in the community. Additionally, spirit sickness, such as those due to soul loss, intrusive spirits, or loss of one's spirit powers, was common.[123] Between 1942 and 1969 the Upper Skagit experienced a decline in Skagit culture: by 1969 many no longer spoke the language, baskets were no longer noticeable within households, and kinship practices were breaking down as more and more young people moved away for school or work. And there were no "power houses" left: those dances that remained were held in private homes.[124] However, Collins noted in the 1970s that guardian spirit dancing continued, with "some new young dancers," though numbers were smaller than in 1942, and new initiates no longer spoke Skagit.

Despite the evidence that traditional culture seemed to ebb during these years, Collins nonetheless noted that "from 1942 to 1969, religious life was the most resilient aspect of Upper Skagit culture, with most community members participating in the Shaker Church, spirit dancing, and some also joining the Pentecostal church."[125] As Collins concluded: "That people of the present day cling to their guardian spirits, which have come to them from older relatives, acknowledging and boasting of them, is evidence that their parents and grandparents did not discard them."[126] The revival of winter spirit dancing did not begin in earnest until after Collins concluded her research. But by the 1980s ceremonial houses were active once again and could be found on the Lummi reservation (four of them) and at the Nooksack, Swinomish, Upper Skagit, Tulalip, and Skokomish tribal communities.[127] Spirit dancing had begun a powerful revival, which would spread throughout the Puget Sound region and Fraser Valley.[128]

Joining the Dance: Initiation

According to Ron Hilbert Coy and Pamela Amoss, individuals joining a contemporary longhouse take one of two paths to get there: the "natural way" or the "homemade way." A spirit power received through dreams and visions is sometimes referred to as "spontaneous possession" by scholars, or as the natural way by some spirit dancers, in contrast to the "homemade way" of receiving the spirit through initiation.[129] In the former, individuals receive spirit powers through a dream or vision and are assisted by elders in the longhouse to bring out their spirit song. Ron Hilbert Coy described his mother Taqʷšəblu's experience of going out as a young child and seeking a spirit helper in this natural way. When she first asked her parents about how to get spirit power, "They told her that when it was the right time, her sqəlalitut (spirit power) would come to her. They said a person had to bathe in the river to get spirit power."[130] In the homemade way individuals are brought into the longhouse, and after a difficult and at times painful initiation that lasts several days, the individual receives the spirit power and spirit song. According to Michael Kew, initiates are laid down in a partitioned enclosure or tent within the longhouse. They are carefully supervised as they abstain from food and water for four days. Each morning they are carried around the longhouse, but are otherwise kept lying down, covered in blankets throughout the four days. During this period of seclusion, often on the third night, an initiate may receive a song in a dream. On the fourth morning the initiate bathes, is given new clothes, and later receives ceremonial regalia, including a cedar bark or mountain goat wool headdress. Later they sing their spirit songs and dance their spirit dances "according to directions also given in the dream." All new dancers remain under supervision for the remainder of their first dance season and are referred to as "babies." Throughout this first year in particular, each new dancer is careful to observe certain restrictions on behavior, and each morning they bathe in freshwater streams or pools, accompanied by an attendant.[131]

Initiation into spirit dancing has some parallels with initiation into the Indian Shaker Church. Individuals demonstrate some kind of sorrow or spirit illness prior to conversion, as the spirit power or Holy Spirit begins to work on them.[132] Both traditions also require a purifying process before one can fully encounter and demonstrate spiritual power. As one spirit dancer noted, "When the power first strikes you you feel empty and sick for a long time. The flesh is impure but the breath of God is pure, so while renewing your body, the ordeal is painful."[133] In both traditions, initiates are instructed to wear a particular garment to sing the song that has been taught by the spiritual power.[134] And both kinds of initiates demonstrate their spiritual power by public performance, during which the new initiate appears out of control. As Collins observed regarding a new Shaker, "The uncontrolled behavior of the novice reminds one of the new spirit dancer who must be watched lest he break loose and injure himself."[135]

According to Collins, spirit dancers and Shakers also share certain styles of spiritual performance. Shaker songs follow the same pattern that spirit songs do: one sentence repeated four times.[136] Songs are accompanied by percussion: drums for spirit dancers and hand bells or stamping in time to the song for Shakers. Both traditions have a long service; spirit dancing can easily go on from dusk until dawn, and even an average Shaker Sunday service can go from early morning into the afternoon. Religious gatherings are nearly always followed by a meal, and if guests are present, people are seated by local affiliation. Among the Upper Skagit Lushootseed the salutation to welcome guests is the same, though its English translation might be different. A spirit dancing master of ceremonies might welcome "my relatives," while a Shaker elder might welcome my "brothers and sisters." Shaker services do not incorporate potlatching, as spirit dancing often does, but gifts are still often given to guests and honored relatives.[137]

And for both traditions, healing is the "chief area of concern." As Amoss has noted, "health or the lack of it, seems to be a subject of general and continued interest; people are always talking about it," and "healing is a major function of both Spirit Dancing and Shakerism."[138] In both traditions, "health" does not distinguish between physical and spiritual ailments: the two are inseparably connected. *When* healing occurs might differ between the traditions (while Shakers offer healing ceremonies on a regular basis, healing within spirit dancing primarily occurs through the initiation process or through participating in the spirit dance itself), but healers manifest the healing process in similar ways.[139] And particularly in the contemporary context, both traditions strongly oppose alcohol and drugs, making sobriety a substantial focus within their practice.[140]

For many, the two traditions are not merely superficially similar but are complementary parts of a cohesive Salish spirituality. Amoss notes that during the 1970s more conservative Shakers (especially among the Yakama) did not approve of Shakers participating in winter spirit dances.[141] Yet she also observed that among the Nooksack "the healing power of the Shake is complementary to the healing to be found in Spirit Dancing."[142] Scholars working with Upper Skagit and Sto:lo communities have noted that the two traditions are seen as being entirely complementary. Collins noted in her study of the

Upper Skagit during the mid-twentieth century that "when one becomes a Shaker, his guardian spirit leaves, but returns later as his Shaker help."[143] One individual explained that when it returns, the spirit is "lighted. It has a different song, almost like it, but it is a little bit different.'"[144] Among the Upper Skagit, "Shakers never say that one must have a guardian spirit in order to become a Shaker, but they infer that the only Shakers who possess strong power are those who have ancestral guardian spirits 'behind them.'"[145] Guardian spirits were thus not necessarily "thrown away" when members joined the Shaker Church, but might rather be transformed into a Shaker power, remaining a valuable tool for healing. Winter spirit dancers understand their *syowen* (the Coast Salish term for spirit power; see chapter 8) to be an entity made by the Creator and tasked with offering spiritual power and help to human beings. With such an understanding, it is perhaps not surprising that the Creator's gift of spiritual power could be manifested both in the longhouse and in the Shaker Church, albeit in different forms. The Shaker Church thus gave many Native people "a means whereby the guardian spirits could be maintained under a new guise" as well as "a means of effecting curing."[146] Jay Miller agreed with Collins, noting that when Lushootseed Coast Salish join the Shaker Church, "their spirit powers convert with them, thus continuing the ancestral religious tradition."[147]

Joint membership and participation in Shaker Churches and Coast Salish longhouse traditions is considered acceptable and complementary within many communities. Vi Hilbert has noted that her Upper Skagit parents were both active members of the Shaker Church and longhouse spirit dancing.[148] And Collins has noted that "practicing Shakers may sponsor winter dances of the old type without losing their Church membership," while at the same time Shaker power can also give individuals the ability to refuse a spirit power safely, if they should so choose.[149] Participating in both traditions is aided by the complementary nature of their calendars.[150] As Bierwert notes regarding the Sto:lo in British Columbia, "some healers may participate in the longhouse during its winter season, in Shakerism during the spring, and in Christian fundamentalism during the summer and on Sundays throughout the year."[151] Collins notes that burial practices are an arena where multiple traditions are successfully brought together: the Catholic priest may attend the burial, after which mourners gather for a potlatch, and finally, the Shakers may then hold their own service.[152]

Whether or not the traditions are seen as complementary, however, they both serve similar social functions within contemporary Coast Salish life: providing social solidarity and locating the individual within an extended network of kin and community.[153] Both traditions "are important parts of what it means to be Indian" within a neocolonial context, where Native people continue to wrestle with and negotiate a means of maintaining a distinct identity, even as they live lives fully engaged with the dominant culture.[154] Both the Indian Shaker Church and winter spirit dancing provide "ethnically legitimate ways of bringing Indian people together and stressing their solidarity by emphasizing a unique spiritual heritage."[155] In an era of increased social isolation, spirit dancing longhouses and Shaker churches provide a new kind of shared, communal space.[156]

Both traditions also play a key role in empowering individuals to fulfill their working identity within their community. Despite the fact that contemporary spirit songs are not tied to specific vocations as they once were, Suttles has argued that one's relationship with a spirit power remains a key factor in shaping individual identity. One's song may not announce, "I am a gatherer," or "I am a hunter," but they do mean, "'I am an Indian.'"[157] Bierwert agreed, observing Sto:lo dances in the 1990s and noting that whereas in previous generations "the spirit familiar was an indicator of the dancer's identity as a fisherman, canoe maker, weaver, and so on, the identity of the dancer during this [contemporary] period was that of Indianness."[158] Participating in religious activities serves as a source of personal pride; demonstrates that one has access to supernatural assistance; and brings good health, the power to overcome hardship, and the support of a strong community. While Kew and Harmon have argued that the principal draw for many to British Columbia dances in the 1960s was "status enhancement," John Wike, observing the Swinomish in the 1930s, and Pamela Amoss, observing the Nooksack in the 1970s, argued that the purpose of attending dances was "not so much to boost their status in traditional ways as to express their individuality in a supportive context."[159] As Kew and Harmon have argued, large ceremonials "stressed kinship ties and a shared dedication to maintaining Indian traditions," and these themes "reflected participants' desire for inclusion and recognition both as Indian individuals and as members of particular Indian families or communities."[160]

"Continuity in Substitute Forms": Thinking about Tradition

This discussion of religious change raises key questions about the nature of tradition, and how one defines what "authentic tradition" is. It is an immensely complex question and a particularly difficult one when dealing with religious practices that have been battered by the loss of land, the imposition of another faith through the removal of children to boarding schools, and the systematic suppression of Native traditions through federal policy.[161] Every cultural and religious practice changes over time. Beliefs change, responding to political, social, and material needs. There is no such thing as pure, unchanging, ahistorical culture. And yet we talk about cultures. We need to identify them in some way, and indeed one goal of my study is to trace some kind of continuity throughout Coast Salish and Chinook cultures, to locate what it means to be a healthy self within these communities, and how that view has changed over time, but also how it has remained consistent.

If one is to argue that Coast Salish spirit dancing is "traditional," what does that mean? Contemporary practice certainly differs from historical practice in many ways, yet clear continuities can also be seen. But continuities with what? With when? With nineteenth-century practice? Is that "traditional"? Even deciding to refer to indigenous cultures as they existed at the time of contact with Euroamericans as the definition of "traditional" is deeply problematic, for it suggests that indigenous cultures were static and unchanging prior to the arrival of Europeans. Trying to find some historical moment of authenticity leads one on an endless journey, for indigenous cultures have always changed, evolved, adapted. And yet falling into sheer relativism is also unhelpful. For there is *something* that we can call Coast Salish culture. There is *something* that we can point to and say: that is traditional. But how do we determine what that something is?

The definition of tradition within scholarship has likewise changed over time. While "salvage ethnographers" of the late nineteenth and early twentieth centuries did indeed look for some pure, authentic, static "tradition," scholarship since the 1960s has begun to see tradition "as a more dynamic, processual phenomenon, open to strategic (re)interpretation within larger social dialectics, and most certainly not the conceptual antithesis of modernity."[162] Such scholars have argued for a sense of tradition that is not in conflict with change. Focusing on tradition as a cultural construct can be useful in revealing power struggles and political agendas. But deconstructing "tradition" out of existence is also profoundly unhelpful, particularly when it runs the risk of simply dismissing Native articulations of their tradition as "mere political rhetoric."[163] Indeed, deconstructing the idea of tradition has been challenged by Native people, who see such efforts as undermining the very claims of identity that they are trying to rebuild. When scholars see all tradition as sheer cultural construction, when they reject categories like "Coast Salish" as having any objective reality, then Native people lose a major tool for reconstructing a coherent identity and articulating a clear claim to political autonomy.

Aaron Glass suggests that it can be more helpful to look instead at how tradition is actually used. "People invoke concepts of tradition and culture to define, validate, and legitimize contemporary practices regardless of their actual historical pedigree." As he argues, tradition may need to be understood as "usefulness . . . to current projects, their affectiveness and effectiveness in fostering in people a sense of historically anchored identity and political agency."[164] In many ways tradition can be seen as a selective reconstruction of the past "as a means of justifying and explaining mobilizations of culture." Change and creativity, innovation within religious practice and belief, thus need not be seen as the antithesis of tradition, but rather tradition can be seen as the "legitimator of innovation."[165]

In her study of Jewish ritual Penina Adelman makes a compelling case for thinking about tradition as "a process of interpretation, attributing meaning to the present through making reference to the past."[166] For Adelman, tradition is not a list of canonized behaviors and practices but rather "a process by which cultures are transmitted." She suggests that Jewish tradition is composed of an unchanging warp (the written text) and the weft (the oral texts and practices interpreting that text). This weaving metaphor is a useful one, in that it heads off accusations of a near nihilistic relativism. Tradition is not whatever we fabricate in the moment but is deeply tied to an unchanging framework upon which contemporary interpretations and applications are woven. Such unchanging features, she suggests, are the sacred stories, symbols, and core values that define a people and their origins.[167]

Other scholars are also helpful in getting us to think beyond tradition as a fixed, ahistorical category of authentic practice. As Paige Raibmon has argued in her discussion of Kwak'waka'wakw efforts to recreate ceremonies for the Chicago World's Fair, "the authenticity of Aboriginal life lay not in the mindless, mechanical reproduction of age-old rituals but in the fresh generation of meaningful ways to identify as Kwakwaka'wakw within a changing and increasingly modern age."[168] The key issue here is the role of tradition within individual and collective identity. As Marcell Mauze has argued, "Reference to tradition is a metaphor for identity. This means it encompasses and illustrates a past, a present, and a future. It is not only the memory of the past frozen in time that reemerges; it is also a reference necessary for elaborating a vision of the contemporary world. . . . Tradition is primarily a political instrument for regulating both internal and external relations."[169] And within the contemporary context, American Indian identities are strongly influenced by understandings, recollections, and reconstructions of tradition.[170] Tradition can also be seen as a key mode of resistance within the neocolonial context. Choosing to engage with one's "traditional culture" is a far cry from retreating or withdrawing from the larger world. It can be a means of "engaging, confrontationally-evasively, this larger world."[171]

Jay Miller has pointed out that while Coast Salish communities may not show many outward signs of "traditional" culture, a closer look can reveal "continuity in substitute forms." Certainly many overt signs of Chinook and Coast Salish cultures are gone. Traditional clothing is worn only on ceremonial occasions; few speak Salish or Chinookan languages; few go on vision quests; longhouses are more likely to be community centers than familial dwellings; and canoes are more likely ceremonial than purely functional.[172] But it is also true that "the cultures of the Indian people did not disappear; indeed, they displayed an amazing ability to persist in the face of massive introduced change. They accommodated their structures and beliefs to introduced elements and assimilated aspects of outside culture that were perceived to be adaptive."[173] Examples of this can be seen throughout Coast Salish life. For instance, while outward forms may have changed, functions and intentions may remain continuous with historical practice. Hearths may have been replaced by cast-iron or electric stoves, but the site of cooking remains the center of the home, and upon entering the house a guest is immediately provided with food. Couches in living rooms may have replaced benches in longhouses, but couches are still "preferred to chairs because each can hold more people and double as a bed, much like the ancient inside platforms."[174] Roads and trucks may have replaced rivers and canoes as primary modes of transportation, but they have provided increased opportunities for maintaining kinship relations by visiting other villages and reservations for winter spirit dances, powwows, potlatches, or summer gatherings and, in doing so, have "helped, not hindered, native interactions along very traditional patterns."[175]

Such notions of evolving tradition extend to approaches to healing as well. As Jay Miller argued in his 1999 analysis of the soul recovery ceremony, while the ceremony itself has largely ceased to be practiced, the ailment it sought to cure, soul loss, continues to afflict

Coast Salish individuals. And Coast Salish continue to seek remedies through alternate means: private healing ceremonies, spirit dance initiation, or prayers from Shakers or Pentecostal ministers. As he explains: "What seems an apparent loss or lapse, therefore, on closer examination is actually continuity in substitute forms, both traditional and Christian."[176]

Miller makes a suggestion that should perhaps be self-evident: that we consider how Coast Salish people *themselves* use the term *traditional*. What do they mean when they use it? While Coast Salish people present a wide array of interpretations of this term, Miller argues that a common notion emerges when Coast Salish people use the term. They often mean "anything that supports the continuity of the community."[177] To put it another way, it can be helpful to think about tradition as a tool for collective cultural survival, rather than as culture itself.

For a people who have always lived along watersheds, the notion of tradition as a thing in motion can make immediate sense. Rivers move, they change, they shift their courses, erode their banks, flood villages, and run dry. They can look very different from one season to the next. But they remain the same river. The spirit and life of the river is the same. In a similar fashion, tradition can be used to refer to continuity, tying past to present to future, even in the midst of cyclical change. Tradition can be seen as a thing in process, an emerging vision for self and collective identity.

As this chapter shows, cultural change is "traditional," having a long history among Native communities of this region. Throughout the nineteenth and twentieth centuries, core values, beliefs, and approaches to healing remained continuous, in the midst of accommodation and adaptation. Spirit power traditions, prophetic movements, the Indian Shaker Church, and contemporary spirit dancing, while taking very different forms, maintained common ways of viewing the embodied self and the healthy working identity. In the chapters that follow we see that this ability to integrate new symbols and modes of spirituality and healing continue to play an important role in the well-being of South Puget Coast Salish and Chinookan communities. Alongside a great deal of creative adaptation, key features remain consistent: a view of illness as an inability to embody one's working identity, a sense of the healthy self as an autonomous individual within a kin-based community, and an understanding of healing as the restoration of human, spiritual, and ecological relationships through collective, embodied practices.

5. Both Traditional and Contemporary

The South Puget Intertribal Women's Wellness Program

> Healthy relationships are the basis of healthy communities.
>
> —*South Puget Intertribal Planning Agency Annual Report,* 1999

> The Creator has put a blueprint inside each of us, a blueprint of who we're meant to be, what we're meant to do. But we have to actualize the blueprint that the Creator put in us. Become what we're meant to be. That's what wellness is.
>
> —CECILIA FIRETHUNDER, keynote speaker, South Puget Intertribal Intergenerational Women and Girls' Gathering, 2001

This chapter discusses efforts by tribal communities in the South Puget Sound to bring traditional approaches to wellness to bear upon contemporary health concerns.[1] It continues to address two central questions raised throughout this book. First, how can contemporary tribal communities integrate non-native approaches to health and wellness while still honoring Coast Salish and other indigenous understandings of the embodied subject and a healthy working identity? This is closely related to a second question: how can such multiple, complex identities exist in a way that maintains a meaningful sense of self? In the previous chapter I argued that Coast Salish practices in this region have a long history of hybridity and change, while maintaining consistent approaches to healing and the embodied subject. Coast Salish and Chinookan communities were not merely acted *upon* by history, but actively shaped their experience, creating and revitalizing religious movements that gave them tools to "participate in and think through the meaning" of their experience, and to "create on a symbolic level" a means of resistance and freedom.[2] While cultural and religious expressions in the region have varied widely, the traditions share a sense of what it means to be a healthy person in community. This is a history of creative negotiation and adaptation, responding to and integrating elements of Euroamerican culture, religion, and medicine so as to preserve communities and Native identities.[3]

At the beginning of the twenty-first century contemporary approaches to health in Native American communities are continuing to draw upon this rich tradition of adaptation and creativity. In this chapter I argue that while contemporary approaches to health and wellness may seem quite different from those of the ancestors (as they now incorporate biomedicine and alternative health care), their internal philosophical structure remains the same. I would suggest that by bringing traditional approaches to health and the body alongside biomedicine, these communities are not so much straying from "tradition" as affirming it.[4] Through an analysis of an intertribal women's wellness gathering, I explore what it means to have a healthy working identity for contemporary Native women in the South Puget Sound. What emerges is a sense of health and wellness that draws upon a traditionally consistent view of the embodied subject: healthy individuals require healthy communities, and healthy communities require individuals able to fulfill their roles and obligations within those communities. Health requires having a clear sense of personal identity and individual autonomy. And at the same time, it requires that individuals find their place within a balanced web of reciprocal relationships: human relationships, spiritual relationships, and ecological relationships.

Moving toward Sovereignty: Local Control of Care

In 1975 the Indian Self-Determination and Education Assistance Act was passed, a landmark legislative move that instructed the Bureau of Indian Affairs and the Indian Health Service to begin turning over management of tribal services to those tribes who requested local control. In the last thirty years that process has accelerated as more and more communities have moved toward local governance of social services, including healthcare. The result has been a radical transformation in medical care for Native people, from a consolidated "single national . . . directly operated federal program" to one "under the control and direction of the local Indian community."[5] The result has been a remarkable shift toward culturally relevant care that integrates elements of traditional indigenous cultures and spirituality within programs for health and wellness.[6]

Indeed, earlier paternalistic policies guiding the Indian Health Service have been dramatically reversed. Instead, we find "the integration of traditional medicine and Western medicine," particularly in alcohol and substance abuse treatment programs. Such integration might be as dramatic as employing or contracting with Native healers or as simple as disconnecting smoke detectors so that patients can be smudged with burning sage. The Indian Health Service as a whole continues to struggle with how best to integrate traditional practitioners and is working to develop "policies and procedures for credentialing traditional healers, granting them privileges, and paying them," as well as other practical concerns, such as how to manage medical records, third party billing, and liability.[7]

It is helpful to consider the history of Cushman Hospital on the Puyallup reservation as a model of how this shift toward tribally directed and culturally integrated healthcare programs came about. Founded in 1864, the hospital was originally Cushman Trade School, a boarding school admitting Native students from throughout the United States and Alaska, to learn vocational trades. A hospital was built onsite to treat sick students, though it was always poorly funded and occasionally not available, such as during World War I, when the hospital was used for wounded soldiers. In 1939 the school was bought by the Department of the Interior and became the largest Indian healthcare facility in the United States. Until the 1950s it would be the only Indian hospital in the Northwest, sometimes requiring the severely ill to travel hundreds of miles to receive medical care.[8] Many Native people within the region feared the place and avoided it at all costs, arguing that it was "the place where people went to die."[9] Cushman was turned over exclusively to the treatment of tuberculosis in 1954, and it was closed in 1959. In the years that followed the Northwest had no Indian hospital at all.

As Native communities began mobilizing politically, they turned their attention to community well-being. In 1958 the American Indian Service League was founded, making an explicit link between political mobilization and traditional culture.[10] In 1960 an Indian Center opened in downtown Seattle at First and Vine, offering community services for the diverse local indigenous population, and providing a voice to protest federal policies such as termination and removal, calling attention to their negative impacts on reservation and urban Indian communities alike.[11] In 1970 Puyallup activist Bob Satiacum led the occupation of Fort Lawton, a U.S. Army post located in northeastern Seattle, in cooperation with United Indians of All Tribes. As a result of the occupation a deal was negotiated with the city of Seattle, securing sixteen acres of what would soon be known as Discovery Park. The Daybreak Star Cultural Center was subsequently opened in 1976, providing community services and cultural events.[12]

It was within this context of growing political activism that the Puyallup tribe occupied the Cushman campus, intending to reclaim the site as an Indian healthcare center. An "armed but peaceful occupation" took place in 1976 and again in 1980. Finally, a federal district court ruling decreed that the site was indeed property of the U.S. Department of the Interior but had been held in trust for the Puyallup tribe. Shortly thereafter, Cushman was transferred to the tribe. On the site the Puyallup opened the first tribally operated medical clinic in the United States, the Indian Community Clinic.[13] The facility struggled under poor funding and high staff turnover, particularly of physicians. Federal budget cuts in 1986 further challenged the facility and brought with them new restrictions on eligibility for access to healthcare at the federally funded clinic. New budgetary regulations imposed on the Puyallup clinic limited who could access service: an individual had to be a member or eligible for membership in a federally recognized tribe, have one quarter ancestry, and live within the health service delivery area.[14]

The Indian Self-Determination and Education Assistance Act of 1975 opened up possibilities for local control of healthcare, prompting other tribes to follow the example set by the Puyallup. In the decades since then more and more tribes have sought to gain local control over healthcare.[15] In 1994 a Tribal Leaders' Summit on Health Care Reform was held in Washington State, where leaders made the case that the best route to ensuring culturally competent care would be for tribes to manage their own clinics and wellness centers. They concluded that the shift to direct tribal control over personnel and policies "has worked exceptionally well and many patients who formerly have received less than adequate treatment now have access to culturally sensitive health care services."[16] Surveys submitted in the early 1990s to tribes with locally directed programs also found that such programs were faring better than federally directed healthcare. They were more likely to have added new programs and facilities, prevention programs, and community-based health programs than were federally run clinics.[17] Most respondents felt that services had been improved, wait times lowered, and more people served.[18] The shift has been embraced at the federal level as well, and since 1995 the Indian Health Service has changed its approach from "direct and control" to "support."[19]

Enormous challenges still remain. Elder care remains an unachieved goal for most tribes: in 1993 only twelve reservation communities had onsite nursing homes, only one of which was in Washington State (the Colville).[20] As casino revenues have increased, other tribes have invested in elder care, including the Puyallup, who have recently completed a new elder center, The House of Respect. The House of Respect includes spaces for indoor and outdoor recreation, meeting rooms, a library, banquet room, health and wellness center, massage, hydrotherapy, and a traditional healing room for ceremonies. At the same time, poorer reservations with less access to private funds continue struggle to provide on-reservation support for the elderly and chronically ill.

Healthcare for American Indians and Alaskan Natives who live in cities remains underfunded and poorly organized.[21] While 56 percent of Native people live in urban centers, as of 2000, Congress continued to allocate scarcely more than 1 percent of the annual appropriation for Indian healthcare to serve the entire urban Native population.[22] Urban communities face other challenges as well. While reservation communities struggle with poverty and geographical isolation, urban Native people can struggle with social isolation, "a major contributor to mental and emotional problems."[23] While challenges remain great, by the early twenty-first century urban Indian communities and groups like United Indians of All Tribes (UIAT) have made substantial achievements. UIAT in Seattle, for instance, offers foster-care advocacy, Head Start classes, outpatient substance abuse treatment, culturally appropriate mental health care, housing referrals, and GED courses. The Seattle Indian Health Board provides dental and medical services and assists with access to traditional healers, while another group (Queer Oyate) provides support to Native people who are HIV positive.[24]

This chapter presents a case study of one tribally directed program: the South Puget Intertribal Planning Agency (SPIPA) and its Women's Wellness Program. SPIPA is a cooperative effort of five South Puget tribes, the Chehalis, Nisqually, Skokomish, Squaxin Island, and Shoalwater Bay. SPIPA's Women's Wellness Program works to increase awareness of health concerns among Native women of the five-tribe coalition through a variety of services and events, including free breast and cervical cancer screening, cancer survivor retreats, counseling and assistance for cases of domestic or sexual violence, and the publication of a magazine that highlights health concerns of Native women and carries interviews with women from the five tribes discussing basketry, oral traditions, healthcare, mammograms, and their personal struggles with breast and cervical cancer. SPIPA as a whole also works with local tribal health centers and social service offices to facilitate a variety of events and programs, including vocational rehabilitation, drug and alcohol counseling, and a food distribution service, including participating in the Women, Infants and Children (WIC) supplemental nutrition program. The Women's Wellness Program sponsors a series of meetings and gatherings throughout the year, including an annual Intertribal Intergenerational Women and Girls' Gathering, a primary focus of this chapter.

Data are drawn from ethnographic observations and conversations conducted during my volunteer work with SPIPA's Women's Wellness Program, from 2001 to 2006, and from publications produced by SPIPA, the Women's Wellness Program, and the five tribes. This organization and the Women's Wellness Program in particular are good places to focus attention, because they stand as strong examples of what tribally directed, locally controlled organizations can do. Their efforts to construct culturally relevant modes of addressing health and wellness have achieved a great deal. While these communities continue to face enormous challenges, this intertribal cooperative effort has made great strides toward addressing those challenges.

SPIPA also provides an ideal setting for considering the profoundly *intertribal* nature of Coast Salish cultures and communities. Indeed, the notion of "tribe" is a recent innovation: prior to the reservation era Coast Salish communities consisted of autonomous villages, which were linked together by a web of kinship relations and shared cultural practices and language but were not identified by a single overarching tribal affiliation. Given this extended kinship network, which continues to connect contemporary tribal communities, the ability to work jointly and share resources and support systems makes sense both practically and culturally.

Finding Common Ground: Cultural Diversity in Western Washington

One challenge faced by SPIPA, as well as by programs geared toward urban Indian communities in the Pacific Northwest, is how best to serve a population marked by enormous cultural and religious diversity. There are twenty-nine different reservations in Washington State alone, and within the urban context of Tacoma and Seattle things become even more complex.[25] The Seattle Indian Health Board noted that between 1989 and 1999 individuals from 238 different federally recognized tribes received healthcare from their facilities.[26] Puget Sound's cities are profoundly intertribal places, having drawn indigenous people from all over the Northwest and the nation seeking out employment and other opportunities. During their relatively brief history, these urban centers, Seattle in particular, became "part of an annual cycle of migration, leading to the formation of a multiethnic urban Indian community," where Native people from other parts of the country soon outnumbered members of local indigenous communities.[27] In the Puyallup tribal health center, for instance, only 22.7 percent of patients are Puyallup, 47.8 percent are members of other Washington tribes, and 29.3 percent are from other tribes or bands from throughout the United States and British Columbia.[28] As many as 75 percent of the tribe's inpatient drug and alcohol treatment programs' patients are originally from another county or state.[29]

Even if one considers only Coast Salish communities, it is virtually impossible to define any singular "Coast Salish" identity. There are twenty-five reservation communities in western Washington State (most of which are Coast Salish, and virtually all of which are home to some Coast Salish), not to mention the numerous Coast Salish reserves in British Columbia. Each community has its unique history and religious and cultural traditions. And of course each individual within these communities has a particular sense of what it means to be Coast Salish. Some communities have integrated into Euroamerican economic systems, while others have remained largely outside such systems.[30] And there are no clear demarcations between groups. With a mobility shared by their ancestors, Coast Salish individuals continue to move from one village or reservation to another and from reservation to urban center.[31] As Alexandra Harmon has concluded in her study of Coast Salish communities in Puget Sound, the descendents of western Washington Indians have remained "diverse, dispersed, and of many minds about government conceptions of them" and have "perpetuated the diversity and ambiguity that had long characterized Indian identity in their region."[32]

Scholars have long disagreed about what might be considered a foundation for Coast Salish identity. Marion Smith (1940) limited his scope to those who were descendents of treaty signers. Wayne

Suttles (1987) emphasized being part of a kin-lineage with its accompanying resource rights. Others have focused on association with modern tribes, though as Harmon points out, tribal entities are a relatively new creation in this region, only in existence since the late nineteenth century. Jay Miller (1997) has suggested that identity is fundamentally about "complex personal social identities," based on "patterns of affiliation." Ultimately Coast Salish identity may be about relations—relations to "immortal beings regarded as ancestral kinfolk," relations to immediate kin and to a wider circle of relatives based on increasingly dispersed interlinkages between households and communities, and to relations with a place expressed through kin-based use rights, habitation of a particular watershed, and a sense of responsibility for particular resource procurement areas.[33]

One challenge for SPIPA and other organizations seeking to meet the health and wellness needs of Native communities in the Pacific Northwest has been wrestling with this diversity. Health and wellness providers are committed to providing culturally congruent care, and yet how can such programs be appropriately developed given such a widely diverse clientele?

Since incorporating traditional approaches to spirituality into health and wellness programs is an important goal for SPIPA, the religious diversity of their clientele poses a particular challenge. Contemporary Coast Salish families continue to employ strategic and flexible affiliation, so as to include many religious options. As Miller has argued, many Coast Salish maintain an ecumenical approach, believing that "the more religions you have, the better for you. Thus, while families continue to attend winter ceremonials to welcome the return of spirit partners, on Sunday they devotedly attend Protestant, Catholic, Bahai, or other services."[34] Some people identify themselves with local smokehouse spirit dancing traditions; others are members of the Shaker Church, while others are devout members of Christian congregations of various stripes. Others move freely among these three arenas, and still others reflect the spiritual makeup of the Northwest itself, famous for being the least-churched and most spiritually independent region of the United States.[35] Today Natives in the region are "highly varied in their spiritual beliefs," and "perhaps a majority are involved in some combination of traditional Indian and Christian religion."[36] Many individuals and communities also incorporate elements of what are sometimes called "pan-Indian" religious practices, which are strongly influenced by northern Plains traditions, including the Sun Dance, pipe ceremonies, talking circles with eagle feathers, cleansing ceremonies with burning sage (smudging), and the use of a sweat lodge.[37] Even among those who might identify strongly with traditional Coast Salish religious practice, such as longhouse spirit dancing, traditions vary widely from family to family and community to community.

As they work to provide resources that are culturally congruent and that incorporate indigenous spirituality, SPIPA's staff must locate those beliefs, values, and worldviews shared by the majority of their constituents. What kind of spirituality will be broadly acceptable, broadly recognized as "traditional," and will draw upon shared, central beliefs and values? Within such diversity, how can one begin to articulate what might be a common worldview or ethos of Native communities of the region? As Guilmet and Whited have argued, "The building of individual identities based on recentering the person within his/her ethnicity requires the development of a pan-Indian and Alaska Native cultural ethos capable of unifying individuals representing diverse native cultures."[38] SPIPA and its intertribal Women's Wellness Program have worked to do just that, seeking to locate those commonalities that bring women of the region together and to implement them within publications, workshops, and cultural events.[39] Hence intertribal organizations such as SPIPA share with urban Indian health centers, such as the Leschi Center Medical Clinic in Seattle, similar challenges of locating a common, shared identity and worldview while also respecting the personal autonomy and unique needs of individual clients.

Native people throughout the region, for instance, shared a common historical experience, including residential schooling, the great depression, military service, and political mobilization. Such experiences contributed to the emergence of a complex layered identity, which included both local identities and a regional or national Indian sensibility. Harmon has noted the role that residential schools played in this process. While maintaining a clear sense of their particular tribal affiliation, most Native children also came to embrace a second layer of "pan-Indian identity that provided a basis for affiliation with other tribes." While federal residential schools worked to remove Native young people from their homes, cultures, and languages, the schools also gave students a chance "to pool memories and myths and thus to develop a standardized lore that became a common heritage" of Native people throughout the Pacific Northwest, and to "present their complex web of social relations in a simplified form."[40] Other contemporary concerns have also united communities throughout the region, including fishing rights, which often serve as common ground for tribal communities and as a place to "fashion a collective Indian history." As Harmon argues, "If they shared nothing else with other Indians, they at least shared a love of fish and a unique relationship—defined by treaty—to the powers that be in America."[41]

In their study of the Puyallup tribal health center, George Guilmet and David Whited identified a series of key shared values held by patients and tribally affiliated staff members: "value orientations towards fishing and hunting, personal power through information or knowledge, a dependence upon extended family and kin based social organization, a spiritual respect for ecosystem and ecology, the continued practice of ascribing individual responsibility to children and adolescents, the emphasis towards cooperation versus competition within the in-group, the tendency to perceive oneself as part of a whole (whether group or part of the community of nature) rather than as a discrete and isolated competitor." Guilmet and Whited concluded that this set of shared values served as "examples of the continuity and survival of the traditional value orientation in the face of accommodative and assimilationist change."[42]

Within the remarkable diversity of Indian communities of the Pacific Northwest, there thus remains a set of shared values and worldviews that, when considered in light of the historical and ethnographic record, can be said to be "traditional." These include a strong emphasis on personal autonomy, locating the individual within a strong kin-based network, an emphasis on cooperation, and a keen sense of interrelatedness with one's human and ecological community.[43] Native identities and worldviews remain a viable and important part of life for South Puget tribal communities, and as viable meaning-making activities they have expanded, contracted, and transformed over time to meet the changing needs of their changing communities. As the present case study shows, Native women's approaches to health and wellness have incorporated Euroamerican biomedicine and eastern holistic care alongside their indigenous traditions, without compromising cultural integrity. How? In part, this is because the expressions and modes of healing have changed, but an underlying indigenous understanding of health and the embodied subject remain.

The Intertribal Intergenerational Women and Girls' Gathering

Within SPIPA's Intertribal Intergenerational Women and Girls' Gathering, staff and volunteers seek to cultivate those shared values and concerns. Held each summer, it is open to Native women and girls from throughout the South Puget Sound region. The goal of the gathering is to further Native women's health and well-being by drawing on "traditional" resources, community ties, and intertribal support systems. Plans for this annual event first began in 1995, when women representing the five tribes met to reflect on what such a gathering should entail. The result was a mission statement: "We the women and girls of the Nisqually, Chehalis, Skokomish, Shoalwater Bay and Squaxin Island tribes believe that women are the backbone of our communities. We therefore have a mission to empower women and girls of our tribal communities and prepare and enable ourselves to be strong leaders. We endeavor to do this by learning more about holistic health, improving relationships, and our tribal cultures and histories."[44] Since that time, planning for the annual event has remained in the hands of the communities, so as to be responsive to the interests and voices of the women they serve. Each year, monthly planning meetings are held at local tribal centers. These meetings involve a meal, a craft, and conversation about what women would like to see at this year's gathering. Feedback is also solicited from the women at the gathering itself, and responses are carefully considered. Tribal staff devote care and energy to ensuring that the gathering is consistent with Native women's perspectives and priorities. Because of this, the gathering provides insight into how South Sound women understand what it means to have a healthy working identity.

In recent years the event has taken place at a 4-H camp centrally located in the South Puget Sound. The setting provides opportunities for quiet reflection in a natural setting, for canoeing, swimming, and walks around the lake. The days are also filled with workshops and classes geared toward teaching women about Native culture—medicinal plants and herbs, basketry, beading, drum making; health and wellness—diabetes, cardiovascular health, HIV/AIDS, domestic violence, and sexual assault care and prevention; opportunities for clinical care—free mammograms, pap smears, and diabetes screening; and alternative care—acupuncturists, Reiki practitioners, reflexologists, and yoga and tai chi instructors are on-staff for the weekend. Talking circles, drumming circles, a sweat lodge, and a giveaway ceremony provide spaces for indigenous approaches to spiritual healing, reflection, and affirmation of community, while keynote speakers address indigenous culture, spirituality, and health and wellness. Free childcare and children's activities provide mothers and other caregivers an opportunity to rest, reflect, and enjoy themselves. The following discussion explores this annual event in greater detail, considering it within its broader historical, cultural, and social context. Doing so demonstrates the ways in which contemporary Native communities have crafted approaches to health and wellness that integrate biomedical and other non-native modes of care within a context and intention that is distinctly Coast Salish and Chinook.

A central goal of the Women's Wellness Program has been to bring traditional modes of healing and community well-being alongside biomedical responses to contemporary health risks. At the heart of their efforts is a sense of health and embodied subjectivity that reflects Coast Salish and Chinook worldviews and traditions. The embodied subject here is one that is defined by relationships with community, with one's ancestors, with spirit powers dwelling in the landscape, and with the natural world itself. In this context health is demonstrated by the proper expression of one's identity-within-community, in which relationships are honored and obligations are met. This means taking care of one's body and spirit, cultivating a strong sense of self, so as to be able to be the daughter, mother, or elder that one's community needs. The variety of programs and activities tribal women at SPIPA have worked together to create all have in common a sense of health and wellness that is dependent upon this sense of *interrelatedness*. As is noted in one SPIPA document, "Healthy relationships are the basis of healthy communities."[45] Health is achieved through the restoration of strong relationships between individuals and their communities, between individuals and their indigenous landscape, and between individuals and their ancestors. The result of this restoration is a resolute sense of collective identity and of individual calling: one's unique contribution to one's community. The healthy self is not one that is subsumed within relationships. Rather, healthy relationships require a clear sense of individual autonomy and purpose, a strong sense of personal identity from which one is able to honor one's place within a kin-based world.

Tradition: A Path toward Healthy Communities

In the discussion of the idea of tradition in the previous chapter, Jay Miller suggested that we think about tradition as "anything that supports the continuity of the community."[46] Women's voices at the Women and Girls' Gathering and in SPIPA publications mirror this view, suggesting that "traditional" activities are those that draw upon the cultural heritage of the community, its oral traditions, arts, and wisdom, but may also have been adapted, modified, and applied in ways that may appear quite different than they did in the nineteenth century. The programs and the literature that SPIPA publishes for the local communities also make a clear association between traditional activities and *healthy* activities.

Being "traditional" is synonymous with being healthy. A 2001 article in the Women's Wellness newsletter reflects this argument. Alysha Waters of the Native Foods Project argued:

> Only a hundred and fifty years ago, the ancestors of this region were the healthiest of any group of peoples living upon the earth. Cancer was very rare and diabetes and heart disease were virtually unknown. For thousands of years Pacific Northwest tribes had food production systems in place that sustained healthy communities. These food systems were rich in tradition and ceremony while connecting integrally to trade, commerce, and sound environmental practices. . . . The health and nutrition of Indian peoples has been greatly affected by the destruction of the sustainable Native American food production systems. Currently, diet is the biggest threat to the health of Native Americans resulting in high rates of obesity, heart disease, high blood pressure, stroke, cancer, and diabetes. In order to successfully address the serious health and nutritional concerns of Native peoples whose diets were recently westernized to industrially processed foods, it is imperative to return to a diet similar to a traditional one. Recent research and traditional ways and knowledge both indicate that wherever native peoples live, eating local indigenous foods is better for our bodies, our communities, our economies and the land itself.[47]

Indigenous modes of food gathering, community cohesion, ceremonial activity, and traditional medicines and lifestyles are all presented in these pages as healthy alternatives to modern lifestyles. And these programs demonstrate ways in which these "traditional" modes of living can be adapted to the contemporary experience.[48]

Concurrently, social ills and physiological illness are viewed as *nontraditional*. SPIPA's publications point to the fact that cancer is not a traditional illness, arguing for instance that "cervical cancer was not common among our ancestors since they practiced protective behaviors: fewer lifetime partners and using tobacco for ceremonies. Today's Native women don't live the healthy lifestyle of the ancestors."[49] Such health risks facing Native people are perceived by community members as "nontraditional" and stemming from the imposition of colonialism. In a 2006 article diabetes is described in similar terms by Skokomish tribal member Sheri Peterson-Hale: "Like the measles or smallpox, this is yet another western culture disease that we must develop resistance to if our culture is to survive. The once-active lifestyle of our ancestors has been lost to modern conveniences, a sedentary lifestyle, and a high fat diet creating expanding waistlines and leaving a legacy of diabetes for future generations."[50]

Similarly, comments were made by 2001 Women and Girls' Gathering keynote speaker Cecilia Firethunder, who has spearheaded successful programs to combat domestic violence on the Pine Ridge Reservation, where she said domestic violence is estimated to play a part in seven out of ten homes. Domestic violence, she argued, is not traditional. Rather, it is indicative of the ways that colonization has disrupted traditional value systems and spirituality.

> Women are valued; women are equal in traditional Indian societies. Lakota spirituality is based on the feminine. It began with a woman. And I think if you look carefully at other Indian religions, you'll find most of them are based on the feminine. Women were the culture bearers, we *are* the carriers, the keepers of culture. . . . Women are the keepers of culture, and yet they are the focus of most of the violence in our communities. When women are under attack, the culture, the community, the future is under attack. If women are safe, children are safe; the culture is safe. Battery of one woman threatens an entire culture. To be well, to be safe, Indian women have to learn to value ourselves as Indian women, to demand that things change, to stand up for each other. . . . Today things are messed up, and that is not reflective of what our communities are really about, what our cultures teach. In our belief systems women are sacred. We're supposed to honor women, not hurt them. If we were really living within our values, we wouldn't be hurting each other.[51]

The very inclusion of speakers such as Ms. Firethunder (Lakota) or Dr. Inés Talamantez (Mescalero Apache) speaks to the processual nature of "tradition" and identity. Nineteenth-century Coast Salish and Chinook communities would not have had any contact with women from those parts of the country. In the twenty-first century such relationships and exchanges are a central piece of community vitality and spiritual growth.

I spoke with several women, both Native and non-native, who work for SPIPA and the Women's Wellness Program about what it means to be traditional. One Native woman who has worked with SPIPA, the Washington State Health Board, and her own South Puget tribe, answered the question by describing several examples of strategies she has employed to bring "traditional" approaches to bear on contemporary concerns. This woman has led several retreats for American Indian youth, educating them about safer sex, STDs, the dangers of drugs and alcohol, and increasing their knowledge and awareness of diabetes, all of which are major threats to Native wellness. She invites elders to speak to teenagers, teaching them basketry, beadwork, and leatherwork, passing on a sense of heritage and connection to tradition. She described one project in particular that effectively demonstrates this adaptation of traditional approaches to wellness to meet contemporary health needs. Accompanying a discussion of sexually transmitted diseases and teen pregnancy at a recent youth retreat, the young people were shown how to make their own medicine bags. They cut and sewed the leather and created a design of personal significance that they then beaded onto the bags. The medicine bags, she said, can double as condom carriers. Acting as a brilliant representation of the merging of traditional culture with contemporary health technology to address current health crises, the medicine bag condom carriers go home with the young people, around their necks, a reminder of who they are and of their responsibility for their own health.[52]

Other events also show this sense of tradition as something adaptable to contemporary circumstances. For instance, in 2003, the Nisqually Women's Wellness Program sponsored two celebration dinners, designed to discuss Coast Salish and Chinook (as well as broader pan-Indian) views of menstruation and menopause. Nisqually

Women's Health Provider Beverly Wright commented that in traditional Native culture the beginning of menstruation is "a celebration. It is not a shame." This gathering to celebrate menstruation invited young girls, their mothers, and aunts to join in an evening together. Participants strung "moon beads": twenty-eight colored beads to indicate days in a cycle, with "a special bead representing ovulation and another for menstruation or *moon time*." Discussions of traditional views of the body and what it means to be a woman were here integrated with biomedical approaches to wellness. Women attending the gathering learned about the value of this time of life within their Native culture as well as the importance of annual medical exams like pap smears. During the gathering to honor menopause or "the change," older women's lives, bodies, and important roles in communities were likewise celebrated, even as women were taught about the importance of calcium intake and regular breast exams.[53] Hence, *tradition* is defined in this context as rooted in Native cultures, as inherently healthy, and also as something that can be easily brought alongside biomedical approaches to wellness. Tradition is comfortable with cultural hybridity.

The Intertribal Intergenerational Women and Girls' Gatherings also illustrate this complex understanding of tradition within their goal of presenting women with "traditional and alternative modes of healing." Midge Porter (Shoalwater/Chinook) was a SPIPA staff member and one of the primary organizers of the annual Women and Girls' Gathering. The event, she told me, introduces women to ways of maintaining their health, dealing with illness, and creating healthy lifestyles. By *traditional*, Midge explained, she meant "first peoples' medicine." This can mean medicine that emerges from "indigenous peoples," medicine that has a holistic approach to healthcare, and recognition of the "whole person," the "person within community." As such, Midge and the other women involved in planning the event have sought out a surprising array of "traditional healers": acupuncturists, massage therapists, qi'gong instructors, Reiki practitioners, and reflexologists, who work alongside Native women herbalists and those running the sweat lodges and talking circles.

The women attending the gathering welcome these alternative practitioners without hesitation. This became evident to me during the first Gathering that I attended, when my task was to keep a log of appointments with these practitioners and to bring the women to their sessions at the proper time. The assignment was a very pleasant one, as it gave me the chance to chat with a wide variety of women at the gathering and to get a sense of their reactions to these alternative healthcare providers. As a whole, the women were thrilled with these Reiki, reflexology, and massage practitioners, seeing a natural continuity and cohesion (though certainly an important distinction) between these alternative healthcare providers and their own traditions. Their holistic approach to health matched the general spiritual and reflective atmosphere of the retreat, and also mirrored SPIPA's message for the weekend, which was to encourage the women to nurture and care for their whole selves.

These massage therapists, Reiki practitioners, reflexologists, and yoga and tai chi instructors continue to play a particularly important role in these annual gatherings, representing the importance of embodied experience within healing. Women seek them out and express excitement over the opportunity to have such personal attention. Just as in traditional healing practices (as well as in Indian Shaker Church healing traditions), touch is a very important part of the healing process. Women who are constant caretakers of others respond positively to being *taken care of* for a change. Touch is a powerful healer, whether it emerges from an eastern tradition like Reiki or acupuncture or a western tradition like massage therapy.

Movement is likewise a central part of wellness. Like historical healing ceremonies centered around dance, embodied practice is an important part of wellness during SPIPA's annual Women and Girls' Gathering. This is seen within early morning walks around Panhandle Lake, or when a large group of women join the tai chi instructors on the shore. The gentle movements of tai chi are such that elders, children, and women who rarely exercise can all join in. As women's responses made clear, it did not matter that this movement came from an eastern tradition, because it shared key similarities with these communities' approaches to "traditional" wellness: integration of body, spirit, and community.

To encompass all these things, to restore these relationships that exist on human, ecological, and spiritual levels, SPIPA and the Women's Wellness Program organizers recognize the necessity of a holistic approach to healthcare. This approach is not limited to SPIPA but emerges within tribally distinct programs as well.[54] Much like the holistic approach present at the various health centers on South Puget Sound reservations, the emphasis here is upon restoring individuals to their full position within their community: as parents, as elders, or as children supporting and caring for their elders. This notion of tradition, as practices that are holistic, coming from first peoples, and that see the patient as an individual-in-community, is an important one. It evokes notions of cultural hybridity, of identities and meanings on the borders, in the spaces in-between. It also reveals important elements of continuity with historically traditional views about the nature of the self. The self is *embodied*, and located within a network of relationships. Put briefly, tradition reconnects to heritage, identity, and a clear sense of one's self-in-community. To be traditional is to be healthy, to reconnect with the ways of the ancestors.

Other tribal healthcare providers in the region have made similar arguments, insisting that successful care must take a holistic approach to individual care. Swinomish Tribal Mental Health care providers have argued that a holistic view "is consistent with most Indian philosophy. For instance, Indian people have long understood that environmental problems such as destruction of natural resources or contamination of water sources can lead to physical, spiritual, or emotional illness."[55] In order to be successful, holistically oriented models must be fundamentally about locating individuals within their community. And to do that, they must be based at the tribal level, located on the reservation, have "organizational ties to tribal social services," and draw upon tribal community members for staffing. For instance, the tribal mental health care project at Swinomish employs "tribal mental health workers": local tribal members trained in care and counseling. But regardless of cultural or ethnic background, effective health and wellness providers must be part of the community they serve: attending tribal functions, spending time developing relationships with community members, becoming acquainted with extended family networks, and meeting the community on its own terms through flexible hours.[56]

Further, according to both Guilmet and Whited and the Swinomish Tribal Mental Health Project, successful models bring "traditional therapies" alongside biomedical treatments, employing both systems as complementary practices. And indeed, as Jay Miller explains, Lushootseed Salish communities continue to make use of both indigenous healing and biomedical systems. "The latter has not replaced the former; the two function side by side because each has separate causative agents, either the ill intent of other beings or invasion by germs."[57] As one Nooksack observer told Pamela Amoss in the 1970s, "There's three things we have to help us, the white doctor, the Shake, and the syowen. If my kids are sick, I go to the white doctor first. If he can't do nothing, I take them to the Shakers; if they can't do nothing, then it's the syowen."[58]

But how exactly traditional therapies can be integrated into a clinical setting is another matter. Guilmet and Whited describe the incorporation of such services at the Puyallup Kwawachee Counseling Center, including "treatments in the longhouse traditions," "the Sacred Pipe Ceremony, sweats," smudging, and Shaker Church healing services.[59] The fact that patients have been interested in making use of such services demonstrates "the persistence of traditional values and beliefs" even when "overt signs of traditionality are absent."[60] In a similar manner the Swinomish tribal mental health center integrates Coast Salish spirituality and worldview by recognizing the interconnection of physical, mental, and spiritual health and by "recognizing the therapeutic value of traditional Indian spiritual beliefs and practices." They provide "referrals, consultants, spiritual support and direct participation in healing ceremonies"; employ "tribal mental health workers who have access to traditional healing systems"; and allow "clients to choose their tradition, helping them contact traditional practitioners, consulting with traditional healers, attending services and assisting when asked to do so."[61]

Cultivating a return to traditional culture and religion has a demonstrated effect upon the health of individuals and communities. For instance, tribal mental health workers continue to emphasize that wellness programs must not only treat individuals for depression but "support tribal communities in overcoming the history of tragedy and loss" that contributes to the individual's depression. They emphasize that "this can successfully be done only by promoting Indian cultural identity and strengthening the Indian way of life. . . . In fact, it appears that the more a person values traditional Indian culture, the less likely they are to become overwhelmed or to decide that they are doomed to meaningless tragedy. Since traditional values seem to offer some protection against an exaggerated sense of personal doom, it may be that a renewal of traditional orientation and building a positive cultural identity may be crucial components in the treatment of this problem."[62]

Guilmet and Whited observed a similar connection within their work at the Puyallup mental health clinic. Those patients with the most successful treatment outcomes tended to be those who were also engaged in the revival of their Coast Salish cultural and religious practices. They concluded that the "relationship between spiritual rebirth and mental health" could not be understated.[63] Tim Byers, the first physician to work with the new Indian Community Clinic on the Puyallup reservation, for instance, wrote in 1979 that "probably the most important positive health factor development has been a rebirth of pride and spiritualism." He noted in particular the example of when, in 1976, "the Tribe decided to reinstate the 'First Fish Ceremony' after 100 years of ignoring the once-important rite."[64]

Anecdotal evidence such as this linking individual well-being with cultural vitality is substantiated in a 2003 study by Michael Chandler, Christopher Lalonde, Bryan Sokol, and Darcy Hallet. Their study of teenage suicide among First Nations and non-native youth in British Columbia describes the "high personal costs of failing to sustain a workable sense of personal persistence," and they argue that "efforts by Aboriginal groups to preserve and promote their culture are associated with dramatic reductions in rates of youth suicide."[65] This has to do, they explain, with the importance of seeing oneself as part of a continuum. "Without some means of counting oneself as continuous in time, there simply would be no reason to show appropriate care and concern for one's own future well-being."[66] Chandler and his colleagues argue that First Nations youth commit suicide at such high rates partly because of their struggle to negotiate a sense of personal, collective, and cultural continuity. A sense of personal continuity, they explain, helps an individual to weather times when life may not seem worth living, encouraging concern and care for one's personal future, in light of a common past and a shared future. Such concern is indicated by efforts to promote and preserve cultural traditions and to manage tribal resources "in ways that conserve cultural identity in the face of acculturative forces." If this is true, they assert, "community level efforts to promote cultural continuity ought to be reflected in the ability of young people to weather the storms of their own identity formation processes."[67]

Indeed, their study found a direct correlation between cultural strength and suicide rates. When "aboriginal communities have succeeded, against mounting odds, in rehabilitating their badly savaged cultures," they "not only apparently salvage their past and harness their future but, along the way, also manage to successfully insulate their youth from the risk of suicide."[68] After an extensive study, they were able to conclude that "in every case," rates of teen suicide were lower or nonexistent in tribal communities that had demonstrated strong cultural continuity through things such as self-governance and locally controlled education, healthcare, and language programs than in those communities that did not.[69]

Many of the women involved in SPIPA's Women's Wellness Program, staff and community members alike, share a sense that returning to traditional spirituality and culture is key to promoting health and wellness and that it will provide women with a strong sense of identity, purpose, and strength. In 2004, during a planning session for the Women and Girls' Gathering, one Nisqually woman explained, "What I'd like to see in this year's gathering is more of an emphasis on spirituality and ceremony . . . because wellness is about having healthy communities, not just individuals. And to get healthy communities, you need spirituality and ceremony. I'd like to see an emphasis on bringing this back in."[70] Megan MacDonald, an undergraduate intern with the Women's Wellness Program, noted in her field notes, "The women of SPIPA have a deep understanding of this relationship [between spirituality and wellness], and are excited to have an underlying spiritual theme at the Gathering."[71] Following the 2004 Gathering one woman noted that the event had helped her remember "there is more than one dimension to things—(there is) a way to be connected to our traditions."[72] A glance through publications issued by the five tribes reveals a similar emphasis on the importance of cultivating traditional wisdom, skills, arts, and language, as a means of restoring and renewing relationships with one's ancestors and with the indigenous landscape. And these relationships, it is argued, are essential for individual and communal health.

The importance of reconnecting with tradition and its potential for restoring a strong sense of personal identity is reflected in an article in the Squaxin Island tribe's monthly newsletter regarding language preservation. Each month the newsletter publishes an article devoted to the tribal language program, offering new words and pronunciations because, as the article makes clear, "through language, people access values, heritage, and culture. . . . By accessing traditional values through language, we perceive our heritage and who we are as an indigenous people. . . . Through articulation of our values, we realize a relationship with our ancestors."[73] Another article followed, describing the community's involvement in archaeological projects, projects designed to strengthen the Squaxin Nation's connection to their ancestral past. As Rhonda Foster, Squaxin Island cultural resources management director, explained: "The artifacts . . . are a physical link between our ancestors, tribal members living now, and our children's children."[74] Maintaining a connection with one's ancestral community has implications for the continued well-being of these nations and their future generations, helping individuals to gain a clear sense of who they are and where their origins lie.[75]

Overall, it is this sense of a return to tradition (however defined), but more specifically a restored sense of identity as "Native women," and Coast Salish or Chinook women in particular, that is seen as holding the key to health and wellness within these communities. Throughout the comments of various women attending a talking circle at one Women and Girls' Gathering, wellness and healing were described as inherently linked with a strong connection to one's traditional identity and culture. For instance, one woman expressed hope for her son, who had gone through troubled times but was now living with his uncle on a central Washington reservation and learning their traditional ways. Another woman spoke tearfully about the importance of reconnecting to her Native heritage and identity and the impact this has had in her work as a healthcare provider for Native communities. A third woman reflected upon how she dealt with the death of her son by returning to traditional spirituality, by transforming grief into a passion for her culture, and by building a sweat lodge that she was able to make available to her community. In other conversations women repeatedly responded that a return to traditional culture and spirituality had enabled them to become sources of personal strength and community healing.

Healing the Self in Community

Tribal mental health care workers argue that healing has to do with restoring relationships and, in particular, with resituating the individual within the collective. Healthcare workers with the Coast Salish Swinomish tribe have explained that while mainstream mental health programs may focus on cultivating "individual autonomy, moving away from home or forming an independent nuclear family," an overemphasis on these goals "may be unrealistic, undesirable and unhealthy for many Indian people," for whom health may be about having "a deep commitment of service to one's people," the ability "to accept responsibility and leadership," and "to give and take."[76]

The goal is not simply to heal the individual, but instead, healthcare providers working with Coast Salish and Chinook communities need to recognize that "the true 'client' is the tribal community, not only the individual. . . . Services should be aimed at helping individuals to live in, rather than be removed from their communities."[77] While traditional approaches to healing vary from family to family, practitioner to practitioner, and tribe to tribe, they share in common a goal of "correcting imbalances between the person and the social and spiritual world."[78] As they explain, "The idea of balance or of being in right relation to the world, and especially to one's family, kin, and significant others, is of central importance" in Coast Salish culture. "To be 'well' means keeping the right balance in all things. . . . Illness may be caused by a mistake or misdeed on the part of the ill person, their family or some other person. Conflict with others, wrong or disrespectful actions or unintentional mistakes may all cause dangerous imbalances and lead to illness or other misfortune. . . . Bad feelings, social conflict and unresolved tensions can make a person ill. . . . Negative thoughts or emotions can have dangerous energy of their own."[79]

Causes of illness are thus often traced back to breaks in social relations. Jay Miller's study of Lushootseed illness and healing made a similar case, arguing that "bad relations ("breaches") with the cosmos, the community, the family, and the self were manifest in particular diseases."[80] Given that healing in this context has everything to do with restoring an individual to that person's place within kin and community, it should not be surprising when mental health workers argue that "the importance of the Indian person's extended family cannot be over-estimated. An Indian person is carefully trained in family relationships and traditions, and his/her social place is largely determined by family connections. Fulfillment of family obligations and a comfortable adaption to family interactions is crucial for Indian mental health."[81]

The Intertribal Women and Girls' Gathering also reflects this strong emphasis on healthy relationships and the interconnectedness of healthy selves and healthy communities. Indeed, speakers during the annual gatherings emphasize restoring relationships within the community as a key means of solving the problems that plague tribal well-being. Alcoholism and domestic violence, it is argued, can best be fought through strong community cohesion and support. Throughout various conversations and workshop sessions, it is repeatedly emphasized that community well-being is dependent upon individual well-being, and vice versa. Communities need their women to be healthy, as elders, as mothers, as responsible daughters. Individual imbalance, expressed through alcoholism, violence, or illness, causes the entire community to suffer.

During the 2001 Gathering one woman, a Yakama elder visiting the gathering, mused on this idea. She recalled that when she was a child, "there was this man called the Whipper. He would go around and knock on your door, and ask if any kids had been bad. He didn't just whip the bad one, though. If any of us had been bad, we all got in trouble." Other women hearing this story laughed and nodded their heads in agreement. It had been the same in their homes. If one child was naughty, they were all spanked. This idea of collective responsibility and collective well-being is present throughout the annual gatherings and is a philosophical given in much of SPIPA's work. Health and wellness are never an individual affair. Wellness depends upon individuals-in-community, all fulfilling their working identity.

The meals at the gathering reflect the importance of strong communities and interpersonal relationships as well. During the 2001 Gathering, for instance, meals were served "Shaker-style," following the traditions of the Indian Shaker Church. Before and after meals prayers were said, bells rung, and the meal officially "opened" and "closed." At these times Shaker leaders spoke, sharing their own life stories, how they had come to the Church, and how it had enabled them to live healthy, sober, drug-free lives. Once the food had been blessed through songs, prayers, and bells, we were told that the food was now considered "blessed food," food that was empowered with divine energy, providing the strength to live and work, to be well and do the right things in life. The Shaker woman who was serving the meal explained why food was served in common bowls rather than individual servings: the mode of serving was intentional, to convey a sense in which each person shares food from a common source, drawing life and strength from that common source. We were also encouraged to speak during the meal, but to do so in a Shaker way. Each table had a leader, an elder. We were told to look to this elder and once, acknowledged, to feel free to stand and speak from the heart. Several women did this throughout the course of the weekend, each time speaking as they felt inspired to do by the Spirit, from the heart. The meals themselves, in the way they were served and how the food was blessed, thus further invoked this sense of community and interconnectedness with one another.

Likewise, the giveaway ceremony that dominates the final day of the gathering is another reminder of the importance of community and reciprocity within traditional Puget Sound cultures and ethics. Each woman brings items to give away, many of them handmade. Beginning with elders, individuals are honored, and then (in descending order of age) everyone is welcomed to select a gift and surplus food to take home. By the end of the day, everyone goes home loaded down with goodies. As one participant later wrote about the giveaway, "the idea was to redistribute the goods amongst our friends and family, which is a very traditional concept many times lost in the throes of consumerism and capitalism. This redistribution of goods echoes the values of reciprocity and balance so ideal to traditional Native culture."[82] As a contemporary reenvisioning of traditional potlatches, the giveaway is a way to honor elders, to thank those who have done something on one's behalf, a way to reestablish relationships and cement intertribal friendships and commitments of mutual support. This practice is seen as being intrinsic to the overall goals of the weekend, insofar as it stands as a clear reminder of tradition, reciprocity, and community.

This sense of wellness as a community affair was also immediately evident in a talking circle on health and spirituality held during a recent gathering. While the original topic of the circle had been "Coping with Cancer," the conversation quickly shifted away from a focus upon cancer prevention and survival to a more general (and perhaps more revealing) discussion of wellness. In contrast to what one might expect in a similar Euroamerican setting, the conversation almost immediately moved from individual life stories and illness narratives and focused instead upon women's concerns for the health of their children and communities. Several women reflected upon the death of children or siblings, and their fears regarding the threats of drugs and suicide that so many young people faced. As one woman talked about the death of her daughter, there was an immediate sense of shared grief and support. As she spoke, she explained that the challenge was not simply her own grief but also the impact of this loss on her other children. What struck me at the time was how quickly an invitation to talk about one's own health and wellness (something many people are eager to do) immediately evoked discussion of the well-being of others and the network of relationships that tied people together.

Knowing Who You Are Meant to Be: Finding an Identity-within-Community

If healthy communities depend on healthy individuals, the implication is that a healthy self-in-community must know who she is, what her responsibilities and obligations are to those around her, and she must be whole in order to fulfill that calling. Coast Salish cultures and communities place a high premium on individual autonomy, granting status and respect to individuals who have found their calling and honor their personal gifts and responsibilities to others. Because this keen individualism is expressed within an intensively kin-based communal culture, individuals come to understand their role, their purpose, and their significance (their *working identity*) through understanding and honoring their relationships to kin and community. SPIPA's Women's Wellness program emphasizes both these concerns. Personal wellness is conceptualized as a necessary means for creating strong communities. A sense of interdependency with and responsibility toward one's kin and community is a dominant theme at the annual Women and Girls' Gatherings.

To that end, cultivating one's identity-within-community was an important element for 2001 keynote speaker Cecilia Firethunder (Lakota). As she spoke about wellness and domestic violence, Firethunder explained that "the Creator has put a blueprint inside each of us, a blueprint of who we're meant to be, what we're meant to do. But we have to actualize the blueprint that the Creator put in us. Become what we're meant to be. That's what wellness is."[83] Realizing that identity and fulfilling the role one is meant to have in one's community are difficult, she said, particularly in communities riddled with alcoholism and domestic and sexual violence and where individuals carry the scars from such experiences. Firethunder's comments are important, underscoring key ideas expressed throughout various gatherings. Such remarks emphasize the intricate tie between individual wellness and community wellness. They also reflect a sense that each person within community has a vital role to play—and that one's own healing enables one to step into that role for others.

Offering events that nurture a sense of personal spirituality through reawakening a commitment to Native traditions is central to the gathering. While biomedical care is available in the form of free breast exams and mammograms, traditional sweats are also held in a sweat lodge at dawn and sunset, and talking circles, storytelling, drumming, and a variety of crafts all provide opportunities for elder women to teach aspects of Native culture to younger women—basketry, beading, and making baby moccasins, masks, and felt shawls. These opportunities to become reacquainted with traditional culture are described by women not simply as educational but as valuable opportunities to become reacquainted with the things that convey a sense of personal identity and affirm Native women's roles and obligations within their culture and community. Within this setting, the cultivation of relationships, identities, and obligations toward their communities are vital for a sense of health and well-being.

Indeed, a key theme found throughout women's comments is that the gatherings and events inspire them to come to a better understanding of their personal worth and their value as unique individuals. One woman left the gathering with a new commitment to "meditate, contemplate, and apply the recognition of my body as a creation of unique design." Another said she had been inspired "to regard my body as a unique gift." Another woman said that the four-day gathering had inspired her to consider mentoring young girls, and as one woman put it, she had been reminded of "the importance of teaching my daughters that women are so important, and that womanhood should be celebrated."

Programming and publications work to send a strong message about the importance of taking care of one's own health and wellness. For instance, articles in SPIPA and other tribal publications have described tribal women who devoted themselves so wholeheartedly to promoting wellness in their communities that they neglected their own health, succumbing to cancer. The narratives are important within a context where responsibilities toward others are keenly felt. Obligations to others, the women are reminded, also mean an obligation to one's own health. A speaker at the 2002 Gathering reflected this focus as well when she discussed the role that spirituality has played in her recovery from alcoholism and domestic violence. The essential aspect, she explained, was learning to have pride in herself and her Indian heritage, learning "that the Great Spirit loves me, and so I can love myself." For this woman, health and wellness are not just about healing relationships with her family and community (though that plays a vital role as well), but also in developing a relationship with the "Great Spirit" and, ultimately, with herself.

At the same time it is argued that cultivating one's health is not a self-centered activity but part of fulfilling one's responsibilities to others. In order to fulfill one's obligations within a community, one's body and spirit need to be well. An image on the back of a newsletter circulated at the gathering illustrates this well: a grandmother from one of the five tribes is seated in the middle of her laughing granddaughters. The caption of the photo reads: "Don't have time for a mammogram? If not for yourself, then who? Remember: early detection saves lives."[84] The implications are important: women are responsible for others, and hence are responsible to ensure their own health, so that they are able to fulfill those obligations to community. This dual message of one's own intrinsic value and one's responsibility to care for others has had a strong impact on some women.[85] Various women's reactions at the conclusion of the 2003 and 2004 gatherings supported this notion. After the 2004 gathering, one woman commented that the weekend "taught me to take better care of my body and the world." Another wrote that the gathering "made me aware of how important it is to be a strong politically active Native woman."[86] As one woman wrote after listening to other elders speak about their struggles and community commitments, "I am now determined to be a strong elder." Emphasis upon women's roles as the preservers of culture and protectors of community inspired other women to say that they wanted "to help my sisters, mother, grandmother, and nieces engage in preventative breast care," and that they wanted to "reach out to women in my life and insist on prevention and early screening." Another woman replied that she wanted to "take care of myself, not just for me, but also for my family." While such perspectives might seem to burden women with the expectations of being perpetual caregivers, they are reflective of Coast Salish and Chinook understandings of the healthy self: a strong sense of personal identity and individuality, expressed through reciprocal obligations to kin and community.

Of course, the other implication here is that women depend upon the community for support and encouragement. Women's comments from various gatherings and SPIPA literature imply that for individuals to heal, they need healthy communities that offer their love and support—and part of what makes the annual gathering so important for them is the opportunity to be within a community of Native women with common cultural and social backgrounds, women who understand and support one another. As one woman in recovery from breast cancer said: "Part of the medicine is having people say to you, 'You look good.' Or, 'It's so good to see you.' Or 'You are welcome here.'"[87] Another woman new to the area described the difficulties she experienced without the strong support of the community she had left behind on her home reservation, and her gratitude for the support and kindness she found at this gathering. One woman in a talking circle spoke strongly of the need for women to join together and support mothers as they care for their children and deal with loss. Others said that they deeply needed opportunities to share, with vulnerability and openness, in a supportive context such as this. Others agreed, saying that they were often praised for their strength and resilience in the midst of crisis, but that they needed this safe space to express pain and concerns. This woman-only space where it was safe to share grief was unique in their experience, they said, and necessary.[88]

This sense of solidarity with other Native women repeatedly emerged as an important theme within each annual gathering. Women pointed to this power of community and sisterhood in facilitating health and wellness.[89] In postevent evaluations, women wrote that they appreciated "getting to know women from other tribes," "female bonding," the expressions of "love and caring," and the "connection of women," as powerful contributors to a sense of spiritual, physical, and mental wellness and said that this time had helped them discover "the power of being a woman," as well as "the similarities between women from different tribes." By connecting with other Native "women of power," one participant said she felt she had been able to "regain a sense of my power, and strength" as a Native woman and thereby to experience a sense of "collective empowerment." Others were inspired by the wealth of wisdom, skills, and knowledge that emerged when "we all come together and teach each other what we know."[90]

Healing the Relationship with Place

Native women involved in SPIPA and the Women's Gathering do not limit these vital relationships to human relationships. Rather, they also emphasize the necessity for cultivating relationships with their ancestral landscape. Various activities, speakers, and publications suggest that Native women can regain a clearer sense of personal identity and cultural continuity by cultivating and renewing these relationships with place. They are able to rediscover the "blueprint" of who they are meant to be. Many of these activities center upon connecting women with their indigenous land base, its plants, and its resources. For instance, at the 2002 Gathering one group of women met to make traditional herbal teas. As they were taught about the plants' medicinal properties, women combined the herbs and put the teas into bags that were then distributed at the giveaway ceremony on the final day.

At the 2001 Gathering the importance of knowledge about the natural world was strikingly illustrated in the presentation of a local elder and herbalist who spoke to women about traditional medicinal plants. The discussion took place in a spacious room, lined with large windows looking out on Panhandle Lake, where children were swimming and playing in paddleboats. In the same room, behind us, older women were teaching younger girls and women how to make baskets and do beadwork. And next to us, a woman sat at a table providing information on breast self-exams. The presentation was so striking that I present a great deal of it here. The speaker explained:

> [Traditionally] we were so connected with Mother Earth, Nature, that when women had babies . . . the fathers were responsible for burying the afterbirth, with prayers to Mother Earth. It's so simple, this is how you want your life to go, your future to be better, if you could just follow it. It's so simple. A lot of our young people are getting away from it, from our culture, our traditions. But these things that bring you a good life, these traditions are so simple. If you really want to know about medicine, you have to look at yourself. What do you want? It's about spirituality. As you walk on Mother Earth, do so with a prayer. Medicines come in dreams, with prayers; they are very sacred . . . Begin to relax, and you'll find out that answers will come to you. You'll feel good, get into the spirit of nature, and nature will tell you, she'll tell you through the wind in the trees, through a feeling in your heart.

She went on to comment on the importance of a patient's spouse or children or parents gathering herbal medicines on their behalf.

> The strongest prayer a person can get is from their spouse or their children. It's good to have your spouse or children gather for you, because

> plants need to be gathered with prayers. The key to these medicinal plants is prayer, listening with love in your heart. . . . Spirituality is the most important thing. All of these plants have a spirit. That's the medicine. Prayer. Listening. Take a look at nature. Enjoy its spirit and your connection with it. . . . We need to be still. Learn to be still. To listen. Medicines and herbs will teach us what to use, and how to use it. Listen and learn what to use to take care of our own little families. . . . You don't need to learn all the medicines at once, you don't learn ten all at once: just get to know one. Be still, listen, let that one plant *choose you*, and *let you* get to know it. Other medicines will come because they'll like your spirit, they'll come to you because you're willing, because you're wanting to learn. But just start with one. Medicines are revealed from prayer. . . . Medicines are prayed for, and they reveal themselves to a person's spirit. It's their *spirit* that makes them effective. It's the relationship with the plant that makes them work. God created everything to be medicine. We just have to pray for it to come into our lives. I thought that was just an old bush, a shrub, that that plant over there was just a weed. But no, I learned, God put spirit in everything, and it's the spirit that heals.[91]

This woman's words point to the sentient nature of plants and the herbalist's work as being essentially a process of relationship building. Words such as this reflect a view of "traditional wellness" that involves developing a spiritual awareness of and interaction with plants and the natural environment. This spiritual nature of plants also makes human relationships all the more powerful: the intensity of human relationships affects the power of prayers, and the prayers directly impact the efficacy of the plant. Within this view, "God," the deity recognized by Indian Shaker Church members, Christians, and many traditional Native people, has endowed *everything* with "spirit." And it is not just the chemical properties of plants that heal, but this unifying spirit, the sentient awareness that is shared by plants, animals, ancestors. The use of traditional herbs requires a relationship with the plant in question. Such a perspective helps to shed light on the notion within Coast Salish and Chinook communities that *health* is often a *relational condition.* It can be the end result of one's ability and commitment to cultivating and honoring spiritual and human relationships.

One woman with whom I later spoke reflected on this aspect of the weekend with excitement. Her words illustrate the powerful way such a perspective of the sentient and relational nature of plants can impact individual Native women's sense of self and identity. As a Native woman who did not grow up as part of her community or knowing her heritage, she explained that she had often felt left out of such cultural activities. "I feel kind of hollow when I'm around other Indian women, women who know who they are and where they came from. But I appreciate the openness here, the welcome," she said. She went on to express her appreciation in particular for the sessions discussing herbalism, prayer, and recovery.

> Because these sessions, what people are talking about, let me know that I can reach a sense of my Indian identity through spirit, through prayer. What she was saying about Devil's Club really got me, because I was just out hiking with my friend, and I saw that plant, I really saw it for the first time, and I said, "Wow! What is that!?" And my friend said, look, it's all over the place, you've seen that plant a million times before. But it was like I saw it for the first time, like it *wanted* me to see it. I was just so excited about it, it was so beautiful, so amazing, those full leaves, and the spines, so intricate. And then she [the session leader] started talking about that plant, and I realized it was the same one. I really felt like there was an important connection there, you know?

For this young woman, the idea that plants might know her, remember her and her ancestry, even if she cannot, opens the door to a personal healing, cultural healing, and the rediscovery of a sense of her indigenous identity. Sessions such as these provide valuable spaces for meaning making, for reflection, and reaffirming one's own sense of identity and purpose.

A similar sensibility can be found in the Native Women's Wellness newsletter, where Squaxin Island tribal member Charlene Krise reflected on her own family's traditions of gathering plant resources.

As in the preceding example, Krise views plants as a tactile way of maintaining a spiritual and relational connection with her family and heritage. For her, she says, the smells of plants are an immediate and visceral connection to her ancestors. When gathering plants she reconnects with their presence.

> Memories of my grandmother, Annie Jackson Krise, and grand-aunt Elvina are easily awakened by the sight, smell, touch and taste of traditional plants. I remember as a child being taught about the importance of traditional plants, which ones were used for medicinal purposes, and which ones were used for food. The traditional way of gathering as a group has continued through the generations of my grandparents, parents, aunts, uncles, cousins, siblings, and myself. . . . I remember my uncle and the strong smell of yarrow. . . . My dad gathered wild roses. . . . I still gather food and medicines from the forest. Gathering reminds me of my loved ones who have passed. Every time I pick a berry, I remember my ancestors. Every time I smell yarrow, I remember my grandmother. Every time I drink Indian tea, I remember my uncle. The activity of gathering keeps these memories alive.[92]

For Krise, her relationship with plants and the embodied process of gathering is a relational activity. Through it she maintains an interactive and reciprocal exchange with her ancestors and the plants and landscape that have supported her family for thousands of years. These relationships serve as a mode of cultivating health and wellness and a strong sense of identity and memory.

Just as the sentient awareness of plants is acknowledged and discussed, so too is the awareness of salmon and other traditional food resources. In 2001, when salmon were brought into the dining room, Yakama women visiting the gathering were asked to sing a welcoming song. As they stood and sang the salmon to the table, the salmon were thanked for their gift, and the women as a whole were reminded of our dependency on the salmon for survival, of our need for them to return next year. Just as annual First Salmon rites in Native nations throughout the Pacific Northwest continue to remind indigenous communities of their dependence upon and interconnection with the health of salmon populations, these prayers of welcoming created a context of dialogue, relationship, and exchange with the salmon people.[93] Such activities emphasize the central role that cultivating spiritual relationships with the natural world plays in the development and healing of Native women's sense of self.

"Healing Is Moving On": Some Conclusions

In 2001 the Women and Girls' Gathering concluded with a talent show, a space for children and adults (though mostly young people) to showcase their talents. The first act was a traditional story, narrated by a young woman and performed by a group of younger children, most of whom were dressed in pow-wow regalia or woven cedar hats and button blankets. The story was about Mount Rainier, who had decided to leave her unfaithful husband, Mount Adams, because he had been having an affair with her sister, Mount St. Helens. She departed, taking along her newborn baby and her dowry—which consisted of sockeye salmon, medicinal plants, and a variety of berries. As she traveled, however, she dropped portions of her dowry, leaving them behind as she went. She dropped the salmon, the plants, the berries. And, it was explained, this is why the sockeye swim in the rivers between Mount Adams and Mount Rainier, and why berries and medicinal plants grow so abundantly in the area. When Mount Adams realized his first wife had left, he erupted in fury at her departure. At the sound, Mount Rainier turned to look back, removing her hairpins and dropping them. Where they fell, the hairpins formed the Cascades, the mountain range separating Rainier from Adams and St. Helens. At the conclusion of the story, the young woman narrating the story spoke to the gathered audience: the story, she explained, is about the importance of letting go of sorrow, of hurt, of pain.

> We can be injured by things that happen to us in life. . . . In this story, it is injury caused by men. But this story explains that when we let go of pain, that that grief brings life. We don't just leave it behind, but the grief and pain and loss give birth to new life, to good things. Her pain

> is why we have the sockeye, and the berries, and medicine. The story is about healing, and why it's important. We seek it in different ways, in church, in the longhouse, the smokehouse, the Shaker Church, the sweat lodge, but we need to let go of those hurts, in order for them to turn into something new, to grow into healthy things, that will bring life to other people. Healing is moving on, and it benefits others, the whole community, when you do it.[94]

Following several days of discussions about domestic violence, rape, sexual abuse, alcoholism, and the struggle to value and take care of one's health, the story struck a powerful chord. This performance is meaningful for several reasons. First, it suggests that Native women can find wisdom and healing within their culture and its oral traditions. It also speaks to the ability of women to restore a sense of self, and to grow through the traumas and crises that they experience, and it conveys the possibility of not just surviving but *thriving*. Finally, it suggests that individual healing can and should ultimately benefit the community as a whole. Growing through and overcoming one's illness, physiologically and spiritually, enables each woman to return to her community with gifts, abilities, and greater strengths. When one woman moves beyond her pain, it is suggested, the trauma becomes a gift that will make her community and nation a stronger one.

And indeed, as various speakers throughout the years have attested, those able to offer words of wisdom and healing are those who have suffered themselves. At these gatherings, women come forward to share stories of their struggles with cancer, their experiences with HIV, with diabetes, with sexual assault or domestic violence. Brave women share brave stories, honoring what they feel to be a call to serve their communities. This stands in close accord with Coast Salish and Chinook traditions where healers are those who first suffered a great illness, a near-death experience, and recovered to tell the story. This long-standing narrative of illness and revival, of personal renewal, is expressed within workshops and talking circles led by women who have managed to find the strength to survive illness, abuse, and trauma. It reflects a key goal of the event: that women will leave the gathering and return to their communities "with new skills, renewed with spirit and in strength."[95] Such stories attest to an understanding of healthy working identities as inherently relational, interconnected with community, landscape, and ancestors. Healthy individuals have particular strengths and spiritual gifts, which they are meant to bring back to their communities.

In addition to this view of the embodied self, the gatherings also attest to the ways in which tradition is brought to bear upon community needs. Tradition takes shape within a worldview that is potentially hybrid, flexible, and creatively adaptive. Coast Salish and Chinook identities are affirmed, along with an affirmation of a broader sense of pan-Indian identity as the women and girls meet Native women from other corners of North America. At the same time, they are able to embrace other cultural practices, such as biomedicine, tai chi, acupuncture, and reflexology.

As another example of this, one might also consider the talent show the following year, when two sisters, of Irish and Alaskan Native descent, shared a performance of traditional Irish step-dancing: a beautiful blend of cultures coming together with ease. Or consider a moment in the summer of 2006, when I sat listening to group of teenage girls giving an articulate and entertaining presentation about the dangers of smoking. As the presentation continued, I noticed that only twenty yards away another group of young women had gathered to practice traditional drumming and learn a medicine song. Both events blended harmoniously in the warm August afternoon.

I mention these performances because they offer such powerful illustrations of the dynamic nature of cultural hybridity, of the ways in which multiple cultural modes of expression can exist side by side. Just as the coming together of mammograms, tai chi , sweat lodges, talking circles and giveaways demonstrates the flexibility of contemporary Native identity, so too do examples such as these. They reflect the ways in which Coast Salish and Chinook women in South Puget Sound are negotiating life in the twenty-first century while also maintaining foundational worldviews consistent with those of their ancestors. Here is traditional healing: women gathering together to preserve their cultures and to help each other achieve a sense of safety, wellness, and cultural identity.

Hence the work of the Women's Wellness Program reflects the creativity and cultural hybridity that is found within the religious history of the region. In all these instances Native communities drew upon Coast Salish, Chinook, and broader "pan-Indian" healing traditions, adapting new religious, technological, and organizational structures to meet new demands. By creating new modes through which to achieve this healing, whether through the Indian Shaker Church, a sweat lodge, tai chi, massage, mammograms, or medicine bundles, these Native communities have been able to craft responses that promote the healing of their communities and the survival of Coast Salish and Chinook cultural traditions. While outward manifestations have certainly changed, many of the foundational understandings of what it means to be healthy have remained largely the same. Health and wellness are expressed within an embodied subject that exists within a complex network of reciprocal relationships between human communities, spiritual communities, and the indigenous land base. The *diseases* under consideration may have changed (from smallpox to alcoholism, for instance), but the *illnesses* remain very similar: soul loss, broken relationships, loss of identity, and loss of cultural continuity. These things give rise to the distinct physical manifestations that biomedicine seeks to cure, such as diabetes, cancer, depression, heart disease, alcoholism. But the means of addressing the root causes of these illnesses are still found within "traditional" approaches to wellness and spirituality, and collective gatherings such as this, where personal identity and collective relationships can be restored.

6. Coming Full Circle

Defining Health and Wellness on the Shoalwater Bay Indian Reservation

We are here to celebrate the visions of our elders, their dreams, and their tenacity.

—CHARLENE NELSON, tribal chairwoman, Shoalwater Bay Wellness Center dedication, 2005

Today, we are bringing things full circle.

—TROY JOHNSON, drummer and singer, Shoalwater Bay Wellness Center dedication, 2005

On July 7, 1992, the Shoalwater Bay Tribal Council declared a health emergency, pointing to a staggeringly high prenatal and neonatal infant mortality rate, which the council feared "may exceed 90% in the last two years."[1] The Center for Disease Control (CDC) conducted an epidemiological study of the crisis in 1999 and estimated that from 1988 to 1992, 53 percent of pregnancies on the reservation ended in pregnancy loss or fetal death, and in 1998, 89 percent of pregnancies (eight out of nine on the reservation) ended in child loss.[2] The impact on the community was severe, to say the least. As was stated in a 1994 joint report, "Most families now are too fearful to have a pregnancy; some said they will move away from the reservation to have a pregnancy and raise children. (There has been only one new pregnancy in the past twenty months, when eight or nine would be expected). Grief for stillbirths and infant deaths may never fully resolve; severe grief may contribute to the fear of some Shoalwater Bay Indian Tribe families to start a pregnancy. One member felt that stress and grief were major causes of the adverse events; it is plausible that they played a role."[3]

This moment in history had profound effects upon the Shoalwater Bay tribal community, manifesting in profoundly personal and spiritual ways. As one woman explained: "What a lot of people don't understand is when a woman becomes pregnant, not only does her body change; she changes emotionally, physically, and spiritually. When you get pregnant, you feel this sense of success. When a woman who is pregnant suddenly loses this being that is inside her, she—or at least I—felt this sense of shame. Why couldn't I carry this baby? What is wrong with me? I felt I had let down my husband as well."[4] The grief associated with this period in the history of the Shoalwater community was profound, and it inspired heroic efforts toward cultivating health and wellness on the reservation.

I initially visited the Shoalwater Bay community in 2000 with the idea of exploring the ways in which this pregnancy loss crisis had been experienced and perceived by the community. However, shortly after I began volunteering at the tribal clinic, I was struck by the disinclination of community members to discuss the crisis itself. While most seemed quite interested in discussing health more generally, I quickly gained the impression that it would be inappropriate to ask people directly what their experience of the pregnancy loss crisis had been. I took to heart what one community member told me: "I think I speak for the whole community when I say that we are tired of talking about the losses. Let's talk about the healthy babies. We have a lot of babies here now—more than we've had in a long time." She suggested that energy should rather be spent creating a daycare center and programs for young children.[5] Other documents confirm this impression. When former tribal chairman Herbert "Ike" Whitish sent letters to the tribal community in 1999, informing them that the high rate of fetal deaths had not come to an end, but remained a serious problem, it drew no response from the community. According to former clinic director Gale Taylor, "people could not stand to confront the tragedy again."[6]

The report from the CDC also made mention of this, noting that an offer to present their findings to the community was rejected: the Shoalwater Bay Indian Tribal Council "stated the positive value of the approach, but given past and current community feelings, the council declined a presentation to the overall community."[7] As one tribal member said to the CDC, "The whole community was suffering from a broken heart. . . . I hate to get back to it again, because it just opens up such a big, huge, void. It was too overwhelming. I can't do it. That's what you guys are going to help us do—move on."[8] This historical context, while painful to recall, is also important to consider, for this period of loss drew the community together and inspired concerted efforts toward healing individuals and the community as a whole.

The 2005 dedication of the new Wellness Center, described in some detail in the introduction to this book, was in many ways the culmination of two decades of work by Shoalwater Bay tribal leaders. It is certainly a milestone in their efforts to promote health and wellness, and to do so in a way that embodies a distinctively Shoalwater sense of what it means to be healthy and whole. The Wellness Center is part of a broader effort on the reservation, and indeed, between 2001 and 2005 healthcare and community services for the Shoalwater tribal community improved at a dramatic rate. In December 2002 the community completed construction of a new gymnasium, with a basketball court, weight room, recreation equipment, showers, and kitchen. The community was also successful in completing a Learning Resources Center that houses "a library, the education administrative offices, a lab with 10 computers, and a large activity room." And the Wellness Center, replacing the first clinic (built in 1995), enabled the tribe to house all health services under one roof: "medical, dental, alternative medicine, mental health, and chemical dependency."[9] Services at the center approach wellness from a holistic perspective, incorporating biomedical care alongside mental health and social programs that are aimed at meeting the needs of the whole person. This includes preventative care such as acupuncture, massage therapy, and health-education classes. Woven throughout many of these modes of care is a concern for the spiritual health and wellness of the tribal community. These various achievements, and the stories behind them, stand as a testimony to what a small Native community with few material resources has been able to achieve. Further, it is evidence of the wisdom of granting tribes local control over healthcare and social services, demonstrating that tribal communities know best how to care for their own needs and how to do so in ways that respect their cultural heritage and spiritual traditions.

My main concern in this chapter is to explore how Shoalwater Bay tribal members define health and wellness, how that understanding can be seen in their extensive community-directed wellness programs, and what these definitions might tell us about the worldview and ethos of this community. As I argued in chapter 2, the ways in which illness and the body are perceived, and the language used to construct narratives about the body, provide a means of illuminating the culturally distinct understandings of the self found and produced within a community. Recognizing the ways in which health is understood in this Native community reveals an understanding of embodied subjectivity, of what it means to be a healthy self, that is particular to their cultural and religious traditions. For the Shoalwater Bay tribal community, health and survival mean something very different than they do for official entities like the CDC, the Environmental Protection Agency (EPA), or other federal and state health agencies.[10] As I seek to show, health and wellness for the Shoalwater community are communal concerns, issues that center on re-creating a clear sense of collective identity and community self-reliance. As the community's reactions to health crises demonstrate, for the people of Shoalwater, a healthy self is defined by healthy relationships within the community, with the natural environment, and with their ancestors.[11] I do not mean to suggest in this chapter that all Shoalwater Bay tribal members feel the same way about these issues and concerns. A great deal of diversity can be found within this small community. What is remarkable to me, however, is the way in which the Shoalwater Bay tribe has managed to come to a kind of consensus, locating a common ethos and worldview that has enabled them to accomplish what they have, putting these shared ideals into practice in programs and accomplishments like the Wellness Center.[12]

The way the community has reacted is important, particularly in order to explain how the Shoalwater community defines health and wellness and, from this, how community members conceive of a healthy individual. If CDC and EPA researchers are concerned with the disease at hand, I am here concerned with the illness: how the crisis has affected their lives, their families, their marriages, and their feelings about being pregnant and what these losses mean in terms of their sense of self, of community, and of tribal history as well as their relationship with the surrounding ecosystem. And I am concerned with how people have responded to that crisis by forming mechanisms and spaces for healing within their own community.[13] To understand community reactions to the crisis, and to begin to formulate a sense of the tribe's understanding of health and subjectivity, it is necessary to look at bodily narratives, the discourses of health, wellness, and sickness that various members of the community have articulated around this period of its history, and to locate those narratives within the tribe's history and experience.[14]

Background and Context

In 1994 a joint investigation by the Shoalwater Bay Indian Tribe, the Washington Department of Health, and the Portland Area Indian Health Service (IHS), sought to determine if environmental toxins or lack of access to medical care might be factors in the high rates of pregnancy loss on the reservation. In the "Joint Report" issued by these groups on October 27, 1994, it was reported that ectopic pregnancies in the community were ten times the expected rate, stillbirths were twenty-nine times the expected rate, and infant mortality was twenty-four times the expected rate.[15] Only 42 percent of pregnancies produced a healthy child, compared to 82 percent for the state of Washington as a whole.[16] The tribe's report in conjunction with the Department of Health and IHS called for an investigation into toxicity levels in nearby Grayland Creek (a drainage ditch used by local cranberry growers), air quality tests, and the testing of water and sediment in surrounding Willapa Bay. They found a variety of reasons for concern.

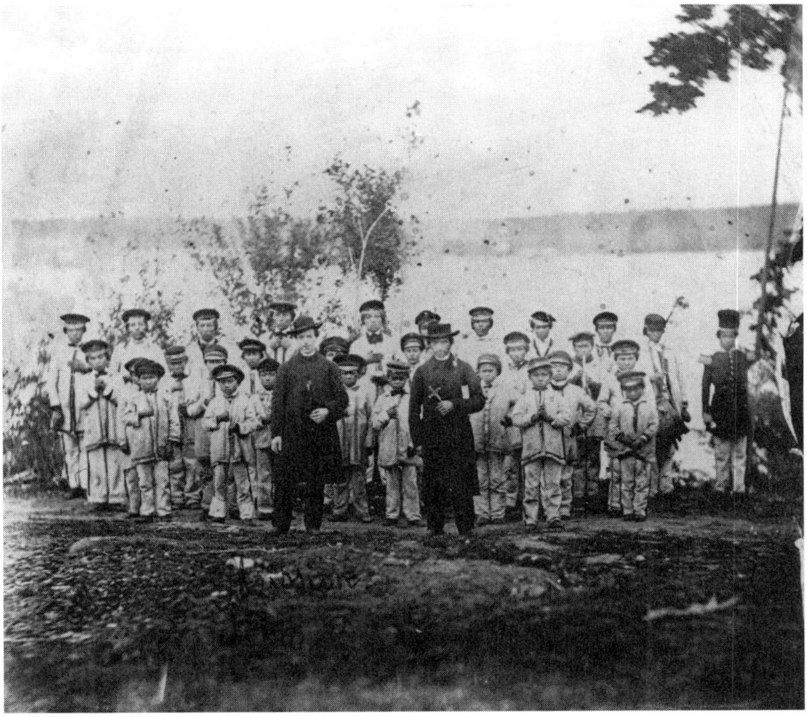

FIGURE 1. Tulalip students in school uniform pose with Father Casimir Chirouse, Tulalip Reservation, ca. 1865. As part of the mission school system, the Tulalip Indian School under Chirouse sought to convert Lushootseed Coast Salish children to Christianity and to instruct them in English and vocational skills. Unlike at many such schools, Chirouse retained the use of the local Native language, preaching sermons in Lushootseed and translating prayers and hymns into Lushootseed. This relatively tolerant approach to the local Native language and culture changed when the school became a federally controlled institution late in the nineteenth century. Reprinted courtesy of the University of Washington Libraries Special Collections, NA 1498.

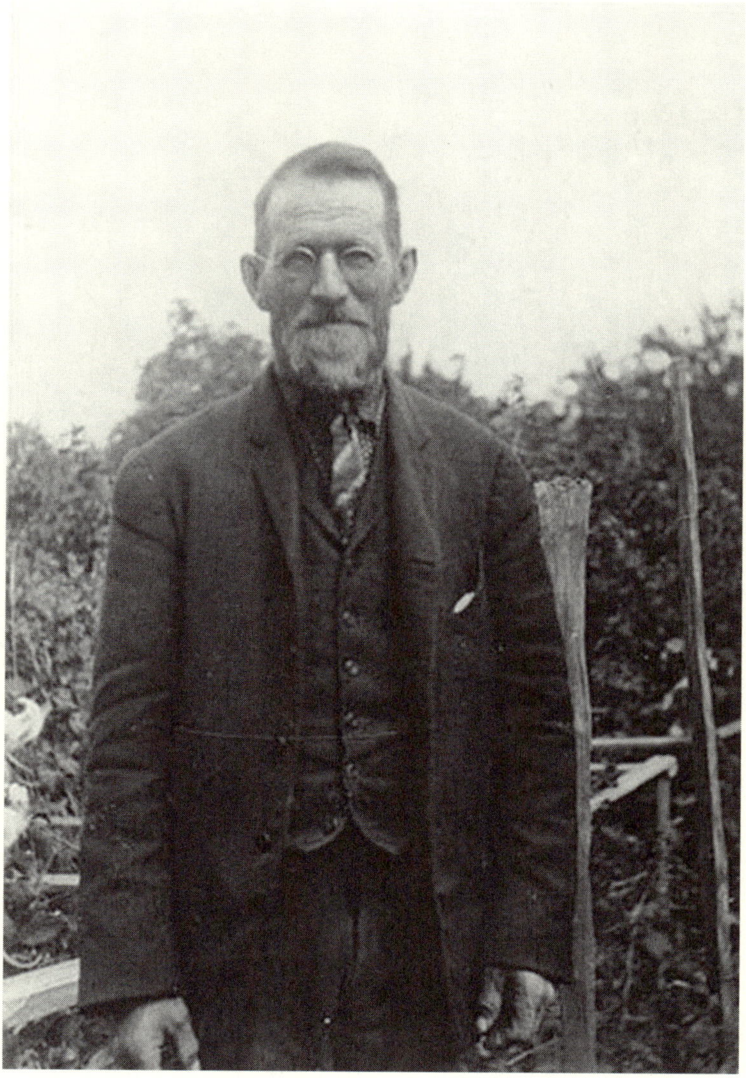

FIGURE 2. Congregationalist missionary Reverend Myron Eells, on the Skokomish reservation, Washington, 1905. Eells devoted himself to the missionization of Coast Salish people in the south Puget Sound. He sought to suppress indigenous religious and cultural traditions, at times imprisoning medicine men and ceremonial leaders, including the leadership of the Indian Shaker Church. Reprinted courtesy of the University of Washington Libraries Special Collections, NA 1170a.

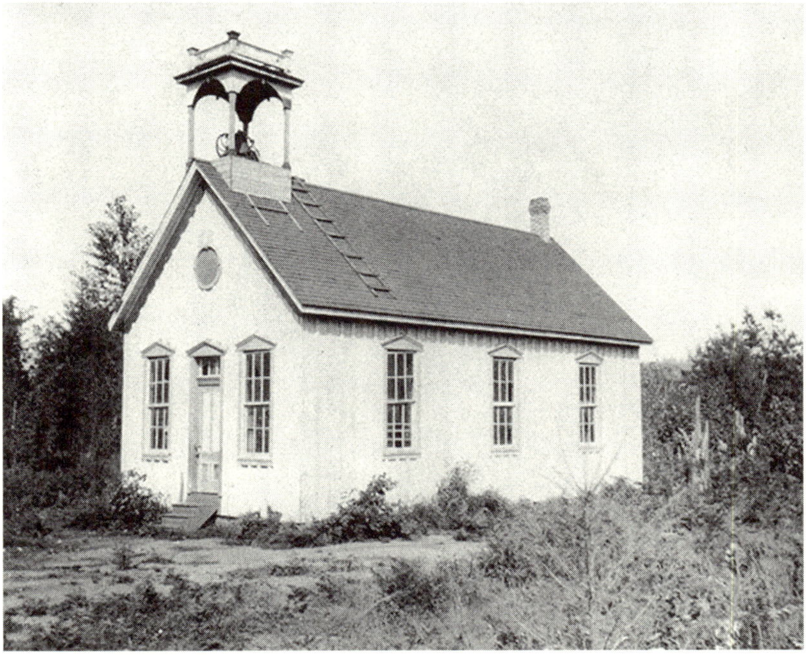

FIGURE 3. Skokomish mission day school and church, founded by Reverend Myron Eells, Skokomish reservation, ca. 1905. This was the site of Eells's weekly church services as well as the reservation's mission school. Reprinted courtesy of the University of Washington Libraries Special Collections, NA 1166a.

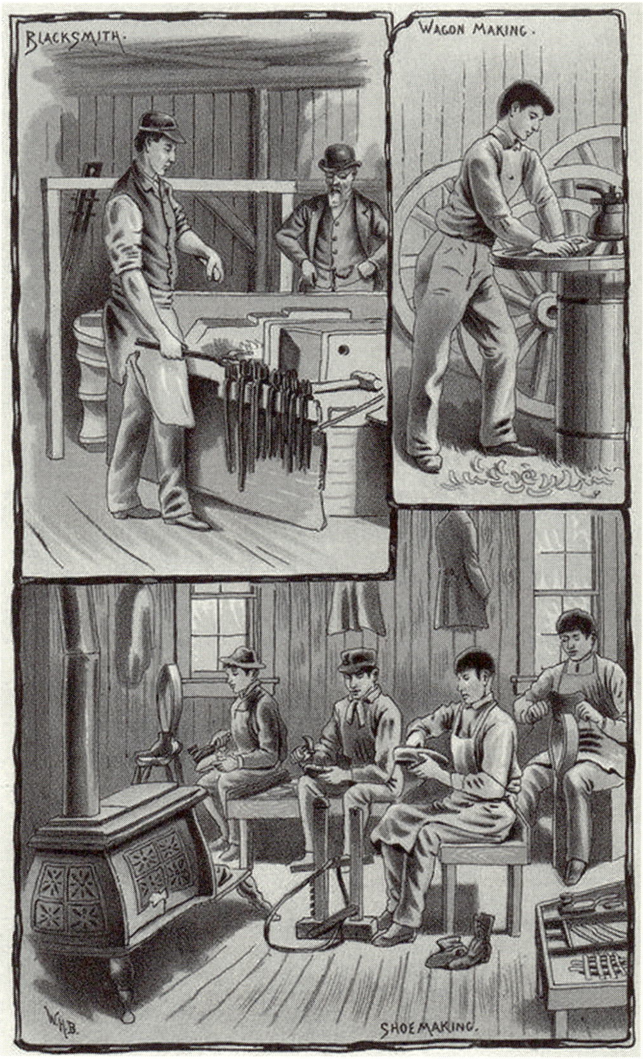

FIGURE 4. Engraving for Chemawa Indian Training School showing boys' vocational training activities, including shoemaking, blacksmithing, and wagon making. Schools such as Chemawa focused on training Native young people into vocational trades. Flyers such as this served as promotional materials, to encourage financial support of the institution. Reprinted courtesy of the University of Washington Libraries Special Collections, NA 4019.

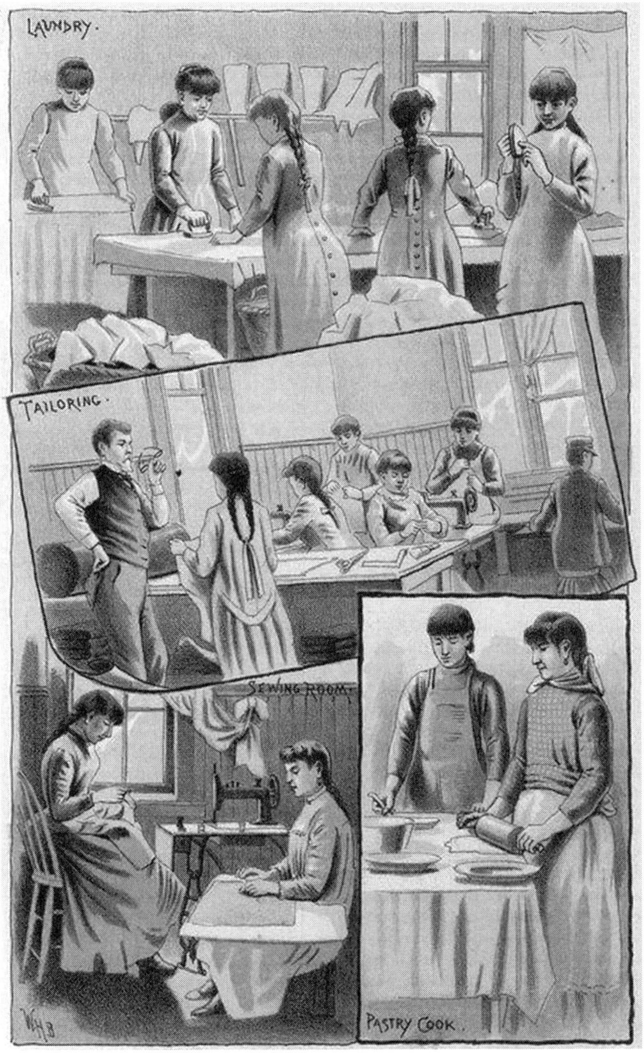

FIGURE 5. Engraving for Chemawa Indian Training School, showing girls' vocational training activities, including laundry, tailoring, sewing, and baking. Students at Chemawa were expected to sustain the institution through their own labor. "Vocational training" meant that students worked for half of the day, doing the farming, wood cutting, sewing, and cooking that kept the school going. Flyers such as this served as promotional materials, to encourage financial support of the institution. Reprinted courtesy of the University of Washington Libraries Special Collections, NA 4018.

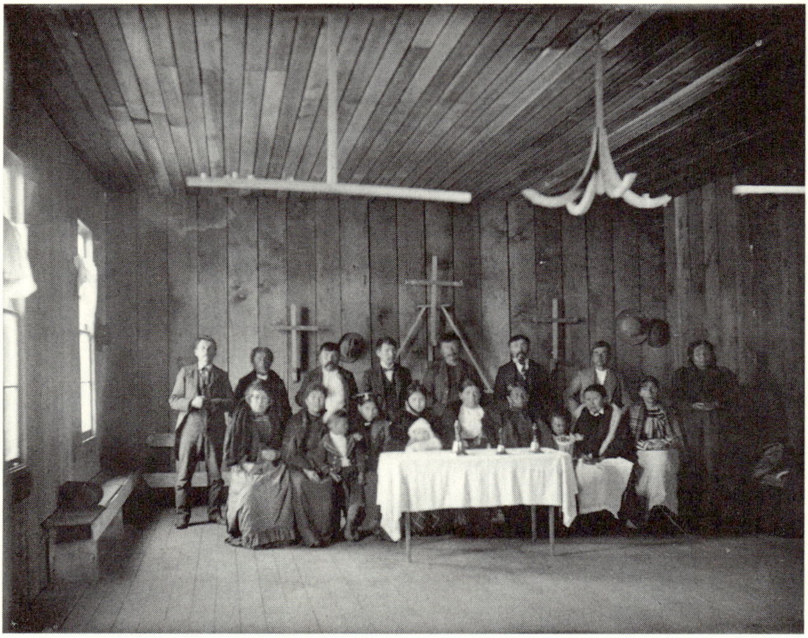

FIGURE 6. Klallam group portrait inside the Indian Shaker Church, Jamestown, Washington, ca. 1903. The Indian Shaker Church combined indigenous religious and healing traditions with Christianity. Note the use of the cross, the ritual number three, and church hand bells. Reprinted courtesy of the University of Washington Libraries Special Collections, NA 1121.

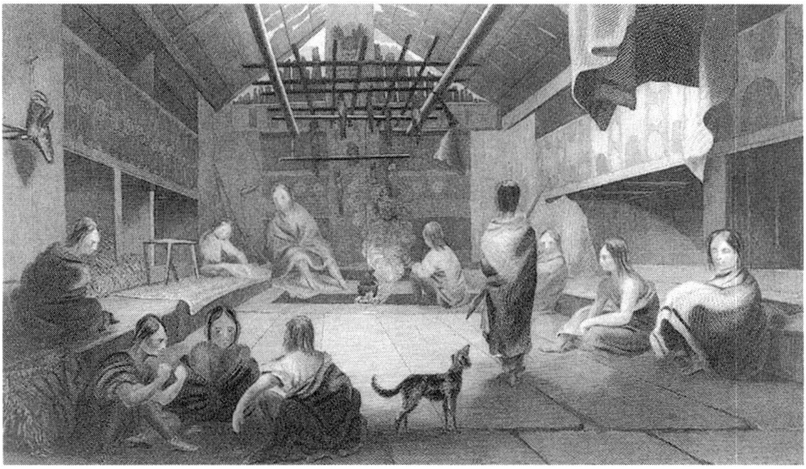

FIGURE 7. Engraving of Chinook group inside a cedar plank lodge, 1841, by A. T. Agate. The engraving gives a sense of what winter dwellings for Native people in this region may have been like. They were warm, dry, fully enclosed permanent structures, with wooden flooring, walls, and ceiling, and decorated with carvings, paintings, and weavings. They provided a comfortable space where extended families could gather throughout the winter months to share stories and engage in arts such as weaving and carving. Reprinted courtesy of the University of Washington Libraries Special Collections, NA 3994.

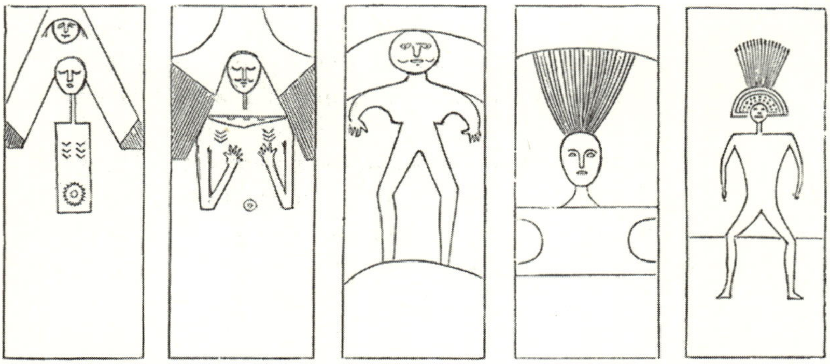

FIGURE 8. Chehalis carved spirit boards, observed along the Chehalis River, Washington. Original woodcut made in 1841 by Henry Eld. These carvings represented individuals' spirit powers and exemplify the unique style of Coast Salish art. Unlike carvings farther north, which were much more formal and stylized, Coast Salish carvings tended to be more abstract representations of personal spirit powers. Images were intentionally obscure, because one's spirit power was a private affair. Reprinted courtesy of the University of Washington Libraries Special Collections, NA 4003.

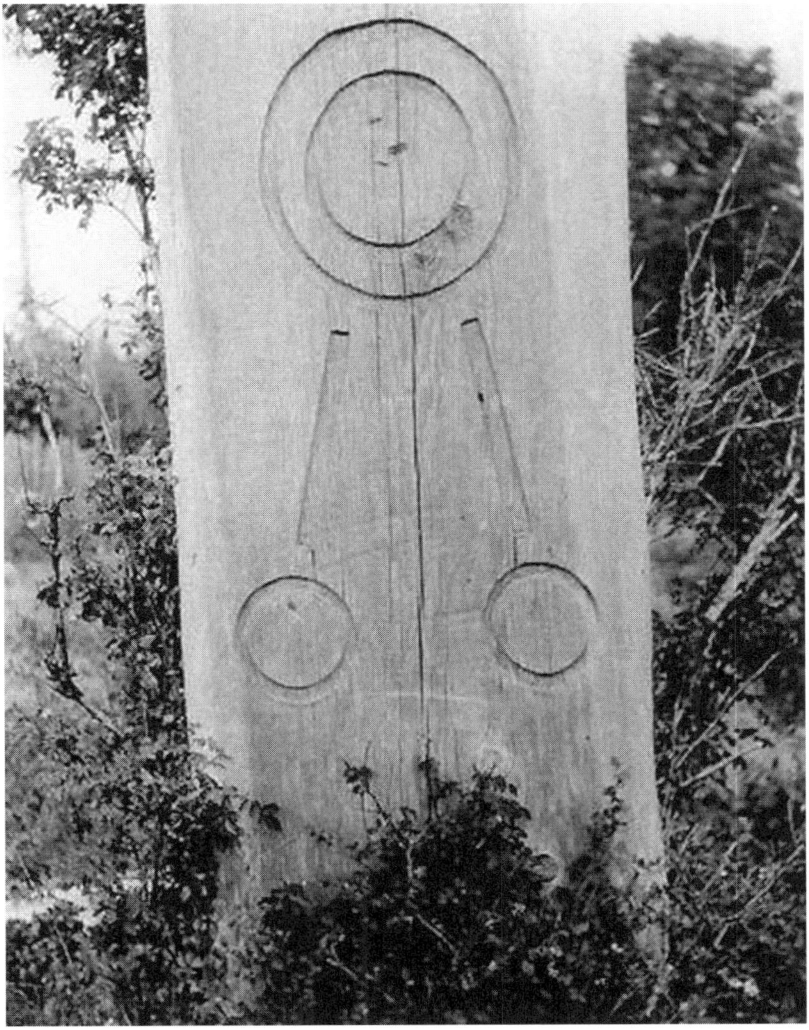

FIGURE 9. Lummi wood carving, from the potlatch house of Chief Chow-its-hoot, Lummi Reservation, ca. 1905. This carving exemplifies the abstract nature of much of traditional Coast Salish art. The image represents a chief's spirit power that enabled him to secure wealth and so host potlatches, but it is intentionally obscure. Reprinted courtesy of the University of Washington Libraries Special Collections, NA 1238.

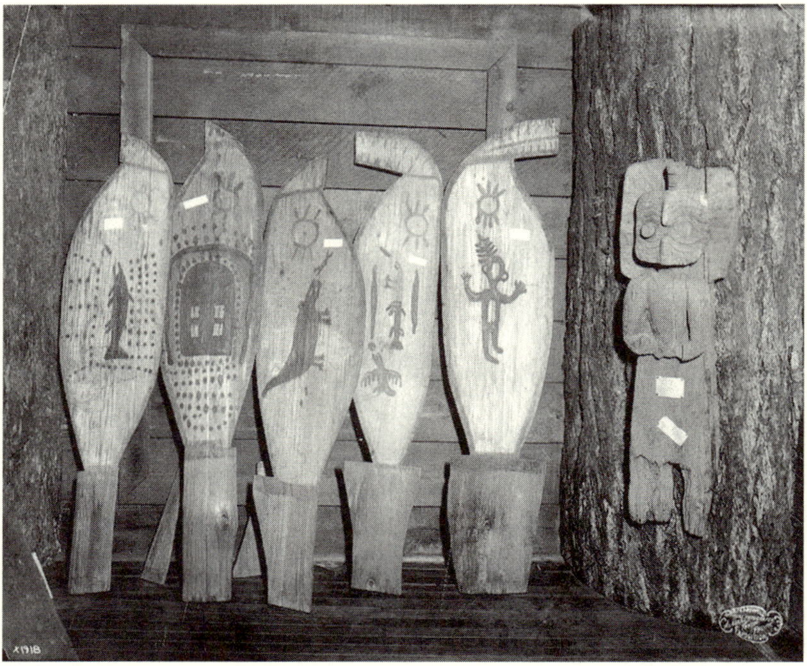

FIGURE 10. Puget Sound spirit boards, photographed at the Alaska Yukon Pacific Exhibition, Seattle, 1909. Likely Duwamish, these spirit boards were collected in 1901 and held by the Washington State Historical Society in Tacoma. Spirit boards such as this would have been used in a soul recovery ceremony. Each healer undertaking the journey to the land of the dead would have painted a spirit board, which would be stood upright in the ground and would accompany him on his spiritual journey. Reprinted courtesy of the University of Washington Libraries Special Collections, NA 679.

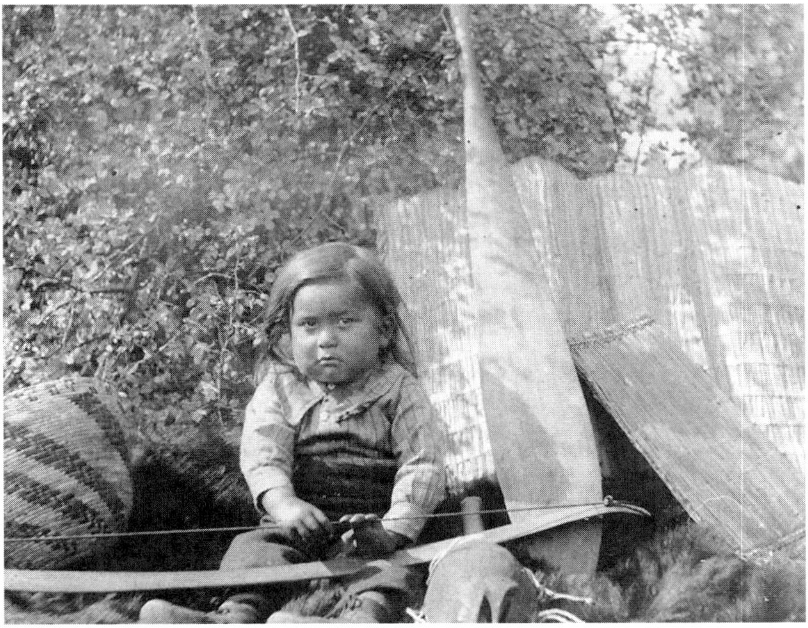

FIGURE 11. Lolota Zickchuse (Snoqualmie), near Lake Sammamish, Washington, 1890. The boy holds a bow and sits near examples of Coast Salish–style baskets, an oar, and woven mats. Reprinted courtesy of the University of Washington Libraries Special Collections, NA 1416.

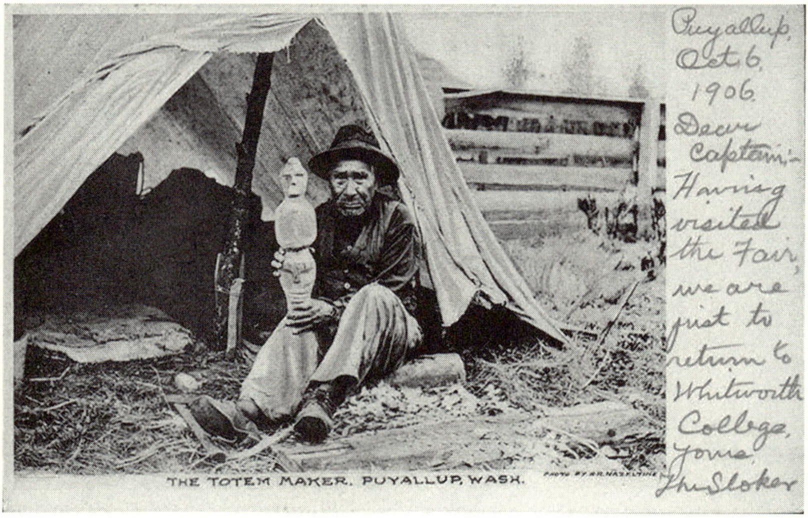
THE TOTEM MAKER. PUYALLUP, WASH.
Puyallup, Oct. 6, 1906.
Dear Captain:-
Having visited the Fair, we are just to return to Whitworth College,
Yours

FIGURE 12. Puyallup wood carver, ca. 1903. The image, captioned "The Totem Maker," was included on a souvenir postcard and provides an illustration of the ways in which Native images were appropriated by Euroamerican tourists. It appears the carver is carving an "earth dwarf," an image used in the soul recovery ceremony. Reprinted courtesy of the University of Washington Libraries Special Collections, NA 1967.

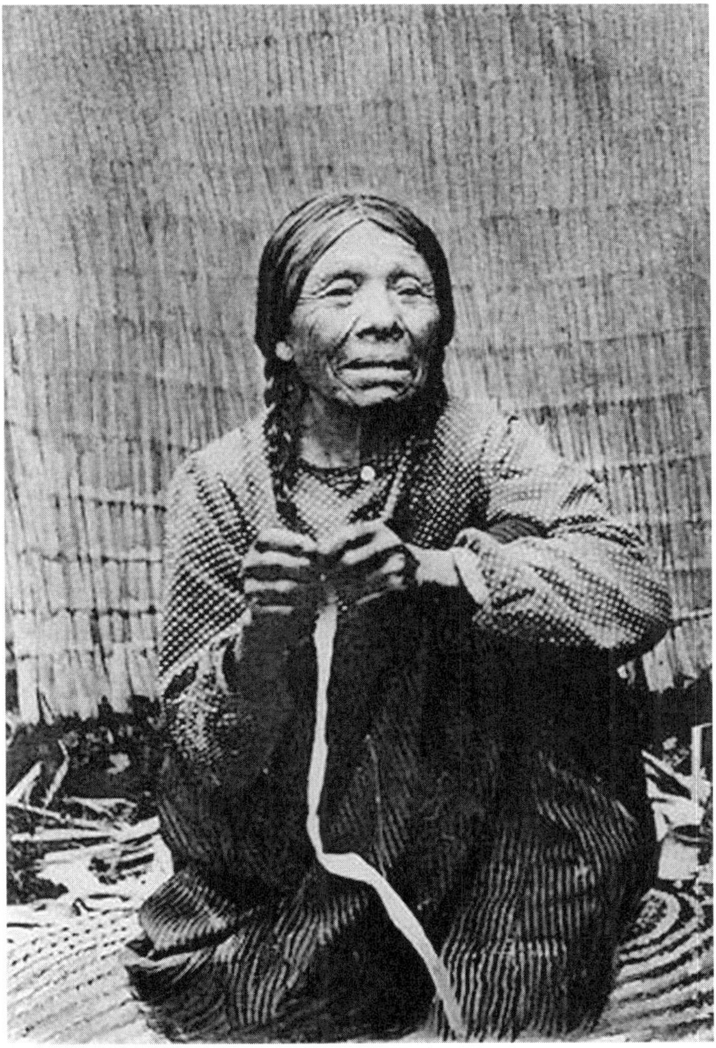

FIGURE 13. Puget Sound Native woman, Mahaly, holding a strand of cattail, used for weaving mats, examples of which can be seen behind her, ca. 1903. Many contemporary Native people argue that their ancestors were healthy, blaming contemporary ill-health on the influences of colonialism. At 106 years old, Mahaly provides a striking example of the longevity and good health enjoyed by Coast Salish and Chinook ancestors. Reprinted courtesy of the University of Washington Libraries Special Collections, NA 1977.

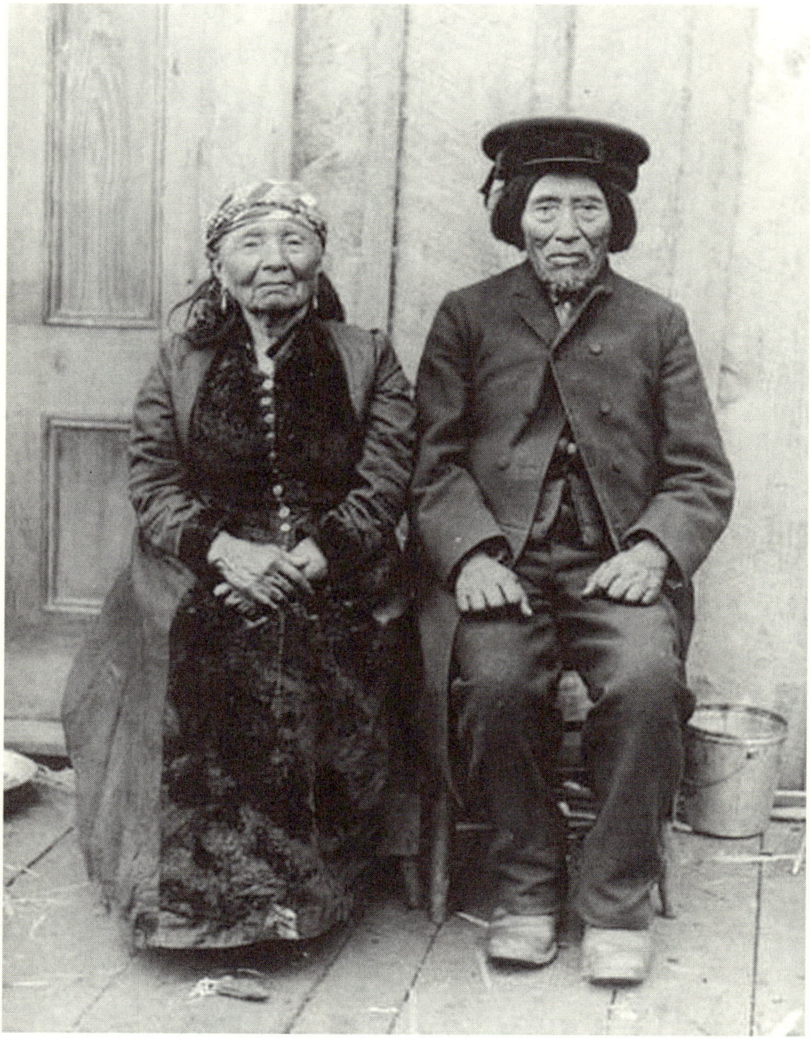

FIGURE 14. Cheshishon (Old Tom) and his wife Madeline, both Duwamish, in front of their home on Portage Bay, Seattle, ca. 1904. Original photograph by Orion Denny. Reprinted courtesy of the University of Washington Libraries Special Collections, NA 591.

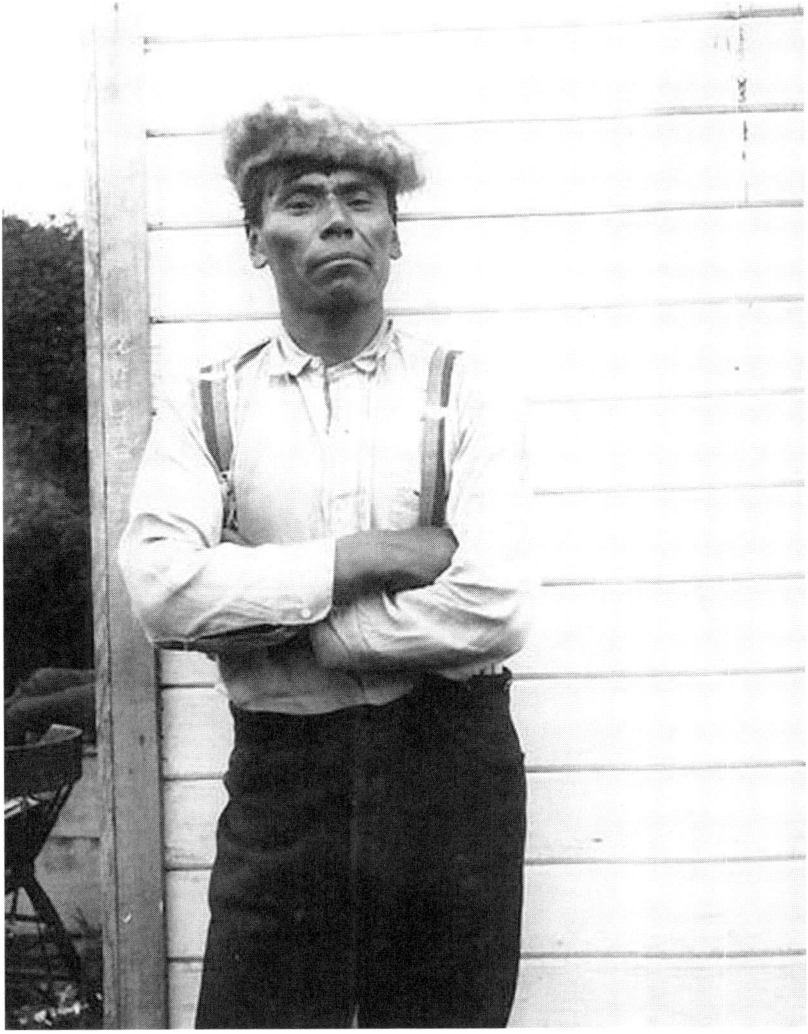

FIGURE 15. Chief George Allen Charley (1864–1936), son of Chief Lighthouse Charley of Shoalwater Bay, ca. 1905. Original photograph by Edmond Meany. The original photo notes that George Allen Charley had his head flattened as an infant, a sign among Chinook communities of one's aristocratic heritage. Reprinted courtesy of the University of Washington Libraries Special Collections, NA 1247.

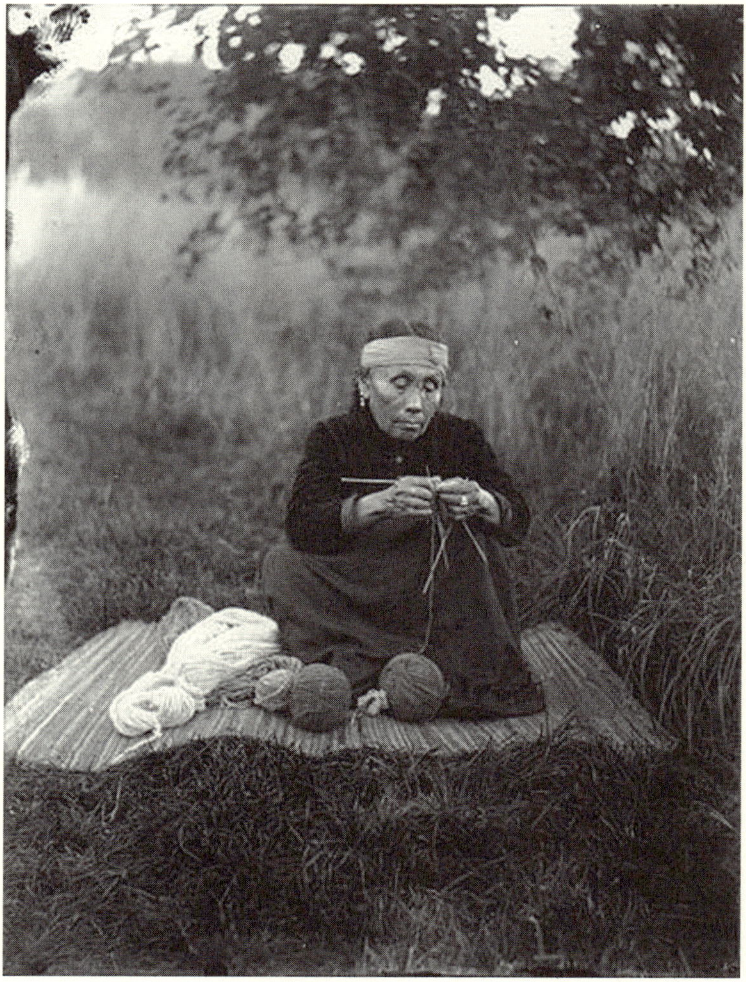

FIGURE 16. Whea-kadim (Magdeline), the mother of Tulalip Chief William Shelton, knitting, Tulalip reservation, Washington, 1906. Original photo by Norman Edson. The image captures a transitional time in Coast Salish history. Whea-kadim wears a scarf that indicates her membership in the longhouse winter spirit dancing tradition, and she sits on a traditional cattail mat. At the same time, the photograph demonstrates the shift toward knitting with commercially available wool and away from older Coast Salish traditions of weaving mountain goat wool blankets on a loom. The traditional Coast Salish style of weaving has seen a resurgence since the 1980s. Reprinted courtesy of the University of Washington Libraries Special Collections, NA 632.

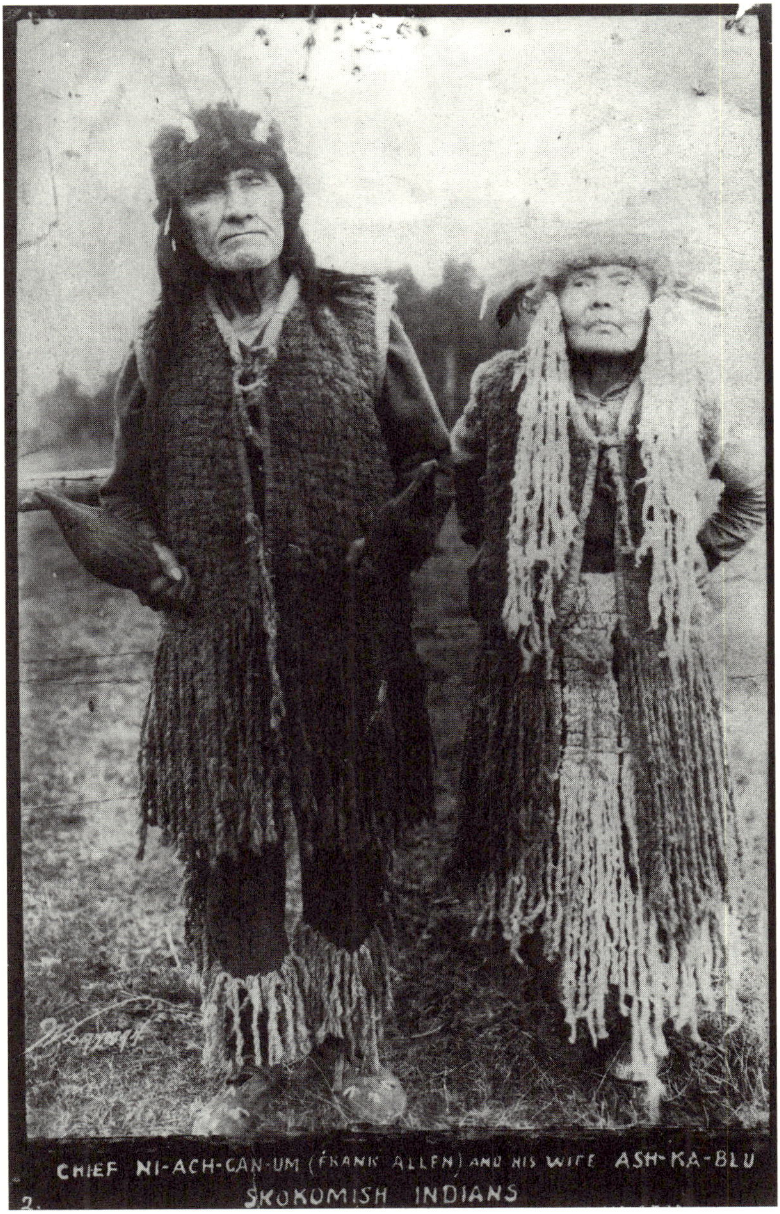

FIGURE 17. Chief Ni'ach'can'um (Frank Allen) and his wife Ash'ka'blu (Lucy Allen) both of Skokomish, in ceremonial regalia, Skokomish reservation, ca. 1930. Reprinted courtesy of the University of Washington Libraries Special Collections, NA 647.

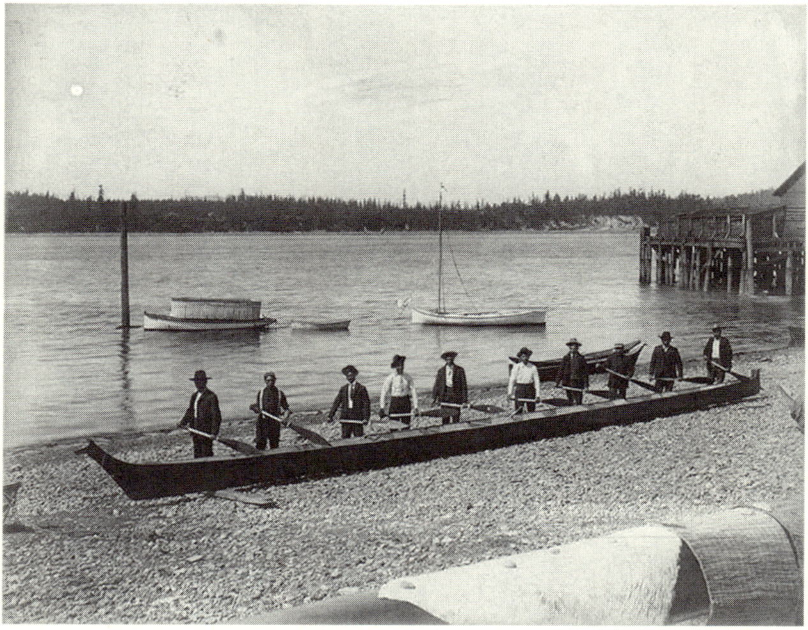

FIGURE 18. Swinomish men with the racing canoe "?" on the beach at La Connor, Washington, ca. 1895. The canoe was famous for its speed and was known to have beaten the University of Washington's rowing team. Original photo by Ole Wingren. The image is striking when considered alongside images from Canoe Journey 2012, which was hosted by the Swinomish Nation, on the beach near La Connor. Reprinted courtesy of the University of Washington Libraries Special Collections, NA 684.

The creek is one and a half miles from the reservation and contains run-off of pesticides from cranberry farms on and off throughout the year. Additionally, herbicides are used on cranberry crops from February to April, a fungicide known to cause reproductive problems in mice is used from February to March, and insecticides are used from May to August. As late as 1995 the drainage ditch flowed directly onto reservation tidal flats, where tribal members swam and gathered oysters and shellfish. Calling it a "drainage ditch" is deceptive, as anyone who has visited Grayland Creek can attest: the creek runs adjacent to and across a stretch of beach north of the reservation before emptying into the Pacific. When I first visited this stretch of beach I was struck by its apparently untouched beauty: it is a pristine stretch of coastline, bordered by an evergreen forest. I was reminded of photos I have seen of the Washington Coast from a century before, and I watched a woman and several children wade through the creek. The stream does not offer any visible sign of being "one of the most polluted bodies of water in the State of Washington," as Gale Taylor, former Shoalwater Bay tribal health director, described it to me.

Along with cranberry farms, the most active economic forces in the region are the production of timber on local tree farms and the farming of oysters, crabs, and other shellfish in Willapa (Shoalwater) Bay. Two chemicals are widely used on Willapa Bay, from Long Beach to South Bend, to protect the oyster beds. One is the insecticide carbaryl, a known teratogen and carcinogen, used against ghost shrimp; Washington is the only state that permits its use on wetlands. And the other is glyphosate, a herbicide used to control the growth of *Spartina* marsh grass. The tribe has also voiced concerns about run-off of herbicides used on tree farms surrounding the bay, intended to prevent the growth of unwanted plant species in timber farms. Water entering the bay comes from the Columbia River and hence is also susceptible to contamination from the Hanford Nuclear Reservation upriver as well as to chemical toxicity from the urban centers along its course: Portland, Oregon, and Vancouver, Washington, in particular. In addition, a World War I munitions dump is located in the hills above the reservation. Its contents, and any possible effects it might have on the water table, are unknown.[17] In September 1998 the Tribal Environmental Testing Laboratory was opened, and the tribe was able to hire an air quality specialist and an analytical chemist to conduct water and sediment testing for possible pesticide contamination.[18]

In addition to the ecological context, the historical context of these people is also significant, for this is not the first time that their existence as a people has been threatened. The Shoalwater Bay Indian Tribe is composed of descendents of forty Chinook, Lower Chehalis, Wakiakum, and Clatsop families, who secured 334 acres at the present location and assigned to the reservation by President Andrew Johnson in 1866. The reservation was established without the benefit of a treaty; it was created in response to demands by Euroamerican settlers in the nearby town of Westport (formerly a Chehalis village), who claimed to be concerned about possible indigenous unrest. These Native people were all from tribes who relied upon both the Columbia River and the Pacific Coast for their livelihoods. Fishing on the Columbia River most of the year, these families returned to the coast and Willapa Bay between salmon runs to gather shellfish, basketry materials, roots, and berries. Gradually, "pressured by the ever increasing settlers," these communities were forced "to abandon their Columbia River villages permanently," and by 1866 "were now residing to the North, on Shoalwater Bay," where the community was led by hereditary Chehalis Chief Keh'leh'uk, also known as Lighthouse Charley Motute.[19]

Many communities had refused to sign the treaty proposed by Governor Stevens at the gathering of Quinault, Chinook, Upper and Lower Chehalis, and Cowlitz in Cosmopolis, Washington, in 1855.[20] Various reasons have been given for why the treaty making ended in chaos. Perhaps most centrally important for his failure was that Stevens suggested the tribes be placed together on a single reservation on the site of the present-day Quinault reservation. Other tribes protested. Throughout their history the Quinault had been occasional adversaries of the Chinook, Chehalis, and Cowlitz. With a smile, one community member told me, "They were historically our enemies. We stole things from each other . . . women, canoes. We're still battling about a lot of things."[21] Another informed me that Stevens brought alcohol to the meeting, hoping to disrupt treaty negotiations and justify taking Native lands outright.[22] In 1864 a 4,200-acre reservation was set aside for interior Chehalis, and in 1866 the 334-acre reservation was created on Shoalwater Bay. As might be inferred from the comments I received, community members reflect on this history with some skepticism. As Shoalwater community member Tom Anderson remarked: "Compare that a single white settler with his wife could attain through the Donation Land Laws 640 acres of land with which to build his home, raise his family, and cultivate his garden, with the fact that thirty to forty families of Natives, descendents of the people occupying the land since time immemorial, were now being required to share a mere 334.5 acres."[23]

By 1934, however, there were only eleven adults living on the Shoalwater Bay Indian reservation. At that time the remaining tribal members voted to reject the Indian Reorganization Act proposed by the federal government, choosing to maintain their own traditional leadership structures. Contemporary members of the Shoalwater Bay Nation are the descendents of these eleven. Chief Charley's son Roland Charley succeeded him in 1935, and in 1958 Roland's eldest daughter Myrtle Landry took the lead. In the 1960s, as part of a larger national effort by the federal government to terminate tribal status, and the reservations and treaty rights that accompanied them, the federal government attempted to terminate Shoalwater Bay's tribal status, arguing that the reservation was deserted. Landry and other community members successfully demonstrated their existence, and the reservation remained. In 1971 the Shoalwater Bay tribe was once again federally recognized, with its own government and constitution.

Access to healthcare facilities is part of this history. Healthcare for the community, until 1995, was vastly inadequate. Tribal members were forced to drive or secure a ride eighty miles to Tahola on the Quinault reservation, or 110 miles to Cushman, the IHS hospital in Tacoma. Several community members recalled feeling ignored, unwelcome, and alienated at both places. "That was a bad situation, because we were treated really poorly there [at the Tahola Clinic]. You'd go, and sit around from 9 a.m. 'til closing time, waiting to be seen, and then maybe they'd just tell you to come back tomorrow. So a lot of people just stopped going. You'd try to take care of yourself, and just hope you didn't get seriously ill."[24] As one woman described her experiences with Cushman: "It was so bad, you wouldn't go if you were sick, that was just the place you went to die." Another woman agreed, saying that the IHS hospital in Tacoma subscribed to the motto "the best Indian is a dead Indian."[25] Such comments suggest that securing funding for their own clinic, and the ability to make their own decisions about healthcare and the form it should take, is very important for the people of Shoalwater and their sense of identity as an independent, self-reliant community.

The first clinic, opened in 1995, was the result of lobbying and careful planning by tribal members and was inspired in large part by the health crises of the 1980s and early 1990s. These trials brought the community together and, led by tribal chairman Herbert "Ike" Whitish, they successfully secured funds to open their own clinic. In 2000 the tribal community had a population of 204, seventy of whom currently lived on or near the reservation. While the population has clearly rebounded from eleven in 1934, it is still a small, tightly knit community, in which everyone keenly feels the loss of every child. This tribal history is important to keep in mind in order to understand more fully how health and wellness are perceived on the reservation today. As noted, the pregnancy loss crisis of the 1980s and 1990s was not the first time the community had had to defend its right to exist. Removed from traditional fishing grounds along the Columbia, nearly forced to share a reservation with a nearby but antagonistic tribal community in 1855, and then narrowly avoiding termination during the 1960s, the people of the Shoalwater tribal community today see their contemporary experience as part of a broader colonial narrative. Threats to their continued existence are viewed within this context.

Defining a "Healthy Self": Person-in-Community

The pregnancy loss crisis challenged the community in profound and painful ways, but it also inspired a renewed sense of determination and a concerted effort to take control of community health and wellness through tribally directed programs. Such activities were aimed at preventing pregnancy losses, but they were also aimed at creating a healthy community as a whole. The remainder of this chapter discusses these efforts and reflects upon what they reveal about Shoalwater notions of a healthy self. The healthy embodied subject articulated within Shoalwater Bay tribal health initiatives is one that exists within a web of relationships: relationships with community, with the natural environment, and with spiritual traditions that link individuals to their ancestors as well as to the broader Coast Salish and Chinook spiritual traditions of the region. The community's response to the crisis is directly indicative of how the community defines health and wellness. Choosing to focus on the living, rather than discuss the whys and hows- of the past, the community has crafted means for reaffirming community identity: connectedness with one another, with the ancestors, and with the landscape.[26] Responses make immediately clear that a healthy working identity is one located within kin and community. This is seen in a variety of ways, which include the communal sense in which the crisis was experienced, a strong sense of collective identity distinguished by a tradition of survival and resistance, and a sense that the path to health and wellness is built upon community cohesion and pride in one's heritage.

Indeed, tribal reactions to the pregnancy loss crisis attest that if there is a collective sense of what it means to be healthy among the Shoalwater, it is that health is a communal and not merely an individual affair. Tribal members describe each pregnancy, and each loss, as taking place for the entire community. Each pregnancy is viewed, to a certain degree, as community property and thus each loss is grieved not only by the woman in question but by everyone in the tribe. While most published studies on the impact of child loss focus on individual women and their partners, in this context it is clear that losses are not simply a matter for individuals alone but for the tribe as a whole. When one baby was born in 1999, her mother remarked that "it is like she is everybody's baby." A tribal clinic employee, visibly pregnant and due within two months, was likewise the object of much attention. "Everyone around here just loves that she looks so pregnant. We are all running around here on pins and needles, looking at her for reassurance. If she comes into work fifteen minutes late, everyone's unnerved. I told her we are going to have to rent a bus to go watch the ultrasound."[27] As one mother commented on her ten-month-old daughter: "This was everybody's pregnancy. She is the community baby. Everybody dotes on her. But you still wonder, where are all the others? Where is the next generation coming from?"[28] And when a baby born in May 2000 visited the tribal center for the first time, "people were fighting to get to hold him."[29] One tribal member, reflecting on the crisis, emphasized that clinical terms and statistics simply do not tell the story. Each child, she emphasized, was deeply loved, part of a family, and part of a community. "Everything that affects one person affects the whole tribe."[30] A distinct sense of community, and a view of the healthy self as one that exists within community, can be seen at Shoalwater. And indeed, it is unlikely that such a view is held to the same extent among non-native communities in the region. For instance, while regional health officials speculate that higher pregnancy loss rates might be found among non-natives in the county, for a long time they could not be sure: non-native towns and cities in the county lack the same degree of communication and cohesiveness, and pregnancy loss statistics are not collectively shared or known to the same degree.[31] Pregnancy loss, while a visible and shared experience at Shoalwater, is generally considered a more private affair among non-native communities.[32]

As an event occurring at the communal level, the pregnancy loss crisis is perceived within the tribe's collective history of epidemics, and as such is seen as another challenge to tribal health brought by colonization. But importantly, within local oral histories of epidemics, the Shoalwater Bay reservation itself is seen as a symbol of tribal survival. As former tribal chairman Ike Whitish explained:

> There's a sense that it's seen as being part of a history of epidemics. There was this huge population decline, and that was due largely to things like smallpox and influenza. This [Shoalwater Bay] was a fishing camp. People would come here during the fishing season. But during the epidemics, everybody ran here. The Chehalis, and the Chinooks, all ran from the smallpox and gathered here, to escape the illnesses, to survive. I've been told by the elders, though I've never read it anywhere, but I've been told that some people went out to that island out there in the Bay to isolate themselves, to keep from getting sick, and that is why so many survived here.[33]

When I asked several older women about this story, while washing dishes together after a community dinner, they readily agreed, saying that their ancestors had retreated to the island in Willapa Bay, thus surviving the epidemics. The land had saved them. This oral history of survival is an important one. The community comes from survivors, originating from a remnant of people determined to outlive the epidemics and resourceful enough to find refuge in the bay. Indeed, the landscape itself, simply seeing the island in the bay every day, serves as a powerful reminder that this is a place of survival.

While maintaining a sense of community identity that includes these histories of survival, there is also a sense that this crisis was distinct. As Whitish went on to say:

> But there is a big difference with the loss of babies. There's a different feeling about it. I wasn't alive back then [during the nineteenth-century epidemics], of course, to know how they felt, but this seems different. It's very frustrating. There's a frustration of living in a so-called pristine area, and yet this danger exists. And it's frustrating to be a small community, like we are, where every child counts, every potential life is so important, and to not be able to do anything about it. It's very frustrating. It's not like we're in the third world, or back in the old days, where vaccines would have helped, but they just weren't around. There is this

> sense that now, in this day and age, in the U.S., we should be able to do something about it. Back then, it couldn't be helped, the influenza and smallpox. But now, no matter what we do, no one is giving us any answers. Nobody seems pressed to look for what the real problems are. They don't seem to really care.

Whitish's description expresses a real sense of being abandoned to their fate by government authorities and indicates that Shoalwater leaders are well aware that there is a clear distinction between the present context and that of the nineteenth century. Their ancestors did not have the resources to fight epidemics of malaria, influenza, or smallpox. But the present-day Shoalwater community *does* have resources to combat this threat and is making use of them.

This creation of a collective identity distinguished by survival in the face of great odds is also evident within written reflections by women in the community. Community efforts for healing have focused on reconnecting to tradition, to history, and to identity and responding to the loss of children by creating a legacy of a different sort: establishing continuity from the past to the present, for the future. One mode in which this occurred was within a Women's Writing Group, which met weekly during the late 1990s to write and share stories. As Judith Altruda Anderson, the writing group's facilitator, described it:

> The act of writing began as a tool for healing, but has grown into something larger. Memories long buried have resurfaced through the process of weekly writing sessions. The act of writing and publicly sharing the stories has been liberating. The past is seen through a different perspective. Pride replaces shame and sorrow, pride in endurance, ingenuity and strength. . . . Our purpose is to write family history in our own words, to honor our relatives and our experiences. By remembering and writing, our past will never be forgotten. We leave a legacy for our grandchildren and all generations to come.[34]

Many of these stories are stories of empowerment, stories that emphasize the strength and endurance of Shoalwater women. These are stories where the women leave home, leave lovers, take jobs, leave jobs, take motorcycle trips across the country or along the Columbia River. These are stories about standing up to husbands—("My husband Max started telling me I *had* to get up and pick cotton. Even at sixteen not knowing much about women's lib, I still did not like to be told I *had* to")—working, supporting themselves, being independent, and returning to community.[35] What emerges is an image of Shoalwater women and their relatives as extremely strong women, determined to survive and to take their families and community along with them. These are active agents, not passive victims to an unseen foe that might threaten their survival. As one woman said: "It makes me proud to have known such an accomplished woman who was a pioneer in Native women's rights without giving it a thought."[36] The same author writes a story of a motorcycle accident. The woman in question, a former flyer and skydiver, was racing along the Columbia Gorge Highway, "missed a turn, and went over a cliff with her motorcycle and landed in the Columbia River. Her parachute days saved her life, because she knew how to roll and tumble when hitting the ground."[37] That message speaks loudly to a community fighting to overcome a pregnancy loss crisis, obstacles to their salmon fishing rights, and the persistent effects of political and economic marginalization. These women know how to roll and tumble when they hit the ground.

This pride in their collective identity was also reflected in comments made at one particular gathering and community dinner. Members of the tribe were invited to comment on what health meant to them and what they felt would contribute to creating a healthy community. Their responses are illuminating. A respected elder spoke first, saying she felt they needed more community dinners, like this one. Tribal members needed to feel like part of a community, she explained, getting together more often, sharing meals. She recalled that in years past the tribe had had frequent cookouts down on the beach. Other women agreed that this was needed. At the time, I was quite struck by this. Having spent considerable amounts of time working in biomedical hospitals and clinics, I had expected suggestions along the lines of additional diabetes screening, an onsite lab, or better access to doctors. Instead, the first and most immediate response was for cookouts or, more specifically, for events that would solidify and promote greater community cohesiveness.

A young man went on to argue that the community needed more activities for children and suggested building a gym, offering martial arts classes, and constructing an off-road-vehicle area. He also suggested creating a week-long wilderness camp on an island in the bay. He and other young adults recalled a similar excursion when they were children, and the young man offered to lead such an endeavor.[38] Others agreed with him regarding the benefits of learning self-reliance, gaining knowledge of and a sense of connection with the landscape, developing friendships, and gaining a feeling of pride from learning how to live off the land. Another young man also suggested building a nature trail around the lake near the reservation. The trail should be paved, he said, so that elders could go there too and teach young people about the plants and wildlife. An elder woman joined in, suggesting basketry classes for young people: elders could take them out to gather materials in the summer and teach them in winter how to weave baskets. Finally, a young adult woman called for increased parental involvement in sports activities:

> If you want kids to be sober and healthy, you've got to give them pride in who they are. Then it won't matter what people out there say about you. And we've got to stop cutting each other down . . . we've got to support each other. We don't have to agree, but we do have to support each other. Teach kids to have pride in their culture and who they are. Give them respect for themselves and their elders and the land. Get them working with elders, learning how to be in nature, how to survive on an island for a week, teach them these things. Nothing will lead a person to drinking quicker than not feeling like they're worth anything.

The meeting points to several key elements in the Shoalwater Bay tribe's understanding of health and wellness: the importance of community, of creating spaces for spiritual and cultural practices, of intergenerational communication and involvement, of learning from and being involved with the natural landscape, and ultimately of creating a strong sense of personal identity and pride in one's culture. That these were the concerns and directives brought forth, rather than demands for further testing of water quality, statistical analysis, or tissue sampling (although tribal members support these efforts as well) is indicative of a view of this community's understandings of health and illness: encompassing the whole person, the community, tradition, culture, history, and landscape.

This same sense that health is achieved through community cohesion is reflected in the way in which the Shoalwater tribe structured its first wellness center, which was opened in 1995. With an eye toward offering complete healthcare, the clinic and its satellite buildings housed not only standard medical and dental care but drug and alcohol counseling, mental health counseling, a dietician, access to a wide variety of social services, and acupuncture, reflexology, massage therapy, and classes in the martial art q'i gong. In 2005 the various buildings housing the clinic were replaced with the new Wellness Center, a structure large enough to encompass within one space all that the tribe had originally intended. Here they are able to offer a full range of "biopsychosocial" care.

In both settings the goal was healthcare that was "traditionally based," with a staff that understood those traditions.[39] While alternative approaches to wellness like acupuncture and reflexology may not be indigenous to the Northwest Coast, it was explained, "they see patients as people-in-community," and hence share a common view of the intersection of health, spirituality, and community. These priorities are also reflected in ongoing efforts to staff the clinic with practitioners who appreciate and respect community-based health, seeing the individual as a whole person existing within a community.[40] Whitish, the individual perhaps most responsible for the establishment of both the first clinic and the new Wellness Center, expressed it this way:

> There's this thing we are as people, with different components of it. All those parts together, in total, is how you achieve health. Spiritual, men-

tal, physical. I don't really like the term, but for lack of a better one, holistic. All those things in balance, means health. Imbalance in any one of those areas leads to weakness, and that can compromise your health. I like to think about this place as a one-stop-shop. You come in those doors down there, and you've got social services, the clinic, the education department if you want help enrolling in school . . . when you walk out of here you've got some hope. Even in the worst of times, hope will get you through. You can survive. When you think about the decimation of tribes, some people can get mired down in depression. If you harbor that anger too long, it starts eating away at you. That defeats the whole purpose. You've got to stay strong. . . . We've been told so long that everything we did was wrong. The women were taken away from the reservation and sent to boarding schools, the men were shipped off to the city, given $600, and sent on their way. They took away our language, our music, to make us nothing, and we started to believe it. Since the '60s, there's been this push to revive things, to remind us that we have good strong traditions, that our past is nothing to be ashamed of.

There are these parts to the self: physical, mental, spiritual. Until we fill this whole circle with positives, we'll always be out of balance. The things we've been taught don't fit. We're walking around in this world where things don't fit . . . and that is part of colonization. That's something that's happened wherever colonization happened. First they try to force religion on us, then they try to break us down, and to do that they take away all that is dear and sacred. That is the philosophy of the government of this country. First it was called genocide. Then they take the women off the reservation and civilize them, stick them in boarding schools. Then take the men and throw them into cities. It is a philosophy of breaking down camaraderie, of breaking down culture, of breaking down community.[41]

This whole-person focus of the clinic is thus geared toward a notion of illness as arising out of the effects of colonization. As such, healing has to address the physiological, spiritual, mental, emotional, and economic needs that have been created by the colonial process.[42] Focusing on the whole person, addressing the wounds caused by historical experience, demands a reconstruction and reaffirmation of identity, of the self-within-community. In this setting, bodies and embodied selves are not simply "culturally constructed" but communally *re*constructed.

The Embodied Subject and the Natural Environment

For the people of Shoalwater, an important part of this process of spiritual healing also involves addressing the community's ties to the natural environment. A healthy individual is intrinsically interdependent with a healthy environment: the health of the Shoalwater tribe and the health of the surrounding landscape are inseparable. Indeed, the pregnancy loss crisis evoked deeply felt concerns about the health of the surrounding ecosystem and the impact colonization has had upon it. This is particularly poignant, considering the oral histories of the locale. Recalling the bay as the place of last resort and determined survival, where their ancestors fled to the island to escape smallpox, malaria, and influenza epidemics, the notion that that bay may not always be a safe refuge is a difficult one to consider. The "Limited Environmental Assessment" report of the EPA described it this way:

> Tribal members were concerned that their natural home, located along the shores of Willapa Bay in southwest Washington, was not safe. Tribal elders spoke of fish and shellfish that no longer inhabited their shores, and of concerns about what might be hidden in the soils of a nearby dump. The Tribe felt their lives were integrally tied to the environment, and if the water, the wildlife, and the fish were being threatened, so might their existence. As Herb Whitish, chairman and tireless spokesman for the tribe argued in a Congressional Appropriations Request, "The Shoalwaters could be the proverbial canary in the mineshaft for the entire Willapa Bay."[43]

Similar concerns were expressed to me directly:

> It's not just the shellfish or the water that is under consideration, but the air too. We could be eating it, drinking it, or breathing it. There are no

> air quality standards out here. We have now gotten a water quality lab up and running, with capabilities to test the water, and we might start testing shellfish. We aim to be an environmental watchdog for Willapa Bay. That makes us very unpopular in some areas, and very popular in others. Whether they're the problem or not, it doesn't make sense to put chemicals in the water and air. It just doesn't make any sense. They call this area pristine. It's not. We've got a beautiful area, but to protect it, we've got to change our philosophy on how we grow oysters, cranberries, trees. We don't want to hurt industries, because those are people.... But when you have several cities, towns, and several industries along a river, and they're each putting things into that stream ... well, it all has to go somewhere. It doesn't just disappear. And we're at the end of that stream.[44]

Such sentiments suggest a sense of the relationship between self and cosmos that is inherently tied to the surrounding landscape, where health and sustained wellness are part of the health of surrounding land and water resources.

Perhaps nowhere else is the ontological relationship between self and land expressed more clearly than in food. Concerns regarding traditional food resources have been particularly difficult for the tribe. Throughout the reservation's history, the primary sources of income and subsistence activities for community members have been salmon fishing in the Columbia River and oystering and crabbing on Willapa Bay. It could be argued that a central element of contemporary Pacific Northwest Native religions and cultures is their relationship to the foods that sustain them.[45] Salmon fishing and shellfish gathering, particularly of oysters and crabs, are key to community identity, are a central part of the economy and spiritual traditions, and are a vivid expression of people's active, daily interaction and interdependence with the natural world. There is virtually never a community gathering at which crab, shellfish, and salmon do not appear, and rarely is there a gesture of hospitality and welcome where these do not figure prominently. When he proposed the present reservation boundaries, W. H. Waterman wrote to the Department of the

Interior in 1866: "These Indians, said to consist of some 30 or 40 families, have always lived upon the Beach and subsisted on fish, clams, oysters, and sea animals. They are unwilling to abandon their former habits of life and turn their attention to agriculture. They desire a place upon the shore."[46]

Given the practical and symbolic roles of traditional food resources, it is not surprising that fishing rights are an important political and spiritual issue for all contemporary Native Northwest peoples. The Shoalwaters were denied access to traditional salmon fishing locations, an injustice that continues to affect tribal members today. As early as 1924 community members were forced to fight for their rights to fish on the Columbia River. At that time Chief George Sa-ah-lin Charley (the son of Lighthouse Charley) and thirty-five other Indian seine fishermen lost a legal battle to establish their right to fish the Columbia. To the tribe, this loss of fishing rights has continued to be a painful reality. Shoalwater Bay tribal member Tom Anderson reflected on the moment: "The story as it appeared in southwest Washington newspapers was simply that the Judge's ruling declared that the Quinault fishing rights were not applicable to the Columbia River. The story that wasn't told is that the state of Washington would not have to suffer 35 non-treaty Indians to take fish in an area occupied and fished by their ancestors for thousands of years."[47] Another ruling shortly thereafter declared Peacock Spit, a traditional salmon fishing ground along Willapa Bay, to be an island and thus subject to state and not federal jurisdiction. As such, it was not covered by federal treaty obligations, thus removing one of the last legal salmon fishing locations from Shoalwater Bay tribal members. Describing this time in their history, Anderson makes clear how deeply connected salmon fishing was and is to the Chinook and Coast Salish when he concludes, "the culture of the lower Columbia tribes was finally broken."[48]

The people have likewise relied upon shellfish as a primary food source for thousands of years, and suggestions that it may be polluted by large-scale industries and subsequently threatening health and wellness are deeply troubling. Oysters, crab, and salmon continue to be served at community gatherings, and there is a genuine reluctance to believe that another staple food, a celebratory expression of interconnection with their history and their landscape, might once again be taken from them. "Everybody around here eats a lot of shellfish," Whitish said. "But nobody is willing to make that leap from ingesting shellfish to an adverse outcome. . . . It's going to take a cooperative look by everyone in this area to find out what is going on. Putting chemicals into this environment is not good for any of us," Native or non-native.[49] "We as a people have had a relationship with the sea throughout our existence. It's hard for us to believe that these chemicals are out there, and that eating these traditional foods can be harmful. These foods and the sea have been a central part of our history and our lives, and it's hard to buy that kind of philosophy, that says that the chemicals in the sea might be affecting the foods. The shellfish are our traditional foods, and they're our traditional economy. It's a hard issue to deal with."[50] Indeed, historians note that precolonial populations in the region were almost never threatened with starvation: the constant presence of shellfish mitigated against hunger.[51] As former tribal health director Gale Taylor put it: "When you have to tell people that maybe the water they drink is the cause, or just walking on the beach is a cause, or that maybe there's no cause at all, that's frightening."[52]

Women's narratives expressed within the Women's Writing Group likewise reflected upon their community's cultural ties to the natural environment through writing about the resources in the landscape: gathering berries and cedar bark as children, deer hunting, fishing, oystering. As Midge Porter writes: "My Uncle Dave was a man of the water," spending his time fishing and oystering.

> Knowledge of the Bay and its channels made him the first man to be able to night dredge to keep up with the quantity of oysters needed for production. . . . He was such a great navigator, he could come back up river in the densest fog. He groomed many a man on the oyster beds to understand how to get quality production off the company's oyster beds. At age 61, he was diagnosed with liver cancer. I'm sure his fatality

> was caused by the chemical "Seven" [carbaryl] that was sprayed on the oyster beds to rid them of ghost shrimp. He had just finished his dream retirement home on the banks of the Naselle River when he found out his fate, he spent his last summer fishing for sturgeon. The fish were so plentiful, they were bumping the bottom of the boat. It was like God's blessing of his love of the water. Uncle Dave died January of 1994. He was a hardworking man who loved his life on the water. I know right now he is on some river doing what he loved most, fishing.[53]

For many at Shoalwater, the loss of access to traditional foods, salmon and now potentially shellfish, is seen as another blow to their physiological and cultural existence as a people. As one woman explained, the pregnancy loss crisis is seen as part of this long history of violence and loss, beginning with the epidemics and continuing with the loss of fishing rights. "So much has already been taken from the Shoalwater people, fishing rights, the right to exist. Now babies are being taken."[54] After a long history of inadequate healthcare, some felt that the State of Washington valued white-owned agricultural businesses more than the well-being of the Shoalwater people.[55] Concerns regarding the safety of traditional subsistence resources thus point to the complex association between self and land, symbolically encoded within foods that have sustained and defined the community for millennia.

The issue is complicated further by the fact that many tribal members feel that government-issue foods, provided under treaty obligations through the Bureau of Indian Affairs to replace traditional (healthy) food resources, have been directly responsible for some of the worst health crises that Native America has faced. When asked what the major challenges to community health were today, I was told that "teaching people how to live healthy, teaching people how to eat, for instance" was of central concern. "Teaching them that McDonald's is deadly, that we need to get back to the traditional ways of eating and preparing foods. Economic problems mean people don't always have the option of just going down to the grocery store, they are living off commodity foods, which are unhealthy, high fat, tasteless."[56] Commodity issue foods tend to be such things as lard, white flour, canned fruit (packed in sugar), processed meats, and other processed foods high in salt and sugar. Most epidemiologists agree that these foods are a primary cause of high rates of diabetes, heart disease, and cancer, some of the biggest killers among Native populations today.[57] Another tribal member told me: "Government-issue food supplies have been one of the worst genocides carried out against Indian people. The foods are the worst things for you they possibly could be."[58] The loss of salmon fishing rights and the potential threat to subsistence shellfish gathering is thus a complicated problem: tribal members are very aware of the loss of these resources to the processes of colonization, and their substitution with commodity foods apparently designed to cause high rates of disease. And the foods are seen within a context of cultural genocide: reflecting the profoundly devastating consequences that efforts to suppress traditional cultures and subsistence practices can have on a people.

With this in mind, it is clear that repairing relationships with the ecosystem as well as defending their rights to subsistence and commercial fishing and shellfish gathering play a central role in the process of restoring a clear sense of community identity, and restructuring the self as an individual-in-community, interdependent with the landscape. The embodied self here is one that extends outward from the individual to encompass a broader array of communal and ecological concerns, and true healing will require addressing those very concerns.

Health and Spirituality: Voices of the Ancestors

This reaffirmation of identity and relatedness is likewise evident in the ways in which the community has worked to reestablish a sense of connection with the spiritual world and, in particular, with their ancestors. This has taken several different forms. Religious life among the Shoalwater people is defined by diversity: there is no single belief or worldview uniting the tribe as a whole. However, spirituality is often talked about in terms of a regional spirituality shared with other Native communities of western Washington, especially Chinookan and Coast Salish communities. At the community dinner previously discussed, for instance, elders emphasized the need to continue raising funds to build a Spirit House. The structure, built like a traditional cedar longhouse, would be used for ceremonies, spirit dancing, meetings of the Indian Shaker Church, and other ceremonial activities.[59] Other elders agreed, also calling for the construction of a sweat lodge. This meeting had been led by the tribal drug and alcohol treatment counselor, and many present agreed that the sweat lodge was an important step in encouraging one another to achieve and maintain their sobriety.

Community leaders have also welcomed religious specialists from a variety of traditions. Religious leaders from the nearby Chehalis and Skokomish reservations have conducted healing, blessing, and naming ceremonies on the reservation. As Whitish explained:

> We've brought in Shakers, and different religious philosophies to help folks deal with [the crisis]. I've tried to bring in Catholics and Presbyterians—it doesn't matter which tradition it is. It's important to have them. For example . . . my wife invited folks down from the north, and we had a ceremony. . . . That was a year ago. I wouldn't call it religion, or religious. Spirituality, I guess. It puts the mind to work; it brings hope. Those things have a role, working with western medicine, the medicine down in the clinic, these things work together. There are no smokehouses here, though I know they're trying to raise the money to build one. And we bring folks in from other tribes.[60]

The Shoalwater people thus draw from surrounding tribal communities, reinforcing and strengthening their relationships with those communities as they discover arenas for spiritual expression. As described in the introduction, this interrelatedness with nearby Native communities was clearly reflected in the dedication ceremony for the Wellness Center. Such mutual support, built upon generations of friendships, intermarriage, and care for one another, has a long history among tribal communities of western Washington.

Working collectively toward survival, with spiritual support from one another and nearby tribes, has been an important part of this process. Shoalwater tribal members have drawn from their ancestral spiritual traditions and adapted them to meet contemporary needs. One striking example of this comes from a naming ceremony that took place shortly before my arrival and was described to me by a woman from a neighboring tribe. In the ceremony a well-known local leader gave Indian names to Shoalwater Bay tribal members. The names had come from nineteenth-century Coast Salish who had died during one of the epidemics of that era and were not survived by any children. The lineages and legacy of those individuals had been halted. But by passing on these names to contemporary Shoalwater tribal members, continuity between these generations and their survival into the present was assured.[61]

Spirituality at Shoalwater is decidedly innovative, flexible, and responsive. While the community does not presently have an official church, smokehouse, or recognized spiritual leader, spirituality nonetheless clearly plays a large part in community life and in the healing process that the tribe has sought. As one tribal member said to me: "People say that spirituality is absent here, that we lack a spiritual base. That is not true. The spirituality is here, but you can't just appoint somebody to be a spiritual leader [laughs]. You can't just point to somebody and say: 'You're our spiritual leader!' When the need is there someone steps forward. There isn't a spiritual leader, but different people with different strengths."[62] Such an approach to spirituality, in which everyone in the community takes part in the cultivation of individual spiritual strengths, and brings them to the community as necessary, coincides with many Coast Salish and Chinook religious practices. It reflects the strong respect for personal autonomy and the expectation that individuals will make the most of their own unique gifts and abilities. At Shoalwater Bay spirituality is not necessarily a formal religious activity but something that is expressed through a variety of activities: community gatherings, prayer, drumming, gathering shellfish, basketry classes, and picking berries.

Indeed, one of the most important ways in which the community has drawn upon spiritual resources to respond to the crisis was with the formation of a basketry group. Women in the community met regularly to gather materials, weave baskets, and share food and conversation. And in 1995 tribal women formed a Women's Healing Group, with the intention of developing ways to express their feelings about the infant mortality crisis. "The women made masks, painted them, then wrote about the meanings or story behind the mask." This experience was what led the women to form the Women's Writing Group. The stories that emerged from this group worked to facilitate healing by reformulating identity, restructuring a sense of a self that is interconnected with the surrounding landscape, with ancestors and children now gone, and with a spiritual world in which those ancestors are continually present with the community of today. Many speak of grief over lost loved ones and, through this writing, work to create another kind of legacy for future generations. These stories and poems reveal women who are consciously and intentionally seeking to explore their spirituality and craft a collective identity that is found through remembering their ancestors, honoring the dead, and finding within those memories a sense of self, of ethics, ideals, and meaning.

Mourning lost loved ones is an important part of these stories: grieving for lost elders and for lost children.[63] As one woman writes, "The worst, most painful separation for a mother is the loss of one of our children to death. Our children are supposed to outlive us. They are supposed to care for us in our old age, and bury us when we die. It's not supposed to be the other way around. I have lost four of my children, all boys."[64] Another woman's poem, "Memories," expresses her grief over a lost child:

> . . . I cannot
> Let go the memory
> Of those first steps nor dim the
> Sight of those
> Last ones down the blue road.
> I miss you
> My son.[65]

Other authors remember people in their community who exemplified their ideals of women and men. One author recalls "Agnes James, A Beautiful Woman":

> There was a lot of beauty in a woman who lived next door to my family on the Shoalwater Reservation. We called her Grandma James. Grandma James made baskets, picked grass out in the Bay in a rowboat. She hunted deer, picked berries, and was a midwife. She raised all her grandchildren by herself. She was around sixty-five or seventy when I first met her and I knew her for about twenty years. She was a very active lady. She would help anyone she could. She made her own butter. She had a milk cow and chickens. She gave butter and eggs and canned food that she canned herself away to families that she heard needed help. She helped mom deliver six of her babies. She was a very short lady. Four feet seven inches, and she was quite round but didn't look fat. She sawed her own wood, split it, and stacked it. She didn't ask anyone to help her. She was still doing all her own work the last time I saw her, about two years before she died.[66]

Narratives like this point to ethical and moral ideals that work to shape Shoalwater women's sense of themselves and their community: hard work, resourcefulness, a reliance upon the landscape and the natural resources within it, generosity, openness, and interdependence with community.[67] One author describes another elder, "Irene Shale": "She'd growl at the snippy tourists nude sunbathing on the beach. She'd say, 'You people lay in the sun for hours trying to get as dark as an Indian.' She had endless wonderful stories to tell that made me laugh. She always wore a dress. A practical dress. She wore aprons and she was always cooking or cleaning or helping someone or clucking about someone's ailing health or misfortune."[68]

As a means by which Shoalwater women have been able to foster memories of the deceased, these stories work to facilitate healing, and to reaffirm identity, through a connection to the community's history and to the very real presence of the ancestors. One author's piece reflects upon welcoming the presence of the spirits of the departed:

> I walk outside and the moonlight draws me . . . pulls me . . . to walk onto the Shoalwater Bay beach and onto the moonlit path. . . . All of my life I have always known there are spirits all around us trying to help us through these hard times. When I pass on, I will join in and help too. I have always had a presence next to me, my Guardian Spirit. . . . In the other place we have fishing rights—no question about it. . . . If I die, when I die, it will be okay. They are there. Here. We will all get through this . . . I want to get through this aware. No drugs. No alcohol. They damage. They prevent us from *hearing*. We are truly strong. Don't worry about the judgments of these people. It is nothing and it will pass away. Learn our own judgment. Listening for the Spirit's judgment is what matters.[69]

This listening to the spirits, acknowledging their presence and listening to what they have to say, has long been a part of traditional southwest Washington religious practices, and acknowledging the ancestral spirits, and cultivating a relationship with them, traditionally and contemporarily, plays a central role in the spiritual practices of the Native people of the area. The author of this piece mentions several aspects of traditional spirituality: cultivating a relationship with a spirit power; the importance of family, and the real presence of ancestors as sources of wisdom, strength, and direction. It is also significant that such religious practice does not necessarily require formal structures or religious leaders to be maintained. As an expression of tradition, of continuity, of connection with the ancestral spirits, and of community independence, projects such as the Women's Writing Group and plans to build the Spirit House exemplify this process of affirming identity and a notion of health as that which emerges from a strong sense of a whole self. As Whitish told me:

> When those things are done, that connection to the other side . . . they deliver messages that aren't always straightforward. It's not like, "take more vitamin C and call me in the morning." It's messages that only that individual might be able to understand. Or maybe even they won't be able to understand it, not right away. You have to think about them, reflect on it. The ancestors are out there, and they will help. It puts you

> in contact with that other side. We have to shed some Eurocentric ideas. Native folks lived in harmony; they had very little sickness before contact. How were they able to do it? There was something they were doing that met their needs . . . as far as spirituality, and food, and whatever.[70]

This chapter reflects upon the ways in which the Shoalwater Bay tribal community has drawn upon their heritage and cultural traditions to craft a sense of health and wellness and then brought these sensibilities, this worldview and ethos, into fruition in the form of community-directed healthcare and wellness programs. The community continues carefully monitoring the health of women and babies, while also emphasizing long-term care and well-being for the community as a whole. They have seen successes in this regard. Since 2001 pregnancy loss on the reservation has dropped to 25 percent: near the national average. Tribally directed programs such as those I have described also work in concert with the South Puget Intertribal Planning Agency's Women's Wellness Program. The Women's Wellness Program provides events such as the "Take Time for Yourself" evening that took place on December 19, 2002, during which Shoalwater women were treated to massage, manicures, healthy food, and health education regarding early breast cancer detection, exercise, and mammograms. Or consider the Women's Wellness Day in April 2004, when women listened to speakers addressing cancer prevention, Alzheimer's disease, and traditional American Indian modes of healing. Good news has also been heard on the ecological front: in April 2003 the Willapa Bay–Grays Harbor Oyster Growers Association signed an agreement with the Washington Toxics Coalition gradually to phase out all use of carbaryl by 2012, an act that will remove one of the most toxic elements currently threatening the region's ecosystem.

It is worth pausing to reflect in this way upon the history and experience of this particular tribal community, in part because it is an exemplar of what community-directed healthcare and activism can achieve. This community continues to face enormous challenges, but it is important to recognize their accomplishments. Such efforts reflect not simply a focus on a *disease* (as Kleinman describes it), with its single original cause, but on *illness*: an experience that affects the whole person-in-community. We might note, for instance, that concerns for political sovereignty take a central role in many Native women's discussions of women's healthcare. And I might call attention to the fact that for the Shoalwater community, the ability to direct their own healthcare, and their own responses to the crisis, has been central to their success. For the Shoalwater Bay community, health has meant more than the absence of disease. It has meant community control of resources, both natural and financial; it has meant community gatherings, basketry groups, writing groups, fishing rights, and a Spirit House.

Ultimately, I would suggest, *health* here is about establishing a clear sense of self, of re-creating a communal sense of identity and cohesion, and addressing the full range of wounds caused by the experience of colonization. Through this community's attention to the living, and their commitment to listening to and learning from the departed, they have crafted a sense of survival based on interconnection between self, community, the natural world, and the spiritual world. Drawing from cultural narratives in which their forebears took refuge from nineteenth-century epidemics on islands in Willapa Bay, and denied twentieth-century government accusations that they had in fact vanished, members of this community tell stories of their resistance and survival—even as some are gifted with the very names of those denied life in a previous century. Passing through a great period of pain and struggle, this community has come full circle. Many healthy babies have been born on the Shoalwater Bay reservation in the past ten years, and accomplishments such as the Wellness Center, Community Center, gym, and Learning Resources Center have transformed this small community in many ways. These achievements reflect the sense of identity found within the poems and stories of the Shoalwater Bay Women's Writing Group, a sense that this community is made of survivors. A poem by Midge Porter, "My Name Is Chinook," reflects this determined struggle for survival in a striking way. Throughout her life she has faced challenges to her existence, the denial of her own Native identity, and has responded by forming a sense of self based on an irrefutable identity as a Chinook woman.

> . . . I know the blood in my veins
> Is that of Chinook
> Yet over and over I have to fight
> The war of existence in a land
> Of false equality and uneven measures
> I am who I am with or without recognition
> The name I will answer to is Chinook.[71]

Four

Person, Body, Place

7. "Rich in Relations"

Self, Kin, and Community

Lady Louse lived there in that huge big house! All alone, by herself.
She had no friends or relatives. Then she took it. And, she swept it.
This huge house. There was lots of dirt!
When she got to the very middle of the house, she got lost!
And that was the end of Lady Louse!
That is the end.

—ELIZABETH KRISE, Tulalip, 1962, translated by Taqʷšəblu (Vi Hilbert)

This very short story about Lady Louse was told on many occasions by the late Taqʷšəblu (Vi Hilbert), who until her death in 2009 worked tirelessly to preserve her Lushootseed culture and language. The story is remarkable in many ways, not the least of which is its ability to speak to many different situations with different meanings for each individual. I begin this chapter with it because it speaks to a core concern within Coast Salish culture essential for understanding Coast Salish views of the self: the central importance of kinship. One interpretation of this story is the danger inherent in isolation. One may have an abundance of personal wealth—perhaps an enormous home all to one's self—but without friends or relatives, one can easily become lost. This story reveals important clues toward understanding Coast Salish and Chinook constructions of a healthy working identity: on the one hand, Lady Louse shows the industriousness and personal responsibility valued within these cultures. But on the other, she lives in isolation, lacking the mooring to kin, to community, and hence to any kind of meaningful personal identity. As Jay Miller and Hilbert have explained, "In Native society, no one should live alone (especially in a large house that is not a lively home), nor be unclean (both physically and spiritually); no one should be kinless and friendless, nor vanish without someone expressing concern."[1]

Throughout this book I make the case that we can define health and wellness as the ability to be one's true self, to have what Jerome Levi has termed a working identity. But to get at particular local understandings of health, illness, and healing, we first have to get a sense of local notions of the self. In this chapter I ask: what does someone with a healthy, a functioning identity look like among Coast Salish and Chinook communities? In particular, I want to get at how the self in these communities exists in relation to others. Considering the arguments put forth by Blackfeather, O'Nell, and Voss in chapter 2, one might be tempted to conclude that all Native American cultures are intrinsically communitarian, where the collective is privileged over the individual; in contrast, Euroamericans are assumed to value individualism about all else. In some ways this is the case, as the story of Lady Louse suggests. But as Chandler and his colleagues have pointed out, there is a danger within such oversimplified dualisms. As they argue, characterizing whole cultures "in terms of broad cultural dichotomies" is "both crude and misleading."[2] As this chapter demonstrates, it is deeply problematic simply to declare: "Euroamericans are individualists! Native Americans are tribalists! Euroamericans are alienated from land and community and honor individualism above all else, while Native Americans are at one with nature and community."

Perhaps in some ways a case can be made that this sweeping judgment holds true for Coast Salish cultures. Respected scholars working with these communities have indeed argued that "all valued life among [Coast Salish] was communal. No healthy, normal person was ever entirely alone."[3] The importance of recognizing the value of the "relational over the individualistic" within mental health care for indigenous people in this region can be seen within a 2003 study of First Nations adolescents living in British Columbia.[4] The authors examined the ways in which young people described "who they were." The authors concluded that Euroamerican youth tended toward "essentialism" while First Nations teenagers tended toward "narrativity."[5] The authors defined essentialism as a sense that the self possesses "some timeless core of persistent sameness, some material or transcendental center," that is "immune to change," a "persistent kernel of existence" that exists apart from context or community.[6] By contrast, the Native youth within the study were far more likely to focus on "process over structure . . . the relational over the individualistic" in describing themselves. Native youth employing a narrative approach to understand the nature of the self were more likely to feel that "that the connectedness of life" could only be understood by the "fashioning of stories meant to integrate all of one's reconstructed past, present, and anticipated future into some overarching narrative structure." Here, selves are rendered "something more like a web or diachronic-patterned relation than an entity, and identities are pictured as more akin to an awareness of process than a test of endurance."[7] This view of the self locates the individual within a process of becoming, one that is dependent upon relationships with others, that gains meaning through those relationships, and is shaped by them. Chandler and his colleagues provide a strong case for thinking about Coast Salish selfhood and working identities in ways that are strongly interrelational and communal.

Additional mental health case studies among Coast Salish communities confirm how vitally important the collective is for constructing one's individual working identity. As Jay Miller notes, "All valued life among Lushootseeds was communal. No healthy, normal person was ever entirely alone, as long as people had their spirit partner(s). Ever aware of other intelligences, any mortal was surrounded by a sentient crowd."[8] In many ways, group affiliation defines and takes precedence over individual identity. Individualism is a key cultural concern, but it is also the case that "a person's identity as part of the group is part of his individuality. He is this person, and part of him is the fact that he is attached to, belongs to, is part of, this particular group. He behaves as an individual, to be sure, but he behaves with reference to his group attachment."[9] Staff at the Swinomish Tribal Mental Health Center agree, arguing that their patients, "value group cohesiveness over individual achievement."[10]

In this context, group cohesiveness means that individuals identify strongly with their larger kin group, and that decisions tend to be made by consensus under the guidance of the wisdom of elders, rather than by individuals acting without concern for others.[11] Cooperating with one's extended family is one of the highest priorities an individual can have, and mental health care workers point to the fact that many patients readily miss a personal appointment in order to help a family member in need of their time.[12] Such an approach that prioritizes human relationships reflects what Vi Hilbert has described as "Indian Time." This "means taking time to be with another person, to visit. It is not something which can be characterized as slow or fast. It is not about coming early or late. It has to do with attention, and attitude, and taking the time to do things in the proper way."[13] In essence, Coast Salish communities are marked by a priority for interpersonal relationships. Locating oneself within a web of human community is essential for living a good and ethical life.

And yet, while Native people in this region in many ways defined themselves by their relationships, they have also been described as "individualists par excellence," with cultural traditions that work to honor and reinforce a clearly individuated sense of self.[14] How do we make sense of this apparent contradiction? To begin to reconcile this potential paradox within Coast Salish views of what it means to be a healthy self-in-a body, I aim to demonstrate that indigenous communities in this region do not fit into a simple individualist/communitarian dualism. Instead, we see cultures that have developed complex ways of negotiating and reconciling both these concerns. The self in this cultural setting is profoundly shaped by kinship, located in a web of relations that give the individual a clear sense of purpose and place. At the same time, as I go on to show, Coast Salish and Chinook cultures also highly value the autonomous individual, creating spaces and means for privacy, personal development, and independent decision making, even within these tightly knit communities. One might make the case that the ideal person in these communities was and is one who cultivates individual identity and self-sufficiency, while remaining moored or anchored to the community that he or she serves.

My Friend Is My Relative

It would be hard to underestimate the central importance of kinship within Coast Salish life. June McCormick Collins's studies of Upper Skagit communities in the mid-twentieth century described this family-centered community: "From birth to death the Upper Skagit person lived in a circle of kin with whom he worked, shared his religious life, and had his recreation."[15] These communities were fundamentally kin-based, where "no one has relations with anyone unrelated either by blood or marriage. . . . One does not enter territory where one has no relatives; if one visits relatives whom one has never met, the first act is to demonstrate relationship by genealogical reckoning."[16] Reflecting on Nooksack communities in the 1970s, Pamela Amoss agreed, noting that "the striking thing about the personal networks of the Nooksack people is how many people in the individual's field of social relations are also kinsmen."[17]

The nearly exclusively familial nature of traditional social life can be found within Coast Salish language. In Lushootseed Salish, for instance, the terms for identifying friends and family reflect this foundational importance of kinship. As Taqʷšəblu and Crisca Bierwert explain, *qwʔsəd* can be translated as "close relatives," and *syəyayaʔ* as "friends." But *syəyayaʔ* "still implies at least a distant relatedness. . . . There is no general word that simply means 'friend' without implying a kind of relative." Further, the notion of family is such a foundational and unquestioned basis for one's social experience that there is no word for "family" in Lushootseed, which instead has various terms for defining particular kinds of kinship relationships. Linguistically, it is simply assumed that some kind of kinship relationship exists.[18]

While kinship was key to social relations, it was also the case that this social system was "fluid and negotiable."[19] For instance, in the early twentieth century Charles Hill-Tout observed among the Squamish:

> The members of these clans were not bound together, as the gentes of the northern tribes, by common totems or crests. They comprised the blood relatives of any given family on both sides of the house for six generations. After the sixth generation the kinship ceases to hold good and the clanship is broken. Under this arrangement an individual's relatives were legion, and he would often have family connections in a score or more different *okwumuq* [subdivisions of a tribe]. Among the present Squamish almost all of them are related in this way to one another, and their cousinships are endless and even perplexing to themselves.[20]

Wayne Suttles made similar observations as he listened to speakers addressing the crowds at contemporary potlatches and spirit dances. As one speaker noted particular individuals in the gathered crowd, he identified them as niece, nephew, auntie, and grandfather, despite their being at best distant relations. As Suttles commented:

> The specific relationship is probably not important; since the terms other than "parent" and "child" are classificatory and extended indefinitely to collaterals, the precise genealogical connection may not even be known. The point is that some relationship can be named, and thus through the sponsors of a big dance most or all of the groups of guests are linked. After several hours of this, one begins to see the whole area as one great kin group embracing several thousand people. When a speaker is addressing the whole house he may use the phrase: "Oh Chiefs, my friends/relatives" (there being no distinction between "friend" and "relative").[21]

Both social structure and the linguistic terminology used to distinguish kinship relations reinforce this sense of a kin-centric social world with fluidly defined family relations. The extended kin group was based on ambilateral descent, being reckoned on both the mother's and the father's side. Reflecting the equal value attributed to each side of one's family, terminology is bilateral: there is no distinction between the kin of one's mother and one's father.[22] Further, Coast Salish kinship terminology reveals a worldview wherein distinctions between relations are less important than the affirmation of relationship itself. For instance, the same terms are used for cousins as for one's siblings; for grandchildren as for grand-nephews or grand-nieces; and there is no terminological distinction made between one's own grandparents and one's great aunts or uncles.[23] Affirmations of familiarity and intimacy do not extend merely to close relatives but also to distant relatives. As Collins noted, "not only relatives who would be regarded as first cousins in our system, but also second, third, and fourth cousins, are called by the same terms applied to siblings."[24] This practice of honoring and counting more distant relations among one's intimate circle has been translated from Coast Salish linguistic terminology into the contemporary English-speaking context as well, according to the Swinomish Tribal Mental Health Project. Just as in the Coast Salish language, likewise in English "all relations of one's grandparents' generation are called 'grandmother' or 'grandfather' . . . relations of one's parents' generation are often called either 'mother,' 'father', 'aunt' or 'uncle' . . . relatives of 2nd, 3rd, 4th, and even 5th degree are often recognized as members of one's family. . . . Indian families are not only larger and more inclusive but are in some ways more flexible. . . . To claim a person as a close relation is a sign of respect."[25]

Family often includes "multiple parents" from various marriages or relationships and in the contemporary context can transcend blood lines, where virtually any older individuals with whom one shares a certain degree of intimacy might be "grandma or uncle or auntie."[26] Within such a setting, parenting often becomes a collective responsibility, as "aunts," "uncles," and "grandparents" of various degrees create what Crisca Bierwert has described as a "a network of diffuse parental authority relationships."[27] Contemporary mental health care workers serving Coast Salish communities have argued for the importance of such a wide network of nurturing adults for the healthy development of children in these communities, explaining that "the psychologically healthy Indian child is generally secure in his/her relationship to a somewhat fluid but nurturing and consistent group of adult relatives." One's identity is formed by participating in and belonging to "the family group" rather than to a particular nuclear family unit.[28]

Despite the seemingly "legion" and "fluid" nature of kinship relations, the ability to identify one's extended family has also been a vital part of composing a healthy sense of self within Coast Salish communities. As one elder explained: "In the past we knew very well who our relatives were, up to our fifth cousins and even beyond that. Because first, second, and third cousins were almost considered to be like brothers and sisters because they shared the same grandparents."[29] This network of kinship relations is, for Coast Salish people, one of the most important factors in shaping individual identity. Consider, for instance, that for the traditionally minded, "the proper way to begin a life story was to recite [one's] lineage, in geographical as well as social and ethnic terms."[30] Each individual named within this lineage becomes what Alexandra Harmon described as another "filament in the net of social ties that defined who he was and where he belonged."[31] Identifying one's place within one's lineage provides a strong sense of self and becomes "an important way of defining who is 'in' and who is 'out' of one's social group."[32] For many contemporary Coast Salish people, "knowing who you are related to and 'what you come from' is an extremely important part of knowing who you are."[33]

Unfortunately, the importance placed upon family identities and loyalties can have destructive tendencies as well, pitting families against each other within tribal communities and creating a history of internal conflict. The high value placed on family autonomy can lead to "atomistic tendencies, especially among reservation Indians. . . . Schisms within the group are common" and can leave one "with the feeling that the elected or appointed leaders have no real power to enforce decisions."[34] Swinomish mental health care workers likewise note this continued potential for conflict, explaining that because "the extended family tends to form the social nucleus in many tribal societies . . . inter-family rivalries, once begun, can be difficult to end. Tension between two people may involve their entire extended family groups . . . a pattern of suspicion and dislike may be perpetuated for quite a long time, possibly for generations."[35]

Coast Salish notions of kinship provide a view of the self that is deeply dependent upon one's extended family. Knowing who you are within this vast network of family, knowing that you *are part of* this vast network, is extremely important. Kinship structure, kinship terminology, and the way in which even distant relations can be included within one's experience of family reflect this. And as community members and mental health workers have affirmed, having a clear sense of place within this fluid and legion web of relations is a vital part of having a healthy sense of self, a working identity, despite the concurrent reality that the high premium placed on kinship can have troubling effects as well, such as the divisions between families that continue to affect tribal communities today. Kinship ties thus clearly reinforce a communitarian view of the self: one that is defined by and strongly identified with one's relations. *Being related* is more important than the specific title of the relationship.

The Village Longhouse: Housing Community

This emphasis on kinship as the heart of one's social life is reflected in traditional residence patterns. Prior to the reservation era, Coast Salish and Chinook communities differed from Native Americans in other parts of the country in that they were not organized into larger tribal groups or formal clan systems; instead, political organization existed primarily at the level of autonomous villages, comprising several extended families living in one or more large longhouses.[36] During the summer months smaller kin groups dispersed to fishing, hunting, and gathering sites that were owned by various families, but during the winter months these families reconvened at their permanent residence.[37] Such winter villages were the heart of social identity. While villages shared a common language with other communities along a particular watershed and may have been deeply connected with such villages through intermarriage, trade, and religious societies, they remained politically independent, and individuals identified strongly with their home village.[38] Such communities tended to be relatively small, perhaps seventy-five people, who were gathered around one elite family with a particularly large longhouse, built parallel to the river or Sound.[39]

In the long, damp and gray winter of the Pacific Northwest, longhouses were warm, dry, and spacious. Longhouses provided an arena for individuals to join together during wet days to work on tasks such as weaving blankets of mountain goat wool, or mats or baskets, cooking or preserving food, or engaging in cultural practices like dancing, singing, storytelling, and religious ceremonies.[40] In the southern Puget Sound region such communal dwellings could range from one to two hundred feet in length.[41] Hill-Tout described such structures in the northern Puget Sound area, where "houses of two or three hundred feet in length were very ordinary dwellings. In width they varied from 20 to 40 feet. The walls too, were of variable height, ranging from 8 to 15 feet when the roofs were gabled. If the roof contained but one slope, then the higher side would rise to 25 or even 30 feet."[42] Longhouses might also be far larger. Keith Thor Carlson notes that "when Simon Fraser visited Sto:lo territory in 1808, he observed a single longhouse at Matsqui (near Abbotsford) that was 192m long and 18m wide (640 feet × 60 feet), or larger than two football fields."[43] Likewise, an 1855 observer described Old Man House, a famous longhouse located at Port Madison in present-day Washington that was 525 feet long.[44] Given their enormous size, such structures could easily house up to a dozen families while also serving as a ceremonial center and religious sanctuary.[45]

Longhouses such as those described here are an important symbol of a key cultural value: the emphasis on a vast and ever-expanding kinship network. As Wayne Suttles has argued, the "slope-pitched shed house" was "aptly suited to the flexibility of Coast Salish and Lushootseed society because it could be expanded at either end as needed."[46] Just as Coast Salish kinship terminology and family structure allowed for a "vast and fluid" network of relations, the longhouse likewise expanded to include relations, even distant relations, under its roof. As families grew, longhouses likewise grew, with additions simply being added, making room for more kin. An extremely large longhouse did not begin that way: rather, it was a symbol of generations of continuity, of families growing and extending the longhouse to accommodate the original inhabitants' descendants and spouses. The value of kinship is thus symbolized in the architecture of Salish longhouses that grew to accommodate the entire family: rather than build additional separate structures, space was made for all one's extended kin.[47]

The interior of the structure also reflects kinship organization. Within the longhouse, space was apportioned by family according to that family's status. The most elite of families occupied the largest and most central quarters, which were also the easiest to defend against attack.[48] But regardless of rank, every immediate family had its allotted space located between support posts along the sides of the longhouse, each with its own hearth. Collins tells us that among the Upper Skagit each hearth was about six feet square.[49] Benches for sitting and sleeping were arranged around three sides, with the fourth open, facing the family's hearth and center of the longhouse. While sharing a single structure, family spaces could be separated from one another by hanging woven curtains of grass or reeds or by wooden planks that could be removed when the longhouse was opened for large gatherings.[50] Support posts in prominent places marked the divisions between living spaces, and were often carved or painted to represent elite families' spirit powers or to commemorate the heroic deeds of particular ancestors. In doing so the posts "anchored certain individuals and families to designated places within the longhouse" as well as within the surrounding landscape.[51]

The physical structure and design of these homes mirrors the creative tension within Coast Salish culture between the individual and the community. The communal nature of longhouse living clearly reinforced a sense of self that was profoundly interrelational. But although longhouses certainly affirmed the communitarian nature of village life, they likewise created private spaces for nuclear families, while carved house posts celebrated individual achievements and identities.[52]

Additionally, longhouses were only seasonal homes. Throughout the long winter, and one must live in the Northwest to fully appreciate this, the community was gathered in one place: one did not need to venture out into the cold and wet in order to find community.

Living together during such a time would strengthen one's sense of communitarian identity, locating one within a large network of kin and community. But during summer months individuals and smaller family groups left on their own, setting up temporary shelters along favorite fishing, berry-picking, hunting, and root-gathering sites. During these months individuals demonstrated their particular skills at subsistence activities, even as they worked cooperatively with close kin to gather resources needed to survive the coming winter. As autumn turned to winter, these smaller groups reconvened at the winter village site, joining their extended kin under one roof. The autonomous quality of villages themselves also reflects the independent nature of Coast Salish and Chinook cultures. Rather than identify with an overarching culture group, or even with communities living on the same watershed, these cultures respected and valued the autonomy of individual families and villages.

Bruce Granville Miller has argued that this importance of personal autonomy within Coast Salish culture distinguishes it from that of its northern neighbors. While northern Northwest Coast cultures traditionally tend to place a premium on rank and class, which are shared collectively with one's clan, Coast Salish cultures place a greater emphasis on personal responsibility. This ethos provides a great deal of room for personal decisions regarding one's actions.[53]

Examples of this can be found in Coast Salish child-rearing patterns, where children are encouraged to have a "high degree of autonomy," and in regional approaches to gender roles, which even in the late nineteenth and early twentieth century appear to have been loosely enforced and continue to be so today.[54] For instance, spirit powers often followed general gender divisions, but these divisions were not strict: anyone could potentially inherit any power.[55] And while men typically did some tasks and women typically did others, it was not strange to engage in activities typically associated with the other gender when convenient or useful to do so. Pamela Amoss observed this among the contemporary Nooksack as well when she noted that "lip service is paid to men's work and women's work," but "little attention is paid to preserving the distinctions."[56]

This high premium placed on personal autonomy continues to be found in contemporary communities' strong emphasis on consensus. Consensus may be a feature of a communitarian culture, but in this setting it also serves to reinforce the value of individual voice. Leaders are encouraged to offer suggestions rather than direct orders, and pulling rank is seen as being in poor taste. Ideal leaders are those who are kind, offer guidance but not orders, and provide resources (food and shelter) for their people. Directly expressing disapproval of or correcting another's actions is rare.[57]

Intervillage Relations: A Web of Kinship

At the same time, despite their independent nature, a larger sense of social cohesion could be found among communities living along the same watershed. Traditionally waterways served as the primary means of transportation, linking communities who were often tied by language, marriage, and trade.[58] Aware as people were of the landscape as "a great watershed," drainage systems provided the most tangible and immediate sense of social identity and unity.[59] And indeed, while villages were the central place to which one returned each winter, they were not necessarily one's primary social identification. While the preceding description of village life may suggest a rather insular, provincial approach to life, villages were far from isolated. In fact, many Coast Salish would have identified strongly with a larger kinship network that extended to other villages, both along a shared watershed and elsewhere throughout Coast Salish territory. Intervillage marriages were often made to create strategic ties between villages (and later between Native and white communities). Such relationships were valuable, ensuring one safe conduct through foreign territories as well as rights to subsistence in foreign territories.[60] While Coast Salish communities tended to be patrilocal, individuals maintained that their maternal relatives living in other communities were equally important to them.[61] A web of kinship relations connected villages, and for many, this "nondiscrete, nonlocalized, property-holding kin group" was more important even than one's village of residence. As Suttles has argued, "it was this group or its head, rather than any of the residential groups that owned the most important ceremonial rights and the most productive natural resources."[62] Such allegiances were particularly important for high-status persons, who as a rule married outside their local village. Harmon has described this "broad web of family ties," which was established through intermarriage and enabled the elite in particular to forge "social bonds that transcended local loyalties."[63] Such "wide-ranging social connections and multiple or layered group affiliations" continue to characterize Coast Salish communities into the contemporary era, in which "webs of kinship" are extensive and individuals continue to reckon their lineage bilaterally.[64]

Villages were also tied to each other by relationships established through cultural or religious societies and other class-based privileges. Such societies (particularly religious secret societies) "were the most complexly structured of all the types of social groups . . . they involved special relations between communities, social classes, and kin groups, which were expressed in complicated ceremonial patterns."[65] Coast Salish social life, while centering on particular winter village sites, was thus fundamentally structured by "a region-wide system of intercommunity relations," where "overlapping kin and social ties linked residents in each winter village directly or indirectly to residents of other villages." Hence—despite the independence of local villages—networks of kinship, intermarriage, and cooperative economic and ceremonial events transformed the Coast Salish social landscape into what Harmon has called a "social continuum."[66]

Maintaining intervillage ties was vitally important for both physical and cultural survival. The Coast Salish ecosystem provides abundant food resources, but such resources tend to come in concentrated bursts: enormous amounts of salmon, berries, roots, or game might be available at any one time but not at another. Hence one village could have an abundance of food one month, and yet potentially find themselves with few resources the next. Intervillage relationships provided a vital means of resource exchange, ensuring that villages always had sufficient food. As Michael Kew has argued, "while the habitat was undeniably rich, abundance did not exist the year round but only here and there and now and then . . . such temporary abundances—though they may well be a necessary condition for population density and cultural development of the sort seen on the Northwest Coast—are not sufficient to create them. Equally necessary conditions were the presence of good though limited food-getting techniques, a social system providing the organization for subsistence activities and permitting exchanges, and a value system that provided the motivation for getting food, storing food, and participating fully in the social system."[67] Villages were not self-sufficient social entities but rather depended upon intervillage relations and the ongoing gift economies that sustained them.

Formal gift giving itself was rarely practiced within one's own village. Rather, gifts were intended for those in other villages as a means of cultivating these long-distance relationships.[68] Importantly, as Suttles notes, "food was not classed as 'wealth.' Nor was it treated as wealth. There is some evidence that food was seen as a gift from the supernatural; xEʔxE sʔíɬən, 'holy food,' a Semiahmoo informant called it. It should be given freely, he felt, and could not be refused. A person in need of food might ask to buy some from another household in his community, offering wealth for it, but food was not generally offered for sale."[69] Extended family exchange networks thus provided a key means of redistributing wealth and guarding against hunger, by providing members of one village with the means and rationale to visit distant villages and exchange locally procured food and other material goods.[70]

While this emphasis on intervillage relations certainly suggests a communitarian view of the healthy self, such networks were also important in shaping individual identity and personal prestige. For instance, social status was earned through creating and maintaining bonds with other communities, which were established through demonstrations of generosity.[71] The ceremonial greeting that begins each formal speech at Upper Skagit potlatch gatherings is indicative of the role of potlatches for establishing individual status and identity and reaffirming intervillage ties: "ʔuɬí swawálus da ʔíšəd: Oh, my distinguished relatives," the master of ceremonies begins.[72]

This ritual greeting serves to remind the audience of the relationships, however distant, that bind them together. As Paige Raibmon notes, the importance of intervillage ties for maintaining personal social status was adapted to changing market conditions during the late nineteenth and early twentieth centuries. During this time individuals continued to visit kin in other villages and reservations, giving gifts and demonstrating their generosity so as to accumulate personal status. The new impetus for travel, she notes, was seasonal labor in newly flourishing hop fields. Traveling for such seasonal work provided many Coast Salish with both the opportunity to visit distant kin and the financial resources to demonstrate their generosity. Such visits were important because social status required regular validation before intervillage audiences. As she goes on to explain, migratory labor in the hop fields may have been new, but seasonal travel to visit extended families was not. Because "the 'upper class' was an intertribal community . . . travel had *always* been a prerequisite for maintaining Coast Salish status."[73] These ceremonial gift exchanges thus served both private concerns, such as establishing one's rank and status, and public social functions, such as reuniting distant relatives and renewing old relationships.

Colonialism and its imports, such as seasonal wage labor, have transformed many of the particulars of how intervillage ties are maintained, yet in many ways the essentials remain the same. As Suttles has argued, "in spite of a century of missionary and government policies that have indeed tended to isolate Indian villages—now reserves—from one another, Native principles of social organization persist in systems of intervillage ceremonialism."[74] Today intervillage ceremonialism primarily occurs through winter dances, summer sporting competitions, and gatherings of the Indian Shaker Church.[75] Winter ceremonials, often referred to as the longhouse or smokehouse tradition, combine potlatching and spirit dancing. The Shaker Church is most active during the spring and summer months, when Shakers often travel from community to community, visiting other churches, offering their healing services, or meeting together for annual conferences.[76] Summer months are also times for familial and tribal gatherings (sometimes at particularly popular fishing sites) for first salmon ceremonies, canoe races and sləhal (a traditional gambling game, also known as the bone game or stick game).[77] These pan-Salish ceremonial activities all provide opportunities for contemporary Coast Salish individuals to interact with a wide segment of their extended kinship network.[78]

A powerful example of this is the Canoe Journey, a variation on nineteenth- and early twentieth-century canoe races. Since 1989, when Emmet Oliver and Frank Brown conceived of the first Paddle to Seattle, growing numbers of young Native people have spent the better part of the summer training for the Canoe Journey, which takes place in July and August. Tribes prepare and send out a traditionally carved canoe, paddled by a "canoe family," often consisting of young adults and especially teenagers. During a journey that may last two to three weeks, canoes meet nightly at prearranged village sites along the coast and around Puget Sound for enormous campouts, feasts, and ceremonial gatherings that include the sharing of songs, stories, and dances. At its conclusion, canoe families and their supporters meet at the final host site for a week-long gathering and celebration. The Canoe Journey has grown to be an enormous event, now known as Tribal Journeys. As one of the most important events of the summer it is an ideal place to renew intertribal and intervillage relationships. Canoes arrive from far-flung tribal communities all the way from northern Vancouver Island to southern Washington, all having made the long and difficult journey. While in some ways a secular activity, the Canoe Journey is filled with ritual, protocol, and sacred symbols that have helped to make it a profoundly spiritual event for many individuals who participate.

Paddling canoes is strenuous work that demands a great deal of an individual in terms of stamina and commitment; it also reinforces one's affiliation with a tribal group. Canoe races and the intertribal Canoe Journey allow each community an opportunity to "re-identify itself in relation to other local groups." As Suttles has argued, the principal participants are not individuals but "crews of canoes," thus reinforcing within participants both a renewed sense of individual identity and achievement and a clear sense of belonging to a group—both one's tribal group and the larger Native community of the Pacific Northwest.

The Canoe Journey and the Tribal Journeys event are clearly a modern adaptation of earlier practices. Prior to the twentieth century, villages made canoe journeys to visit one another during the summer months, and when they approached the beach they were welcomed with ritual and protocol similar to what greets them today. Historically, of course, such visits were not organized and facilitated by means of a website and email list-serve, nor were the feasts occasionally sponsored by local Methodist or Quaker churches. And given the historical animosity among some tribes, this large-scale intertribal gathering is certainly a new thing. In 1993, for instance, more than thirty canoes and three thousand people gathered at Bella Bella, British Columbia, some having paddled from Washington State. It was the first time in history that all those peoples gathered together in one place.[79] Intervillage summer canoe journeys obviously did not have support boats or ground crews that followed them in trucks and set up tents anticipating their arrival. But such modern modifications are beside the point. As Suttles has pointed out regarding similar events: "that canoe racing is really an old Indian tradition may be doubted. But the intergroup gathering certainly is, and the intergroup ties may well be what the speakers [at such events] are insisting must be maintained."[80]

Intervillage ties are the essential strands that weave together the large and fluid Coast Salish kinship network. Because of such ties, the definition of family can remain a fluid one, where relationships with extended kin provide opportunities for mobility and the option of moving to different villages, tribal communities, or homes.[81] As adults, individuals likewise may move seasonally, visiting favorite fishing spots at one time of year, hunting areas at another, or returning to another for winter ceremonial events.[82] With marriage, one's field of relations expands even further, providing "a bond with reciprocal economic rights" for each of the families involved. Couples might move at any time, living with the husband's family part of the year, and the wife's family during the rest of the year. And of course their children have the opportunity to make their home with either.[83] As Yvonne Hajda has noted, among the Coast Salish of the southern Puget Sound, an ambilateral kinship structure combined with a tradition of village exogamy provides children with multiple homes and a wide network of nurturing family. Having relatives in other villages and on other reservations provides opportunities for additional change and mobility, and many children travel back and forth between communities a great deal, a practice contemporary communities share with their ancestors. Individuals can thus "belong to more than one 'community' simultaneously."[84] Despite the mobility that such relationships afforded, Amoss has argued that most individuals generally chose the most advantageous living situation and, once settled, remained there. While they were careful to maintain relationships with more distant kin, "people had a deep and genuine attachment to their villages and to the kinsmen by blood or marriage who lived there."[85] But regardless of one's loyalty to one's home community, this tradition of a large and fluid kinship network, of autonomous villages tied together by complex intervillage relations, has created a legacy that Alexandra Harmon has described as "a sophisticated, far-reaching, and versatile social system," which has provided its members with the tools to cope with the impacts of colonialism through having "more than one possible place to belong." Their ability to survive through the onslaught of the nineteenth and twentieth centuries, she argues, is testimony "to the considerable power of *inter*connection."[86]

In many ways, it is this interconnected and versatile social system that has continually challenged Euroamerican agendas and policies for the region. When Governor Isaac Stevens set out to establish treaties with Washington tribes in 1855, his goal was to create reservations and open land for settlement. To do this, he went looking for "tribes": clearly differentiated communities, made up of individuals with unambiguous loyalties to a single group. Instead, he met with independent villages made up of individuals who might change their village affiliation at any time, joining their kin in another settlement nearby, along the same watershed or many miles away. This "flexibility of residence . . . led to confusion as to the actual affiliation of individuals" and left government officials without a clear sense of how to proceed.[87] In *Indians in the Making* Harmon provides an analysis of this challenge and its implications for future tribal communities. As she explains, the reservation system was premised upon the assumption that Native people were easily identifiable and born into particular tribes. But for the interconnected villages of western Washington, it was simply impossible to make such clear declarations of identity. Coast Salish individuals did not stay in one place or identify with only one group. "For them, identification has more to do with interpersonal relations" than with geographical location.[88] Complex kin networks led Edwin Eells, Indian agent at the Skokomish Agency in the late nineteenth century, to declare in frustration that "half of those he listed as Klallams were 'intermingled with eighteen other tribes' and many had the 'blood' of three or four tribes."[89] Attempts to create enrollment lists were confusing and rarely successful: even people from the same immediate family identified with different tribes.[90] And since treaty rights were equally applied to tribal groups throughout the Sound, most individuals lacked the motivation to settle on any one community.

When the Indian Reorganization Act was implemented in 1934, it again was based on a false assumption about the nature of Native tribes and communities in western Washington. The law assumed tribes were coherent entities and "disregarded kinship ties that crossed the boundaries of reservations."[91] When attempts were once again made to compile definitive tribal rolls in 1956, it remained an elusive goal. As Harmon notes, "each organized tribe had criteria for admitting people to membership, but none of the organized tribes employed those criteria to compile definitive rolls of their members. Applying the criteria of membership remained difficult . . . most potential tribe members also had strong reasons to affiliate with other tribes and even with other racial groups" and simply were not interested in identifying solely with one. As Harmon concludes, "the transition from a world of interlinked autonomous villages to a world where Indians belong to a handful of such tribes has been halting and remains incomplete." In the twenty-first century, people's tribal affiliations continue to be "contested or impermanent."[92]

The nature and importance of intervillage relations within Coast Salish communities is thus essential to understanding Coast Salish views of a healthy working identity. Personal identities are tied to one's home community but also comprise a web of extended relations with other villages and tribes. As Harmon has articulated so well, the Coast Salish case defies Euroamerican assumptions and provides us with individuals with multiple alliances, where the same nuclear family might identify with several different tribes, and a single person might carry a dozen personal identifications and loyalties. As Gerald Sider has argued, any notions that indigenous communities consist of "*a* culture, *a* social organization, *a* kinship system," miss the complicated reality of human communities that fail to fit into neat categories.[93]

Ancestral Kinship: Inheriting Spiritual Wealth

Getting a fuller sense of a healthy working identity within late nineteenth- and early twentieth-century Coast Salish cultures requires that we expand our notion of kinship even further. Within Coast Salish cultures, kinship relationships include not only the living but also one's deceased relatives. Jay Miller explains that "in practice, households included three generations of actual residents, along with at least a fourth generation recalled through hereditary names."[94] He goes on to explain that the deceased might be referred to as "cedar root ancestors." Just as cedar roots "grew in every direction away from the tree, sending tendrils throughout the landscape . . . like a network of roots an individual represented a 'coming together and stretching out' of links from many different places. As a tree fed from diverse roots, so the person came from many sources."[95] Knowing one's ancestors and having a clear sense of connection with them continues to be a key part of cultivating and maintaining contemporary indigenous identities. As the Swinomish Tribal

Mental Health Project explains, "ancestors are part of one's family. They determine who one is."[96]

Within Coast Salish worldviews the human self has been described as being composed of four core elements: a material body, the mind (often located in the heart), the soul, and the shadow or reflection. Variations on these divisions exist; for instance, in other Coast Salish traditions the four components can be described as body, soul, breath, and shadow. All share a sense that an immortal soul or spirit continues to live on after death, usually traveling to the village of the dead. While one is alive, however, the soul can become lost or be stolen away, and the individual may gradually sicken or die if the missing soul is not found. One's shadow and one's breath are more closely tied to the body during life, though they can also become lost or be stolen away, causing illness. After death, varying traditions say that the shadow either disappears, or may continue as a ghost, lingering near places associated with it during life.

To these four elements can be added add key components that, if one is to receive them (not everyone does), also become intrinsic to one's sense of self and personal identity: an Indian name and a spirit power or *syowen* (pronounced see-*oh*-when), the spiritual presence that speaks to individuals through dreams, guides them through life, and animates them during the trance-state of spirit dancing.[97] These aspects of the self are certainly not separate components but are profoundly interconnected: a threat to any one of them may in turn affect others. A weakening in one's relationship with one's spirit power, for instance, could manifest in bodily illness. Or, if one were to lose one's shadow, one might become mentally unwell.[98] In his now classic book *Symbolic Immortality* Sergei Kan argues in a similar vein that Tlingit selfhood, or what he calls the "complete social persona," can be said to include ghost, spirit, and reincarnated spirit as well as inherited cultural property such as names, regalia, totem, crest, and *shagoon* (one's origin, heritage, and destiny as tied to one's matrilineal ancestors). While the Coast Salish cultural context differs from the Tlingit both in terms of its ambilateral descent (rather than matrilineal descent in the case of the Tlingit) and in terms of a sense of self that is more individualistic and less tied to clan and totem, I would make a similar argument that certain components of inherited cultural property (names, spirit powers, spirit songs, and rights to certain subsistence sites) also make up a vital part of Coast Salish understandings of selfhood.[99]

Cultural property such as names, spirit powers, songs, or subsistence rights are important components of individual identity partly because they symbolize one's relationship with one's ancestors.[100] Such cultural property—both spiritual and material—functions as a tangible link to one's predecessors. In contrast to prevailing stereotypes that Native people had no sense of property ownership, Coast Salish communities had very sophisticated traditions of property, though these differed from Euroamerican legal definitions of ownership. Property was held by families, inherited from the ancestors. Individuals and families within each generation acted as stewards of the property in question. And unlike in typical Euroamerican conceptions, property was not understood to be limited to material goods (such as land and natural resources) but also included family names, songs, and other forms of spiritual, intellectual, and cultural property.[101] Taqʷšəblu and Jay Miller, for instance, have described an Indian name as "one of the most valuable forms of wealth that a person could own."[102] Possessing such things in the contemporary era has taken on a particularly potent significance, enabling individuals and families to possess a history that clearly links them to their ancestors.[103]

Receiving an Indian name is an enormously important part of one's individual identity. Such naming generally occurs later in life and is formalized during a ceremony with a potlatch. As guests receive a gift, they acknowledge the individual by the new name, thus witnessing the name and publically affirming its validity. Such names bring with them a great deal of responsibility. As Amoss notes, "when a young person was chosen to 'carry a name,' it was almost as if he were given to the name rather than the name given to him. Such names were valuable family property and were used only on very formal occasions."[104] And Hilbert has explained, because names are owned by families, not by individuals, they are considered a living entity and a reflection of one's ancestors. Names come with an attendant history that has been carefully stewarded by the family. When one receives a name, one receives the history of the honored ancestors who have also held that name. Such histories often point back to the name's origin, perhaps when an ancestor was given the name by his or her spirit power. Names are to be worn "with the dignity and respect that our ancestors would naturally expect" and are to be "respected and treasured."[105] To have a name means that one's "actions from that day on would affect the honor not only of themselves but of their families and tribal community . . . name is connected to family," so if the individual were to act in a disrespectful or shameful way, "that family loses respect as well . . . without a name we are destitute and lack resilience."[106] Along with the personal responsibility to live up to the history of the name in question, names are also accompanied by certain rights, such as the rights to family-owned subsistence resources like berrying or fishing spots.[107]

Indian names, in particular, exemplify the complex interplay between individualism and collectivism within Coast Salish cultures: receiving a name is a reflection of one's individual achievement, a singular honor. At the same time, names are "owned" by families, and perhaps most important, they are a direct tie to one's ancestors. Receiving such a name both affirms and expands one's personal identity, defining one as an individual as well as affirming one's connection to previous generations. It is both a "mark of recognition" that "tends to increase an individual's status" and a living reminder that serves to "connect a person to their ancestors."[108] Names are thus simultaneously *not* you and *you*. Names have a life apart from the individual who receives them. And at the same time, they come to be a central part of one's working identity.

In addition to names, one may also inherit the rights and responsibilities of caring for an ancestor's guardian spirit. Coast Salish young people traditionally secured a guardian spirit by venturing out into wild places and conducting vision quests over the course of several days. In the twentieth century it became more common for spirits to be received through dreams (often when one is ill or experiencing great personal trauma) or through initiation.[109] Regardless of how they are received, spirit powers are often inherited from an ancestor. Elmendorf (writing in the early twentieth century) described inheritance of an ancestor's spirit among the Skokomish Twana as "less common." Contemporary observers of Nooksack and Upper Skagit communities, however, have argued that it is becoming increasingly common to inherit one's spirit power.[110] Pamela Amoss, writing among the Nooksack in the late 1970s, noted that "since questing is no longer practiced, any dancer who comes in through spontaneous possession gets his syowen from his family line—he inherits it from some remote or proximate ancestor."[111] And June Collins, describing the Upper Skagit of the mid-twentieth century, writes that whether questing or finding a spirit through dream or initiation, "people usually, if not exclusively, earn spirits which have belonged to one of their ancestors. Since descent is reckoned from both the paternal and the maternal kin, and since nearly every ancestor had one spirit or more, the number available to any one individual is considerable."[112]

Spirit powers maintain a profound and long-term relationship with particular families. At old age and death, spirits depart, preferring "to be recognized by the close relatives of the deceased."[113] Many individuals welcome spirits that belonged to their ancestors, finding within them a deep emotional and spiritual connection with their deceased relatives. And, it is believed, the spirits themselves are in turn drawn to them. As Collins puts it, "not only the descendants want the spirits, [but] the spirits want very much to be recognized by close relatives of the deceased."[114] Jay Miller, describing Lushootseed traditions of the southern Puget Sound, paints a similarly poignant picture: "after the death of the human partner, the spirit is often compared to a lost dog seeking to attach itself to another close member of the family."[115] And Elmendorf relates a similar perspective among the Twana Skokomish:

> When a person dies his power does not go with him to the country of the dead. It has always followed him around like a dog, and after he dies

it is just like a lost dog. Sometimes the power will just forget its dead owner, but sometimes it wants to belong to someone and it comes and hangs around a relative or a descendent of its dead owner. This makes the person it chooses sick, until a doctor can treat him and find out what is the matter and bring the power to him. Then he has to show that power at a power dance.[116]

Spirit powers act as a vital fiber weaving generations together. While one's relationship with a spirit power is deeply individual and private, it is also something that profoundly ties one to one's ancestors. To receive the spirit power held by one's mother, grandmother, or great-great-aunt creates an intimate connection with those previous generations, even as it provides the individual with a strong sense of personal identity, worth, and purpose.

The personal and private nature of Coast Salish religious life can also be seen within the style of Coast Salish and Chinook art. Because most of Coast Salish and Chinook art was motivated by religious sensibilities and themes, it often sought to represent supernatural beings, perhaps in ways that had been indicated by the beings themselves. But while "what one has got" might be guessed at based on the sounds of one's song or the movements of one's spirit dance, trance remains strictly a private matter.[117] Because of this secretive nature of one's relationship with spirit powers, images of them were often abstract, reflecting personal interpretations of a particular being. This "crypticism" has been described as the "hallmark of Coast Salish graphic and performative arts." While Coast Salish art such as painted house posts, spirit boards, or rattles may be used in public arenas, their form remains abstract and meanings may not be generally recognizable.[118]

The significance of this is made clearer when one considers northern Northwest Coast cultures, such as the Tlingit and Haida, where artistic imagery is more formalized. These more easily recognizable images represent the rank and status of one's family or clan, rather than an individualized experience, as is found in the Coast Salish territories. As such, the forms have been developed over centuries, perhaps millennia, becoming highly stylized. Southern and Northern art forms thus differ based on their public and private nature. On the Northern coast images are public and are owned by particular families, clans, and lineages. In Puget Sound images represent a personal and intensely private experience—and hence, such representations tend toward the cryptic and abstract.[119] At the same time, as Bill Holm notes, when Coast Salish images are associated with words or ritual formulae—which are owned by families and passed down through generations—the images might be more literal and stylized.

These differences can be seen in other performative modes as well. The individualized spirit dances of the southern Salish can be contrasted with "the family-owned spectacles of the northern British Columbia tribes."[120] Northern ceremonies and dances, such as those among the Tlingit, Haida, and Kwak'waka'wakw, are intended to initiate individuals (who have inherited the privilege) into secret societies or to celebrate a heritage shared by clan or moiety. The dances have elaborate masks and follow a set protocol and choreography. Ceremonial life among the Coast Salish of Puget Sound, on the other hand, exists primarily to emphasize what Barnett described as "the indispensable expression of the individual dancer's spirit."[121] Each person's dance, while following a shared style and pattern, is a unique and private expression of a spiritual relationship.

Songs, another central form of cultural property, also reflect this creative tension between individualism and collectivism in Coast Salish culture. Songs originate with individuals, and typically emerge from an individual's very personal and private encounter with his or her spirit power. After an individual's death, songs often become the property of families and should only be sung by individuals who have inherited or been given the right to sing a particular song.[122] Like spirit powers, songs are thus simultaneously indicative of spirituality that is both deeply personal and profoundly tied to one's kin and ancestors.

Other forms of cultural knowledge, such as the ability to initiate individuals into winter spirit dances, skills such as basket weaving or storytelling, and intimate family histories are also the property of individuals and families, carefully guarded and gifted down through generations.[123] Such knowledge also included verbal formulae, such as those that might empower herbal medicines to heal, encourage cultivated plants to grow, calm the weather, or ensure good fishing. Such cultural knowledge, along with names and songs, formed what Elmendorf described as "a type of incorporeal, individually exercised, kin-group property."[124] While food resources, in particular, were expected to be widely and generously shared, "kin-group property" such as this was intended to be carefully kept within family lines, stewarded and exercised by particular individuals during their lifetime, but "owned" by their collective kin.[125]

Rights and responsibilities tied to particular pieces of land, and the subsistence resources they supplied are another example of such individually exercised kin-group property. Natural resources were inherited from one's ancestors, and the responsibility to care for them fell to particular individuals. Such resource sites could not be bought and sold, since they were owned not by an individual but rather by one's family line. The responsibility to care for such sites was inherited or acquired through marriage.[126] In the contemporary context, subsistence sites such as favored fishing grounds continue to be considered the property of particular families, not individuals.[127] Such sites may be managed by one family member, who manages and cares for the site but is not the site's owner.[128] Access to resource gathering sites continues to be assured through establishing one's kin relationship to the primary caretaker and respectfully requesting permission.[129]

Just as social life is based on an extended kinship network, so is traditional Coast Salish economic life. The cultivation of natural resources at these fishing, berry-gathering, camas-digging, or hunting sites was a joint effort, involving one's extended family. As Carlson explains, "parents, aunts, uncles, nephews, nieces, cousins, grandparents, great-aunts and uncles frequently operated as a collective whole. To promote the well-being of the extended family, they monitored and regulated family resources, pooled labour and equipment, and defended one another from hostile outsiders."[130] What is important to note here is that individuals inherited both land and resources from their ancestors as well as the responsibility to care for them. Such "property" was held collectively: just as one did not have exclusive right to one's ancestors, neither did one have exclusive right to one's ancestors' property. Individuals within families had preferred positions to care for and manage land, but anyone with a legitimate tie to that lineage could request (and nearly always receive) permission to utilize and steward the resources in question. This notion of property and wealth as something inherited from one's ancestors is a further example of this cultural tension between individual achievement and autonomy and one's reliance upon and responsibility toward one's extended kin network. Responsibility to care for inherited cultural and material property, as well as the privilege of use of them, falls to individuals. But the property itself remains a powerful symbolic link to one's ancestors and relations.

Rich in Relations: Kinship and Wealth

To understand better how property and wealth serve to shape Coast Salish working identities and values, it helps to reflect further on Coast Salish traditions of economic distribution and class. Precolonial Coast Salish communities comprised three classes: slaves, a small lower class, and a large upper class. Wayne Suttles has described this as a "social pear" because most individuals identified as upper class.[131] A high-status person is referred to as "si'Em," in Halkomelem, or "si'ab" in Lushootseed, and can be roughly translated as sir, madam, or my lord or my lady. The polite term for low-status individuals can be translated as "younger sibling."[132] Social rank and wealth provide another important window on Coast Salish notions of the self and what it means to have a working identity, further illustrating the tension between individual achievement and interdependency within a kinship network. Status is held by individuals and reflects individual achievement. But to be a "high-class person" both requires family and demands that one demonstrate responsibility and generosity toward others.

For instance, having high status was tied to one's ability to be generous with food. Suttles argues that "food and high status are directly related. High status comes from sharing food."[133] However, to be able to be generous with food required an extended kinship network. High-status families generally owned access to the best food-gathering sites as well as the cultural knowledge about how best to protect and maintain such sites and how to harvest and preserve the foods gathered there. Elite status was thus tied to cultural knowledge gleaned from one's elders and ancestors relevant to food production. Carlson argues that among the Sto:lo (northern Coast Salish) to be *smela:lh*, or worthy, "a person had to be from a family that 'knew its history.' Knowing your history meant, among other things, knowing which productive fishing or berry picking sites your family owned, legends about the mythological past, special information about plants and other resources, and having a relationship with the spirits of prominent family ancestors."[134] Likewise, among the Nooksack, "to be si'ab was to be endowed with resourceful, knowledgeable family—not just wealth."[135] The ability to procure the quantity of foods necessary to gift to others, for instance, required the cooperative efforts of one's family. As Suttles explains, "one conjugal family working alone had the instruments for equal access to most types of resources within the territory of its community. But some of the most productive techniques required the cooperation of several persons. Moreover, access to some of the most productive sites was restricted by property rights. Not all, but the best camas beds, fern beds, wapato ponds, and clam beds were owned by extended families with control exercised by individuals."[136] Gathering food was necessarily a joint effort. And since the ability to share food and demonstrate generosity marked one as high status, it was the rare individual who could achieve this alone.[137]

In addition to the ability to be generous with food, to be high status also meant that one had been raised well, that one had been taught how to act ethically and properly, and that one demonstrated generosity and kindness as an adult. High-status individuals honored what Pamela Amoss described as the "moral dictum that kin solidarity must be honored above all."[138] Kin solidarity included the importance of pooling resources, caring for dependents, and honoring one's responsibilities within the extended family, even if it should mean compromising one's own individual success or financial security. By contrast, actions motivated by selfishness or those that were wasteful were viewed with the greatest disdain.[139] The ethical conduct of a high-class person thus required, and in the contemporary context continues to require, the ability to identify one's proper place in the social structure, knowing that of other persons, and demonstrating appropriate respect and care, particularly for elders.[140]

Individuals considered to have "low status" were those who had no family, or whose family had become alienated from their ancestors and their extended relations. These were individuals who had "lost their history" or who "had no advice" from elders and relations as they were growing up.[141] As one Sto:lo community member put it: "The lower class people were just people who didn't have anybody. They were from small families. Your richness was your extended family in those times. . . . When you got down to being almost by yourself that was the lowest class family, because you didn't have anybody for support. You didn't have anyone to help you with your game or providing for you or anything when you were the lowest class. It didn't mean you were ignorant; it's just that you didn't have any of the status of wealth; I guess that's what it was. You didn't have the helping people provide for you."[142] Without family to support and educate them, *st'exem* individuals were those who had "lost or forgotten their history." To become "dissociated from their history" was to become "worthless."[143] As these definitions of high-status and low-status individuals indicate, social standing was largely dependent upon having a strong family who knew their history, maintained their traditions, and passed on both cultural knowledge and natural resources to each generation.

"Wealth" in this context is thus not simply the accumulation of material goods but an indication of the strength of one's relationships. In traditional Coast Salish worldviews, wealth was a symbolic representation of one's social ties. As Harmon has argued, "economic activity created, symbolized, and followed from particular social relations. Acquiring precious items was desirable primarily because the items represented valuable personal relationships and afforded the means to establish more such relationships. To indigenous people, social ties were the real indicators of a person's worth."[144] Hence, while material goods were certainly of value, the actual wealth that they constituted was the "intangible social credit" that one earned by giving such wealth within the gift economy.[145]

Wealth not only symbolized human relationships; it signified one's spiritual relationships as well. Within Coast Salish religious theory, success required the acquisition of a spirit power.[146] Hence while particular goods such as blankets, canoes, carvings, etc., were symbols of wealth, the real wealth was not the objects themselves but "the spirit power necessary for the success of any enterprise."[147] Further, spiritual help was most often given to those who were hardworking and disciplined, as demonstrated through undertaking strenuous vision quests as well as the purification rites that they required, and through the expensive and time-consuming practice of honoring such spiritual help at annual winter spirit dances. Those who were loyal to their kin and their village were most likely to receive spiritual help, particularly spirit powers that were inherited from ancestors. Such supernatural help "fueled the productive economy" and the intervillage trade that resulted from it, all of which were "supported by the belief that supernatural powers were demonstrated through wealth and generosity."[148] Because the acquisition of spirit powers provided young adults with the capacity to excel at certain endeavors and these endeavors in turn provided the potential to earn wealth, that wealth became a symbol of the health and power of a person's relationship with a guardian spirit. Having a powerful guardian spirit was thus a necessary part of being an "upper-class" person.[149]

Completing the circle, spirit powers also implied a supportive family. Good birth ensured that one received good training, which was likely to ensure successful quests for spirit power, which in turn would provide individuals with particular abilities that would enable them to earn personal prestige throughout life.[150] Given that spirit powers are most often inherited from one's ancestors, such wealth symbolized not only a powerful relationship with a spirit power but also, by extension, a deeply meaningful tie to one's deceased ancestors, who also shared that spirit power. Hence wealth and personal status provide another example of cultural values that exist at the fulcrum between individualism and communalism. Status is attributed to and earned by individuals. And at the same time, it is virtually impossible to gain that status without the support, training, and guidance of one's kin and community.

Status requires the validation of one's community, and in Coast Salish communities this occurs at potlatches. While potlatches are often described as relatively secular affairs, given the spiritual origins of wealth, the ritual exchange of wealth during a potlatch can be seen as a sacred event—both because the new status being conferred and confirmed through gift giving was of supernatural origin, and because the wealth exchanged represented the spiritual powers with whom individuals had established relationships.[151] Such events honor individual achievement, but to do so requires the active participation and support of a wide network of kin. Potlatches are extremely expensive affairs. Entire extended families pool their resources to make such events possible. Describing traditions in the early twentieth century among the Twana Skokomish, Elmendorf explained that "one could be largely supported in an enterprise of this sort by relatives and yet figure as an individual donor. What was necessary was that someone, somewhere within the group of relatives of 'good blood,' should possess the requisite goods. Loans from within the bilateral kin group were of great utility to any individual sponsor of an expensive social function. . . . The social reputation of an individual reflected on his entire kin group."[152] Indeed, while the "work" of potlatches appears to be the recognition of particular individuals, the events also establish respect and honor for one's entire family. As Suttles argues, "By potlatching, a group established its status vis-à-vis other groups, in effect saying, 'we are an extended family (or village of several extended families) with title to such-and-such a territory having such-and-such resources.'"[153]

Even as they establish the position of the person hosting the event, such giveaways also reflected, affirmed, and created kinship relationships within the Coast Salish social world. This is in part because potlatches required travel: visiting kin and friends in distant villages. And second, the giving of a gift created a reciprocal relationship, an expectation if not of repayment then of mutual reliance and exchange.

When Euroamericans encountered such symbolic social capital, they were often confused. Consider the comments of Joseph Heath, a mid-nineteenth-century settler who was frustrated to realize "that natives . . . expected him to host a feast when his larders were full. To his dismay he also learned that good relations had to be periodically renewed with reciprocal gifts and favors, writing: 'I don't want to have presents made me . . . always pay too dearly for them.'"[154]

The ritual exchange of wealth during potlatches also had the effect of ensuring that wealth objects were continually moved among individuals: one never permanently owned a valuable thing. Rather, it rotated throughout one's kinship network. While wealth was valued for its symbolic significance, the objects themselves were not something to be hoarded or possessed absolutely. Among the Puyallup-Nisqually in southern Puget Sound, for instance, certain wealth objects received in potlatches were stored in mint condition, not intended for use but "only for ceremonial distribution."[155] The effect of this was that ceremonial goods might be widely circulated, gaining value with each gifting, and enabling many people to possess something of value at least temporarily.

Beyond this ceremonial gift exchange seen at potlatches, routine giving and generosity, particularly to those within one's extended kinship network, was a central value in nineteenth- and early twentieth-century Coast Salish culture and remains so today. One can make the case that such an ethic reflects the survival of communitarian values among contemporary Coast Salish communities. For instance, a 1978 study of giving patterns among Coast Salish communities of southern Vancouver Island found that even within urban areas such as the city of Victoria, Coast Salish formed "networks of assistance," made up of "two to nine households each, involving strong sentiments of obligation and dependence." Such households were usually close kin such as parents, siblings, etc. Families shared food, particularly traditional subsistence resources such as fish, game, and shellfish, services or transportation, and "hand-gathered/grown/baked delicacies."[156] Mooney found that such giving did not decrease during times of need but rather tended to increase.[157] Indeed, those who lived closest to poverty were actually those most likely to give most freely. There was a clear link, as Mooney puts it, between "adversity and an expanded sharing circuit."[158] The most affluent Coast Salish families were also likely to share resources widely, particularly within ceremonial gift-giving occasions. "The most and the least fortunate share more widely," she concluded.[159]

Reflecting the traditional emphasis on kinship, such giving appears to have been limited almost entirely to "the family"; that is, to kin who are within one's house or with whom one has a strong ongoing relationship. Giving to nonrelatives, or to kin with whom one did not have a close relationship, was rare and was considered "beyond the call of duty," and giving decreased as genealogical distance increased.[160] Such findings reflect what we know of nineteenth- and early twentieth-century patterns of giving and sharing, where gifts were given first to close relatives, than to more distant relatives, unrelated elders, and finally to needy individuals living nearby. Interestingly, however, Mooney also found that among contemporary urban Coast Salish, a "peculiar quasi-kin" status had emerged for non-kin with whom one had a close relationship. Such an individual "may also be a person to whom one considers oneself related through some unknown links ('we're all relatives here') but who is identified primarily as a friend rather than a relative." Because such friendships in the modern era may become closer than bonds with distant kin, a "tendency toward generosity within one's community" can override "the lack of genealogical connection."[161]

While the emphasis on giving to kin or non-kin may vary, what remains the same is the sense that giving is an ethical imperative. In part this is because giving creates a kind of social insurance. As

Mooney notes, "these more casual neighborly relations answer real economic needs and maintain solidarity as insurance against possible times of greater need, a hope voiced by a number of persons."[162] The underlying ethical principle involved here is what Mooney terms "collectivism"; that is, an emphasis on a "communitarian spirit and co-operation," wherein individuals and families are called to "support kin and friends selflessly, sharing money resources, and skills when needed rather than saving for [their] own narrow gain."[163] This "collective ethic," as Mooney puts it, serves to link the contemporary Coast Salish community with their ancestral past, even as it provides a means of surviving during economically precarious times.[164] Hence Coast Salish cultures continue to be strongly guided by a communitarian ethic of sharing, particularly among one's kin and among friends who have come to be "quasi-kin." Resources, whether cash, a catch of salmon, a ride into town, freshly harvested tomatoes from the garden, or the knowhow to fix a leaky kitchen sink, are meant to be shared among one's kinship circle. Hoarding such goods, knowledge, or abilities is considered enormously unethical.

Sharing and generosity are thus key Coast Salish values and remain a quality identified with being "high class" or simply a "good person." Bierwert described this ethical polarity among the Sto:lo communities with whom she worked in the 1980s as 1990s, who contrasted "Indian ways" with "white ways." As she observed, gestures of generosity "are considered to be part of 'Indian ways.'" By contrast, "white ways" are associated with "stinginess . . . ambition," and economic success that can "make others jealous. . . . Generosity vies with withholding; collective interest with self-interest; modesty with showiness; artistry with mass production; exchange with purchase; manual ("real") work with mental work; seasonal work with steady work." Overall, "living like a white man" is associated with "those who disconnect from familial relations."[165] The ethics of kinship demand that one make the most of one's talents and resources by making them available to those within one's family. This parallels what one Coast Salish individual told Mooney: "Granny told me, even if your worst enemy comes to the door, offer them tea or food. We never keep anything to ourselves."[166] Taqʷšəblu's recollections from her childhood and traditional upbringing are similar: "You never asked your visitors how long they were planning to stay. Every household responded in the same way to welcome guests. A fire was immediately built in the kitchen stove. The woman of the house began preparing something to place before the guests. You never asked, 'Are you folks hungry?'" Failing to show a spirit of generosity was simply bad manners, but it could have negative consequences as well, compromising one's luck or well-being. Failing to share the first catch of spring salmon, for instance, might mean poor fishing for the rest of the season.[167] Failing to share things with those in need could lead to illness or even death.[168]

This communitarian emphasis on sharing and generosity is brought into creative tension with a high cultural value placed on self-sufficiency, though in this case, "self-sufficiency can also be defined as 'family-sufficiency.'" Harmon identifies this strong ethic within the history of Native Americans in Puget Sound. Coast Salish communities, she writes, have crafted an identity that is independent and takes pride in rarely needing government assistance. She narrates a history in which Puget Sound Indians have been both very progressive economically and simultaneously stubbornly resistant to changing their religious traditions or social structures.[169] The ease with which these communities integrated into the Euroamerican economy, she argues, had everything to do with this high value placed on personal responsibility and self-sufficiency. In a sense, making use of the white economic system was a traditional thing to do, appealing to several traditional Coast Salish values, all of which required the accumulation of wealth: self-sufficiency, achieving status through demonstrations of generosity toward others, and caring for others within one's kinship network.[170] This focus on being independent, self-sufficient, and hardworking are part of the "Indian ways" that Bierwert describes. It is a way of living that requires "an energetic response to circumstances, taking initiative, and drawing on natural resources."[171]

This emphasis on personal initiative helped Coast Salish individuals integrate into the colonial economic system, despite the fact that Native and Euroamerican workers were motivated by different things: Euroamericans focused on productivity geared toward accumulating personal wealth, while Coast Salish communities were motivated by a sense of personal responsibility toward community and spirit powers that enabled the accumulation of wealth. And yet, as Miller, Collins, and Harmon have all pointed out, both Coast Salish and Euroamericans shared a belief that material goods confirmed one's spiritual condition. "As prosperity was an outward manifestation of inward grace for some Christians," material wealth was also a sign of one's relationship with supernatural powers within a traditional Coast Salish worldview. With an ideology that sounds a great deal like the Protestant work ethic described by Max Weber, Coast Salish religious practice "supported the idea of industry; in turn the fruits of industry were the signs of both devotion and success in the religious life."[172] The distinction lay in the understanding of the supernatural power behind one's economic success, and in the ends to which such wealth should be put. As Jay Miller put it, "goods were an outpouring of the good and godly, which for Europeans relates to the individual but for natives relates to family, community, and society."[173] In the new economy wealth continued to be viewed as a sign of religious power, though the origins and understandings of that power may have differed.

The literature suggests that healthy Coast Salish working identities exist at the fulcrum between communitarian and individualist ideals. This creative tension is exemplified by the way in which the individual lives within a complex web of extended kinship, one that connects individual people to a vast network of relations. In ways that remain true in the twenty-first century, Coast Salish families continue to be fluid and vast, with relatives of even fifth and sixth degree being referred to as "sister," "brother," "aunt," and "grandparent." And these relationships play a key role in constructing Coast Salish individual identity, where locating one's self within this kinship network is a vital part of mental health. Further, kinship also includes ties to one's ancestors, made tangible in one's life through inherited names, spirit powers, spirit songs, cultural knowledge, and subsistence resources. One's inheritance is not merely about rights but also about responsibilities to *care for* these things, because such things are the property of a family lineage, not individuals, and so (whether one is talking about names, spiritual powers, basketry knowledge, or a good fishing site) one is to steward them for future generations. While individuals receive particular rights and honors such as names, spirit powers, and particular kinds of knowledge, such things are given to only one individual at a time. They are received both because one is part of a particular family and because one has proven one's worth, and as such are particular individual honors. But such honors are also a profound tie to a larger collective: names, spirit powers, or camas-digging sites are not owned exclusively but only temporarily stewarded. Such a rich inheritance simultaneously defines you as a unique individual and ties you to a nearly infinite web of kinship. As healthcare workers at the Swinomish Tribal Mental Health Project argue, the healthy Indian adult "is one who has achieved a balanced and adapted relationship to his/her family and tribe: he/she functions smoothly in the tribal system of shared responsibility and mutual exchanges; he/she is responsive to community opinion and deeply concerned for the overall welfare of the extended family and tribal group."[174]

A clear understanding of the importance of kinship for a healthy working identity is important when crafting best care practices for contemporary Native communities in this part of the world. For instance, because a healthy self in Coast Salish society is so dependent upon kinship relations, tragedies within one's extended family can have dramatic consequences for individual health. As the mental health care providers at the Swinomish community have explained, mourning a loss threatens the well-being of their Coast Salish constituents. "Because of the close family ties, family members of the deceased are seen as particularly at risk, both emotionally and spiritually. People in mourning may lose part of themselves." For this reason having extended family nearby is seen as particularly important for successful healthcare. "Togetherness is felt to be the primary source of strength at the time of a loss."[175] In their study of mental health among the Puyallup, George Guilmet and David Whited argued for a similar approach: "The extended family support system is of ultimate importance . . . extended family are known to provide emotional support, material assistance, physical care, information referral, and mediation in times of emotional need . . . [a] client who perceives him/herself as being isolated and without 'family' to depend upon and interact with may experience much more difficulty in coping with acute episodes or chronic illness."[176] Having the support of one's living family, as well as a clear sense of connection with one's ancestors, is thus a central part of restoring a working identity.

In light of this, it becomes clearer how devastating the historical experience of colonialism has been within Coast Salish communities. Efforts to assimilate Native people into mainstream America targeted the very foundation of Coast Salish working identities: connections to family, ancestors, and place. Policy makers intentionally sought to disrupt the strength of the extended family, through allotment policies and through the at times forcible removal of children to boarding schools. As has been described, communal dwellings and the common holding of land were key elements in affirming and reinforcing kinship ties and relations, to both the living and the dead. Nineteenth-century missionaries and Indian agents appear to have been aware of this, when they targeted collective land and resource ownership, arguing that giving up multifamily dwellings and adopting single-family homes would "undermine the traditional Indian social structure and speed up the 'civilization' process." While Coast Salish cultural practice would have dictated that heads of kin groups managed collectively held villages and subsistence sites, under new systems lands were distributed to nuclear families.[177] While many aspects of traditional kinship structures have clearly survived, the ability to maintain collectively owned resources was severely damaged. Despite this, traditional Coast Salish ethics carry on in modified forms within contemporary efforts toward tribal fisheries and other resource management and within families that continue to care for fishing or berry-picking sites within their traditional territories.

Kinship networks were likewise devastated by decades of federal boarding schools, the official policies of which were to separate Native children from their families and cultures. Given what this chapter has articulated about the importance of kinship within Coast Salish working identities, the impact of such policies cannot be understated. Keeping in mind the utter centrality of kinship within healthy Coast Salish working identities, consider the comments made by one Sto:lo man about his boarding school experience: "I didn't even know my brothers and sisters were there. I didn't really have a close relationship with them. I never had a close relationship with my mother and I never developed close relationships with any of my cousins either, whether they were at home or school or wherever, just because of the way we were raised. The residential school experience resulted in the total destruction of family structure . . . They basically took away the family experiences I should have enjoyed and should have been able to pass on to my kids."[178] Such experiences targeted the heart of Coast Salish identity, values, and social cohesion, and they had drastic effects.

8. The Healthy Self

Embedded in Place

So, our resources are more than just resources, they are our extended family. They are our ancestors.

—KEITH THOR CARLSON, ed., *You Are Asked to Witness: The Sto:lo in Canada's Pacific Coast History*

Having reviewed how Coast Salish communities regard the individual self in relation to others, I turn now to the question of how Coast Salish identities have been shaped by the relationship of the self to place. All human communities build relationships with the places in which they exist, though most scholars would agree that indigenous communities, wherever they may be found, have particularly profound engagements with their landscapes, engagements that have been built over millennia and are deeply rooted in particular places. These are cultures conceived and born of that particular place. But rather than take this truism for granted, one must ask if this is the case for the Coast Salish, and if so, in what ways? And for the purposes of thinking about *healing*, does this help clarify Coast Salish views of what it means to be a healthy self? In this chapter I discuss three ways in which personal identity might be tied to place: first, through ties to particular resources; second, through a sense of ancestral connection to particular places; and third, through personal relationships with spirit powers that emerge from and are tied to the natural landscape.

Coast Salish and Chinook communities are in many ways closely identified with their local ecology. As described in the previous chapter, precolonial villages were typically located along watersheds, and in terms of culture and language had most in common with those other communities living along the same watershed. Elmendorf noted for instance that the Twana Skokomish communities identified strongly with the watershed in which they lived. Prior to the reservation era the Twana were composed of autonomous village communities, but there was also a sense of a shared identity, stemming primarily from "the feeling for a common Twana territory which coincided with the drainage area of Hood Canal."[1] Village site names were often translated as "people of x watershed."[2] Members of the contemporary Sto:lo Nation expresses a similar sentiment by identifying themselves as the "People of the River—not the People *by* the River or the People *near* the River but the People *of* the River.[3]

Salmon: Relative Subsistence

Indigenous communities in the region are deeply tied to place, in part because of an ancient history of subsistence. Prior to the twentieth century, salmon in particular were so prolific that "by working hard for a few weeks, a household could catch and dry enough fish to last the winter." Salmon ran from spring to fall, forming a central part of Coast Salish diet. Dozens of kinds of berries gathered in high altitudes were likewise processed and stored for the winter. Hunting in the fall and winter provided game, and fresh greens and roots were also cultivated for harvest in the spring.[4] This is not merely subsistence, however, but a complex religio-ethical system built upon reciprocal obligations to a sentient world. Hill-Tout, describing northern Coast Salish communities in the late nineteenth and early twentieth century, explained:

> Nothing that the Indian of this region eats is regarded by him as mere food and nothing more. Not a single plant, animal or fish, or other object upon which he feeds, is looked upon in this light, or as something he has secured for himself by his own wit and skill. He regards it rather as something which has been voluntarily and compassionately placed in his hands by the goodwill and consent of the spirit of the object itself. [This worldview demands that individuals show] respect and reverent care in the killing or plucking of the animal or plant, and proper

treatment of the parts he has no use for, such as the bones, blood, and offal, and the depositing of the same in some stream or lake, so that the object may by that means renew its life and physical form.[5]

Fishing in particular took on religious implications for nineteenth- and early twentieth-century Coast Salish and Chinookan populations and continues to do so today. As Bierwert has argued regarding contemporary Sto:lo, fishing "is religious. Fishers make prayers and have dreams that help them in their fishing, just as hunters and basketmakers do . . . a first salmon may be shared among family members, with special thanks for the coming run. . . . Talking to the river is a spiritual practice, a cleansing, prayerful act. Talking to the cedars lifts the weight from one's heart, the spiritual people say. . . . People say they are helped by the river . . . they can see the presence of the river."[6] During efforts to defend Nisqually fishing rights in the 1970s, Puget Sound communities made similar arguments, explaining that "fish and fishing still represent meanings and relationships so old and tenacious that even Indians who no longer fish will fight to preserve the accustomed rights in the rivers and streams with which they are traditionally connected. Fishing . . . is a remaining avenue of close relationship with the natural world."[7] Fishing remains "the center, in a sense the soul . . . of the feeling of relationship to the environment. The fact of fishing as a fundamental aspect of personal and group relationship to what is important in existence is as real for many Indians today as it was for the treaty signers, and for those before them."[8]

Of course, it is not fish in general that are meaningful here, but salmon in particular, and various Coast Salish communities attest to a unique relationship with that species. A Skokomish story, for instance, describes the community as being descended from a young woman, the only person to survive a great fire. This young woman married Chum Salmon and had several half-salmon children with him. Later, Sequalal (Grandmother Cedar) gave her children a song that turned them back into humans, becoming ancestors of the present-day Skokomish people.[9] In a similar fashion, the Pitt River people describe a creation story where the founding figure of their community married a sockeye salmon. Because of this, the spawning sockeye salmon returning to the Pitt River each year are considered "relatives, returning to give themselves to their kin."[10] Another example can be found among the Snohomish, where the nickname for humpback salmon is "Ki'kaya," or "old grandmother."[11]

Other stories directly tie the well-being of human communities to their salmon relatives.[12] Told by a Squamish elder in 1897, one myth chronicles four eras of destruction and renewal, illustrating the interconnection between the health of salmon and the health of the Coast Salish communities that rely upon and are related to them. The story first describes the creation of Kalama, the first man. Transformer gave him a wife, a chisel, and a salmon trap, the vital elements of a good life. He had many children, and the people grew and prospered. But eventually a great flood struck the community, destroying everyone except Kalama's first son, Cheatmuh, and his wife. Slowly, the earth recovered, with the first sign of its recovery being the return of the salmon. Soon, the people recovered as well, growing again to their earlier numbers. During this time "many salmon came upon the Squamish every season, and there was food for everybody and to spare." But later, a great storm came, with tiny snowflakes so small they "penetrated everywhere, freezing everything. Snowflakes came into their homes, and put out their fires, and into their clothes and made them wet and cold." The people were near starvation. "Soon the children and old people began to die in scores and hundreds. But still the snow came down and the misery of those that were left increased. Dead bodies lay around everywhere, dead and dying lying together." They waited for salmon season, "but when this long-looked-for relief came it was found that the salmon were so thin that there was nothing on them but the skin and bones. It was impossible to cure salmon of this description." Again, only two people survived the time of starvation. After a time of grief, this couple began life anew, and the people again recovered, regaining their original strength and numbers. But once again, tragedy struck:

> One salmon season the fish were found to be covered with running sores and blotches, which rendered them unfit for food. But as the people depended largely upon these salmon for their winter's food supply, they were obliged to catch and cure them as best they could, and store them away for food. They put off eating them till no other food was available, and then began a terrible time of sickness and distress. A dreadful skin disease, loathsome to look upon, broke out upon all-alike. None were spared. Men, women and children sickened, took the disease and died in agony by the hundreds, so that when spring arrived, and fresh food was procurable, there was scarcely a person left of all their numbers to get it. . . . Little by little the remnant left by the disease grew into a nation once more, and when the first white men sailed up the Squamish in their big boats, the tribe was strong and numerous again.[13]

This narrative constructs an image of health as essentially and vitally interconnected with that of salmon: when the people starve, the salmon likewise become thin; when the salmon become ill, the people share the same illness. This story provides a powerful illustration of the degree to which the health of the individual is inseparable both from that of the community and from that of the natural world—in this case represented by the salmon.

Salmon act as a potent symbol for American Indian cultures of the Northwest. Their life cycle and the nature of spawning powerfully and tangibly reveal the interdependence of human populations and cultures. Billy Frank Jr. (Nisqually), one of the leading figures in the fight for salmon fishing rights, put it this way:

> That river was my life. You understood it right from when you were a little boy. The winter floods, the spring floods, the low summer water. We lived right on the bank, right near the edge of tidewater. At Frank's Landing you know exactly when the tide comes and when it goes out. And there was a relationship between your life as a little boy and the salmon. You knew that every year the salmon came back. Spring salmon, summer salmon, fall salmon, then the winter run of chum salmon up to Muck Creek. Then the cycle would start over again.[14]

The actions of one group toward salmon affect those up- and downstream: overfishing or habitat destruction by one group directly impacts the catch of those upstream as well as the health of future salmon runs.[15]

Their annual and cyclical return is linked to and reflected within Coast Salish and Chinook ritual, ceremony, and beliefs about the afterlife. Within these traditions, each year salmon give their lives to the people, and each year they return to the sea, are reborn, and return with new life. Salmon as a central food source and cultural image convey an identity that is capable of cyclical renewal—communities that can die, return, and be restored to their former strengths. Like human communities, salmon populations can "fluctuate markedly over time," and can "experience failures from such cataclysms as land slides, flooding, drought, and the like," yet can also "recover in a few cycles. They are resilient populations."[16]

Welcoming the Chief: First Salmon Ceremonies

The importance of salmon for Native communities in the Pacific Northwest, symbolically and materially, is richly attested to within their first salmon ceremonies, which are a key part of ceremonial life.[17] Chinookan and Coast Salish communities throughout the Pacific Northwest all maintained some form of first salmon ceremony. While particulars differed from region to region, common features included a moratorium on fishing for a prescribed period of time and the ceremonial welcoming of the first salmon caught, described as the King or the Mother of all Salmon, which must be cut and cooked in a particular manner.[18] The salmon would then be distributed in a sacramental fashion to the gathered community, and finally the bones would be returned to the river.[19] Oral traditions accompanying the ceremony describe some version of a story in which previous generations of the human community had formed a relationship with the salmon people.[20] According to the Twana Skokomish version for instance, such ceremonies were based on the belief that "there were five races of salmon people, of human form, living to the west in 'homes beyond the ocean.' Each year in the spawning season, the salmon people left their villages and traveled to the Twana country to run up the streams. Each kind was led by a chief to whom the special term was applied, stu'yičad, 'boss of the salmon.' . . . Each ordinary salmon killed during the year was a salmon person whose soul returned to the salmon country and came back as a fish with the following year's run."[21] In return for people treating them respectfully and honoring certain restrictions, the salmon people would come every year, offering their lives so that the human beings might live. If their bones were disposed of properly, they would return to the salmon people's village, where they would be reborn.

It was believed that if these restrictions were not followed, the salmon runs could be threatened. As a result, Native communities hesitated to sell salmon, particularly whole salmon, to traders during the first days and weeks in which they were running. Early Euroamerican observers noted these practices. As Alexander Ross wrote, "When the salmon make their first appearance in the river, they are never allowed to be cut crosswise, nor boiled, but roasted; nor are they allowed to be sold without the heart being first taken out, nor to be kept over night, but must be all consumed or eaten the day they are taken out of the water. All these rules are observed for about ten days. These superstitious customs perplexed us at first not a little, because they absolutely refused to sell us any unless we complied with their notions, which, of course, we consented to do."[22] As Charles Wilson noted, "About the salmon they have a curious superstition, always cutting off the head, and taking out the backbone before they bring it to Europeans, as they consider it would destroy fishing if a European was to get hold of those parts."[23] Proper respectful treatment of the first salmon to come up the river was considered a crucial action in maintaining the health of the species as well as the health of the community. Failing to follow these ceremonial restrictions and activities could result in starvation or illness for individuals or their community.[24]

Since the restoration of fishing rights in the 1970s, Coast Salish communities in western Washington have revived the public performance of the first salmon ceremonies. In contemporary descriptions of the rite the salmon is treated as an honored guest, whose arrival is announced much like that of a visiting dignitary arriving by canoe. Taqʷšəblu and Bierwert describe it well: "Soon a young man arrived. He had some news! It seemed that there appeared to be a very important person coming in to shore. The leader from Tulalip said, 'We had better all go down to the shore to meet our visitor who arrives by water.' Then the leader sang a song and we all joined him. We went down to the shore, singing as we walked. We could see someone coming. He came. Arrived. Yes, it is indeed this very important person. It is King Salmon who is the very important person who has arrived to us."[25] A description of the contemporary Puyallup first salmon ceremony tells us that the first salmon is cooked over an open fire, then "parceled out to all, in small morsels or portions so all can participate. Doing this, all bones are saved intact. Then in a torch bearing, dancing, chanting and singing procession they proceeded to the river where they cast the skeleton of the salmon into the stream with its head pointing upstream, symbolic of a spawning salmon, so the run of salmon will return a thousandfold."[26]

First salmon ceremonies stand out within Coast Salish religious life as one of a very few public rites. Most of Coast Salish religious life centers on private, individual relationships with spirit powers, and while these may be celebrated at public dances, the spiritual event itself is between an individual and his or her personal power. In this instance the collective (human people) are speaking with and cultivating relationships with another collective (the salmon people).[27] As Suttles acknowledges, first salmon ceremonies were likely the closest that Coast Salish societies "came to religious ceremonies for the benefit of a group," since "the spirit dance gathering was essentially a series of individual performances."[28] With the suppression of indigenous fishing and declining salmon runs, first salmon rites grew less and less common, occurring for the most part as private family affairs. But following the 1974 Boldt Decision, which restored long-neglected treaty rights and guaranteed half of the harvestable catch to Native fishers, first salmon ceremonies have been revived, and large public ceremonies are once again an annual event for many tribal communities throughout Washington.[29] The ceremonies are indicative of a political and cultural revival of Native communities in the region, as tribes have once again gained some degree of control over this valuable resource and have been able to reclaim their role as "ecological stewards and protectors of cultural patrimony."[30]

Coast Salish subsistence practices and ceremonial activities thus reinforce a sense of ancestral connection with a particular landscape, its mountains, its animals, and its plants. But the ability to have a relationship with the natural world is also dependent upon an assumption that the natural world has an *ability to be in* relationship. While it is more common within Euroamerican scholarly work to assume that this "relationship" is unidirectional, scholars who pay attention to Native worldviews and take indigenous perspectives seriously acknowledge that from a traditional perspective, this relationship is mutual. And relationships require some degree of sentient awareness. The case for this can be found within Coast Salish oral traditions of spirit helpers that reside in the natural world. Religious traditions, particularly those regarding spirit powers, or *syowen*, helped create a strong tie between Coast Salish people and their place.

"This Country Gave It to Us to Be Like That": Indigenous Views of Spirit Power

SHXWELÍ: LIFE FORCE

One key to understanding Coast Salish relationships to place can also be found in the Sto:lo notion of *shxwelí*, which might be translated as the spirit or life force that animates all things in the natural world. This spirit is shared by all sentient beings and passed on to present generations from their ancestors. Shxwelí might be envisioned as water flowing from a common spring. Each generation's life force comes from and returns to this spring, connecting current generations to the past. Shxwelí transforms the way one thinks about natural resources as well as particular places considered to be sacred. Plants and animals are not simply "regarded as food and a resource" but instead "like an ancestor. There's a connection there, and that connection is known as *shxwelí*. *Shxwelí* is what's referred to as the spirit or the life force, and everything has that spirit and everything's connected through that."[31] More than a philosophical idea, shxwelí is an embodied connection between one's self and one's ancestors. Sto:lo elder Rosaleen George put it this way. With her hand on her chest, she explained:

> "'*Shxwelí* is inside us here.' And she put her hand in front of her and she said, *shxwelí* is in your parents.' She raised her hand higher and said, 'then your grandparents, your great-grandparents, it's in your great-great-grandparents. It's in the rocks, it's in the trees, it's in the grass, it's in the ground. *Shxwelí* is everywhere. . . . What ties us? What ties us to the sturgeon? It's the *shxwelí*. The sturgeon has a *shxwelí*, we have a *shxwelí*. So we're connected to that.'"[32]

Transformer stories help further to explain the role of shxwelí in developing a sense of place. Within Coast Salish oral traditions, in a time before history, Transformer (*xa'ls* in Lushootseed; *xexá:ls* in Halkomelem; *du'kʷibətl* in southern Puget Salish and Twana) moved throughout the landscape, putting the world in order, assigning animals and plants to their particular tasks, punishing individuals who did not demonstrate proper ethical behavior, and rewarding those who did. Within such stories some ancestors of the Coast Salish people were transformed into entities within the natural world. Sturgeon, mountain goat, salmon, mountains, or unusual features of the landscape were thus once ancestors of contemporary people. Wherever ancestors of the Sto:lo were transformed into trees, animals, or rocks, those entities were (and are) considered to have a shxwelí, the animating life force of all living beings. And because human beings share in this common shxwelí, they are materially and spiritually connected to these other beings. As one Sto:lo elder explained: "When you look at *Lhílheqey*, the mother mountain, and her three daughters, *Seyewot*, *Oyewot* and *Xomo:th'iya*: they were ancestors who were transformed into those mountains. The *shxwelí* of those ancestors are inside those mountains and we're connected to it; we need to take care of that place . . . wherever one of our ancestors was transformed into a rock—the places—those are special places! . . . Anywhere where one of our ancestors is transformed into a mountain, there's that connection we have, through our *shxwelí*, to that mountain, and we have to take care of it.'"[33] As another Sto:lo cultural leader explained: "So, our resources are more than just resources, they are our extended family. They are our ancestors, our *shxweli* (spirit life force). Our *shxweli* includes our parents, grandparents, great grandparents, cedar tree, salmon, sturgeon, and transformer rocks. . . . Our Elders tell us everything has a spirit. So when we use a resource, like a sturgeon or cedar tree, we have to thank our ancestors who were transformed into these things. We don't like to think that our ancestors came over the Bering Land Bridge. We have always been here."[34]

David Schaepe explains that when features of the natural world are animated by shxwelí they are also considered to be "*ancestral*; that is, they are linked to the contemporary community through the transformative acts of *Xexá:ls*, the Transformers." Place-based religious practice thus becomes a means to "'link back to' one's ancestors, here found in the resources and the surrounding landscape."[35] When honoring cedar or salmon, then, one may be recognizing it as an ancestor rather than a natural resource, recognizing the shxwelí within it, not merely its utilitarian uses.[36]

SYOWEN: SPIRIT POWERS WITHIN THE LANDSCAPE

This life force takes on a personal and sentient presence within *syowen*, or spirit powers. According to ethnographies recorded in the late nineteenth and early twentieth centuries, traditional spiritual practices of the region centered on relationships with spirit powers, most often acquired just prior to and during adolescence.[37] Nineteenth- and early twentieth-century Coast Salish and Chinook young people went out in search of syowen. As very young children, girls and boys were sent out in the night to collect water or run small errands, in the hope that they might "find something." As they grew older, such outings were lengthened and made increasingly difficult, until during puberty they were sent on vision quests. Young men and women would fast and stay awake and busy through the night, swimming, keeping a fire, or piling rocks, brush, or earth.[38] If they were fortunate enough to receive a vision of their spirit power, they would also be given a spirit song and might receive special instructions as to what to wear, how to dance, or how to honor their power in other ways.[39] Reverend Myron Eells observed these vision quest endeavors among Native communities of the south Puget Sound in the late nineteenth century:

> A father would send his son into the woods or mountains a long way from home, where he was not allowed to eat for a period of from ten to thirteen days, though he was required to bathe often, and keep up a good fire. They say that such fasting would kill a man under ordinary circumstances, but that his tamahnous keeps him alive, though he has not yet seen or found it. At last his tamahnous reveals itself to him in the shape of a bird or bear, which ever afterwards is sacred to him. The women have their tamahnous, which they find in much the same way.[40]

Among the Skokomish Twana, William Elmendorf explained, spirit questing emphasized solitude and ritual purity. Young people purified the body through frequent bathing in streams or lakes and scrubbed the body with evergreen boughs. They sometimes used a sweat lodge, or purified the interior of their bodies with fasting and the use of emetics. People seeking spirit powers were also careful to avoid any contact with semen or menstrual blood.[41] Physical austerity and ritual purity were rewarded with powerful visions. Marian Smith notes that among the Puyallup-Nisqually "the recipient became like a dead body (but did not die), was physically transported to the 'home' of a power, which might be under water but was not necessarily so, received certain information through instruction or observation, and was re-transported either to the same or another spot."[42]

Similar traditions existed among other groups in western Washington and Oregon as well. As one Coos woman described: "Go round outside! Fear nothing! No matter how bad (fearful) it may be, you are to go nevertheless right to it there, (perhaps) to the ocean, (or perhaps) to a lake, no matter how bad it may be, you must not fear it. . . . Even though (they are) young girls, they will nevertheless tell such things to them. And indeed, that is what they (girls) themselves do. That is the way a girl at puberty goes around, swims, and encounters a (luck-power) person indeed."[43] Another narrative in Jacobs's *Kalapuya Texts* mirrors this: "That was the way my people used to be long ago. This country gave it to us to be like that. We went to get our shaman spirit-powers in the mountains, and in the lakes too. That is where we got our spirit-powers. It was in consequence of that that some of the people were powerful."[44] James Swan observed these customs in practice among the Shoalwater Bay Chinook of the 1850s, where young people fasted for from three to seven days, during which time they neither ate nor slept, though they could drink water.[45] Such efforts needed to be undertaken with care and supervision, because to seek a spirit power in an inappropriate way was to risk illness or death. As one individual told Jacobs: "But if he (a person) stole (went unannounced in order to obtain) a spirit-power, something (some one spirit-power) would devour you forthwith, or you (he) would drown in the water. That is the way it would happen in the waters (or) in the mountains should you want instead to steal (secure unannounced) a spirit power. A grizzly would kill you very quickly, or wolf."[46]

Receiving a vision such as this marked the beginning of a relationship between the person and the individual's power, a relationship that must thereafter be maintained and celebrated in a variety of ways. As Jacobs recorded, "Whatever was their dream, that is what became their power. . . . They saw them as persons, and as persons understood their language. . . . Whatever sort of food was their day (spirit power), they did not eat what their day was. They said of it thus, if they should have eaten their day, that then their day would take vengeance on them (causing their death)."[47] Spirit powers might also be honored in carvings upon house-posts, figures at house doors, the prows and sterns of canoes, or upon images left to guard burial scaffolds. These relationships were also affirmed, commemorated, and strengthened by participating in winter spirit dances, in which individuals danced their spirit power, providing a space for communion and reverence.[48]

In return, spirit powers endowed the individual with certain gifts, strengths, and abilities and became an inseparable part of one's identity and personality.[49] For example, Jacobs recorded an instance in which a young woman received fir-power while in a dream. The power then led her to certain medicinal plants, which she was able to use in her curing practice. Another young man likewise described receiving fir-power, which gave him the ability to hunt.[50] As Smith notes, "a strong tie [was] felt to exist between an individual and power: people were strong because of their power and strong people got more or stronger powers. . . . Pride, gruffness, a fondness for berries, any such personality differences, were connected with certain animal or bird powers or inanimate objects in nature. . . . Other traits, such as the ability to remain a long while under water, to be a good hunter or wood worker, were likewise related to similar capacities of animals or birds. These often had specific reference to economic pursuits."[51] Hence certain spirit powers were considered to accompany those with particular traits. For instance among the Puyallup and Nisqually, individuals with wolf power were excellent hunters, someone with a tree power was likely "attractive and a good singer," and likely "to lead on social occasions," while someone with snake power might be antisocial and needed to live apart from others.[52] Alternatively, cedar power might gift one with the power of canoe building, clam power for clam digging; root power might give someone the gift for finding and digging roots, while a spirit of a burial canoe support-post might signal one's gift for retrieving lost souls.[53] Virtually all strengths and weaknesses could be associated with one's relationships with spiritual beings. As Elmendorf wrote regarding the Skokomish Twana, "In this culture all human success and failure, skill and mediocrity, received their explanation in terms of personal relations or lack of relations with supernatural beings."[54]

What is essential to note here is that spirit powers were traditionally acquired through great effort, that every individual of good upbringing would go out in search of such a spirit power, and that such spirit powers then enabled one to fulfill one's role within the community.[55] Spirit powers served material, practical purposes—empowering one to be a leader, a hunter, a healer, etc. One's sense of self as part of one's community, one's working identity, was intrinsically bound up within these spiritual relationships. Sustaining such relationships meant sustaining who one was, and the role one could play within one's community. The loss of such relationships meant the loss of personal meaning, sustenance, and responsibility. Finally, such relationships provided a strong sense of connection and interdependency between an individual and the surrounding spirit-filled landscape: to be who you were meant to be, to have the spiritual power to fulfill your role in your community, required that you maintain these spiritual relationships, and that required being ritually engaged with the natural world.

Spirits of Places: Syowen and Personal Spirit Powers in Contemporary Religious Practice

Forming an individual relationship with a spirit power, *syowen*, was the central experience of Chinook and Coast Salish religious life. Syowen were sought out through vision quest experiences or received through initiation rites. In the contemporary context, many individuals continue to cultivate relationships with spirit powers, honoring them during winter spirit dances. The tradition has certainly transformed in many ways: it is relatively rare to receive a spirit power through vision quest today, according to Bierwert and Amoss, who explain that most contemporary Coast Salish encounter them in dreams or visions, often during times of illness, grief, or emotional distress. And as demonstrated in the previous chapter, such spirits are usually inherited from one's ancestors. For those in the contemporary context who participate in traditional religious practice, these relationships become an enormously important part of one's life and personal identity, providing strength, healing, direction, and wisdom throughout life.

Syowen continue to be associated with specific places and entities within the natural world. When encountered in a dream or vision, spirits can take the forms of plants, animals, natural phenomena, monsters, or spirits of the dead, though all spirits can appear in a human form if they will.[56] Syowen are "strictly localized."[57] Spirits might be found within any number of animal species, atmospheric conditions, or places within the landscape, like lakes or oddly shaped boulders.[58] Because places provide "the abodes of spirits," this tradition is "mostly about place . . . in this world and in the afterworld."[59] This experience of syowen in particular locales reaffirms a people's connection to place.[60]

In a way that appears consistent with nineteenth-century traditions, contemporary Coast Salish do not describe syowen as abstract energy or impersonal forces of nature but rather as having personhood, agency, and hence the ability to be in relationship with human beings. Crisca Bierwert makes the case for this most clearly (in a rhetorical move that is unusual within the anthropological world) when she argues that contemporary Coast Salish social life is not merely a human affair but involves "wholly and unequivocally—relationship to other sacred beings that have agency in and of themselves." What makes her approach so distinct is that she does not reduce syowen to a product of culture or of individual or collective imagination but argues instead that we take Coast Salish perspectives seriously. And such views suggest that syowen are something real, something that exists apart from human experience. To think of syowen as anything other than "autonomous being," she writes, "is to drain it of the vital force that it effectively has."[61] While previous studies have argued that the power of syowen resides in its function as a cathartic coping mechanism (Jilek), or as a tool for social organization (Amoss), Bierwert insists that syowen "figures actively in these stories, not as something to fill a gap, but as something struggling for recognition."[62] Having witnessed the profound effect that spirit dancing can have toward transforming an individual's life, Bierwert was led to conclude that rather than a psychological coping mechanism, syowen is "an autonomous agent. . . . If this is religious solace, it is a personified solace and a personal one, that of an intimate partner. Syowen requires a relationship and attention to itself in exchange for its attention to the dancer." Rather than catharsis, this is "cathexis—that focused, directed attention and love" that requires interpersonal relationship.[63] In a similar fashion Kew and Kew have argued that the power within Coast Salish spiritual leaders to heal "stems from a source that is external to and separate from [the healer] himself."[64] If we take Coast Salish perspectives seriously, we must allow that syowen is not a figment of imagination, or psychological wish fulfillment, but something present and aware.

Importantly, Bierwert also argues that this agency, this awareness "inheres in what we would call the natural world."[65] Hence the landscape itself, animated by spiritual presence, is alive. As she puts it, places can "have agency, intelligence and will."[66] The Coast Salish landscape that Bierwert describes is one animated by spiritual presence, syowen. "The river rocks, the mountains, the salmon runs, the flow of the river itself" all serve as sentient beings to be reckoned with.[67] This view of the landscape as imbued with spiritual presence that is conscious and aware leads Coast Salish individuals, Bierwert writes, to refer to the landscape and its resources as part of their social community.

The use of the term *si:le*, meaning "grandparent," is indicative of this. Si:le is "used by Halkomelem speakers and other Sto:lo elders to describe natural things and beings." For instance, "the mountains are your si:le. . . . All living things, they are all si:le. And the rocks too, even the little rocks. Everything there is si:le, to be respected." When she inquired about the practice of referring to a local mountain as "grandmother," she was told quite simply that "the Mountain *is* a lady" and should be respected as such.[68] It is this "relational sensibility" that marks Coast Salish perspectives toward the natural world. Syowen are persons. And as such they have (as Eugene Hunn puts it) "intelligence and will, and thus have moral rights and obligations as PERSONS."[69]

Reflecting this sensibility is the way in which Coast Salish refer to these relationships with deep affection, as something private and personal. During her time with the Upper Skagit, June Collins described this sensibility as individuals spoke about spirits that had been inherited from ancestors within the same family. Their attitude, she writes, "was not so much one of fear or awe, unless the spirit was displeased, but rather of affection and intimacy."[70] The "central theme" of Coast Salish religious practice, as Collins experienced it, was "the deep, warm, lasting, personal relationship between each individual and his own guardian spirit."[71] This is a kind of intimacy similar to that of one's family. While syowen are not associated with the souls of one's ancestors, they are often inherited from one's ancestors, thus associating them with one's kin relations.

Further, the relationship between an individual and his or her syowen can be described as a kind of adoption: a *created kinship* relationship. Seaburg and Miller note that among the Tillamook (the southernmost Coast Salish culture), all spiritual beings could become "special kinds of human-like relatives by adoption."[72] Amoss noted this as well, explaining that the Nooksack shared in common with other Coast Salish a view that humanity is not "a part of nature but rather is set apart from it. In order to exploit his natural environment successfully a person needed to establish lines of communication with the nonhuman realm," by creating kinlike relationships with sentient beings in the natural world.[73] Describing the creation of a relationship with syowen as adoption into a family is no small thing, in light of the importance of kinship relationships within the Coast Salish world. Such relationships provide emotional and material support, as kinship means a lifetime of reciprocal obligations and mutual care between the individual and his or her spirit power. And it means an insurance of safety to travel into the other's territory. In this case, this means that the supernatural has access to venture into the human realm and the human person may travel safely into the supernatural.

In the contemporary spirit dancing tradition these relationships are primarily maintained through spirit dancing, though some spirits also call upon their adherents to reject alcohol or certain kinds of foods, wear particular regalia, or engage in regular early morning bathing.[74] While individuals might receive a vision of their spirit power in childhood or adolescence, they generally put the experience aside until adulthood, when they might be made ill by spirit sickness. Such illness was a sign that one's spirit power was ready to be acknowledged, and the cure was to demonstrate one's spirit power at a winter dance.[75] Failure to do so could result in chronic illness or even death.[76] *Smíłə*, or spirit dancing, takes place during the coldest months of the year. Small dances may be relatively private affairs made up of close family, while large dances may welcome visitors who have traveled hundreds of miles from far-off villages and reservations. Every dancer is given the opportunity to perform, from the most vulnerable to the least vulnerable: new initiates ("babies") precede veteran dancers. Women precede men. Visitors precede locals.[77] Hosts provide food for all the guests before and after dancing. Elmendorf was told by Frank Allen (Skokomish), that "the real reason why people worked so hard in the summer and put aside all that food—more than they needed—was to feed their c'ša'lt (guardian spirits) when they came to them in the winter."[78] While the food at a winter spirit dance was technically used to feed guests, not the spirits themselves, it was in effect the same thing. The dance itself is what feeds the spirit, and the dance cannot be undertaken without the presence of one's extended community and family, who must be fed. Dancing maintained these vital spiritual relationships, embodying them before one's community and extended kinship network.[79]

In return for being "fed" and honored through winter spirit dances, syowen empowered individuals to achieve their working identity. The ability to be successful in life or in particular endeavors was largely dependent upon one's ability to gain and maintain a "life-long partnership" with a spirit power.[80] Here power is understood not as political or social influence but rather as "a manifestation of largely unspoken human-nonhuman relations."[81] By cultivating such a relationship, through spirit dancing and singing of a spirit song, individuals received gifts that enabled them to succeed. Success then stood as "evidence of good relations with spirits, and people who did attract the favor of powerful spirits expected to be effective in human society."[82] Indeed, "all success involved a spirit and human bond."[83] While particular spirits were associated with particular vocations (woodpecker with woodworking, snake with weaving, etc.), in the contemporary context this is less often the case. Instead, syowen often empower more generally, offering strength and healing.[84] Success, health, physical prowess, and material wealth can signal the presence of syowen in one's life. And, as demonstrated in the previous chapter, such success is made evident through "hard work and abundant provision" for the family.[85]

Preserving a Sacred Landscape

Establishing a relationship with syowen and maintaining that relationship throughout one's life requires access to the natural world. Not only are syowen themselves located within particular places, but the means to honor them ceremonially requires particular resources, such as old-growth cedar. Because the place-based nature of spirit powers requires spiritual practices within the natural world, the well-being of the natural world is necessary for Coast Salish religious and cultural traditions to survive. For instance, Bierwert explains that contemporary Coast Salish religious practices include "bathing, visiting old growth cedar, and finding physical connection in the streams, rocks, and other inhabitants of the mountains that surround the river valleys. The cleansing power experienced in these practices stimulates the cleansing power of longhouse healers. . . . Sto:lo people see these as dwelling places for other beings, and longhouse people consider themselves to be part of this larger community, belonging to it rather than claiming it as their own."[86] Michael Kew makes a similar case, arguing that "a requirement of spirit dancing is wilderness." And indeed, in the wake of the American Indian Religious Freedom Act of 1978, Washington tribes and Upper Sto:lo bands have worked together with Mount Baker–Snoqualmie National Forest representatives to inventory sacred sites so as to enable their protection.[87]

Before his death in 2005, subiyay (Gerald Bruce Miller), the late spiritual leader of the Skokomish Nation, made impassioned pleas for the protection of cedar forests and ecosystems.[88] According to Miller, old growth cedar forests function as holy shrines for the Skokomish and are a tangible connection to their ancestral history. "Because many of the old growth Cedar predate the coming of the white man, they are our link to more pure times before the land was desecrated and razed. . . . We need a place where old growth trees, especially the Red Cedar, live along with young trees; where we know our shrines will be unmolested; where we can obtain Cedar for ceremonial purposes; where we can go for retreat and meditation with our Grandmother, the Cedar; and where we can take our spiritual baths unmolested."[89] CHiXapkaid (D. Michael Pavel), subiyay, and Mary Pavel point out that cedar plays a central role in Coast Salish ceremonial life: the longhouses are made of cedar, spirit dancers bathe in cedar forests, scrubbing their bodies with cedar boughs; they burn cedar as incense to cleanse ceremonial spaces; cedar bark nests are used to house spirit songs; initiate regalia and other paraphernalia are made from cedar wood and cedar bark; and young people are trained about medicine plants in cedar forests.[90] As Miller concludes: "Protecting the environment is essential, because the Skokomish spiritual philosophy focuses not on events but on relationships with entities like the earth, water, air, animals, and plant people. Maintaining this symbolic connection is important to the survival of our traditional culture, because a spiritual relationship with other life forms pervades all aspects of our life."[91]

Amoss has argued that by the end of the nineteenth century, when many communities in Washington had moved away from their home territories and relocated onto reservations, the relationship between religion and place was substantially strained.[92] The loss of ancestral lands brought practical challenges: what does one do if spiritual power is found in places, and one cannot get to those places?[93] Indeed, spirit dancing has survived best where communities were not displaced but able to stay close to ancestral homelands, as among the Upper Skagit and in British Columbia, where Coast Salish communities were often granted small reserves on the sites of their traditional villages, rather than being relocated to larger reservations.[94]

This is not to say that contemporary communities do not feel a keen connection to place. Indeed, this is one of the most common sentiments expressed by individuals at ceremonial gatherings, whether spirit dances, first salmon ceremonies, or welcoming the canoes to shore during the Canoe Journey. Taqʷšəblu herself described her son's questing for power in the late twentieth century, emphasizing that it required a profound kind of interaction with a particular place on the Skagit River. This remained true despite the fact that she and her family had lived away from the Skagit River for most of their lives.

> Everything about the river was spirit help: the ripples in the water, the whirlpools and the eddies. These things were recognized by the people as their help. People would bathe in the river when they were looking for their spirit help. It had to be unpolluted, clear, cold water. My son had to do that even just a few years ago. He'd come up out of that water and his hair would freeze with icicles. So it's a discipline and you have to have a mindset that says, "my body is going to endure this. I'm doing this for a special purpose."[95]

Despite (or perhaps because of) the fact that Taqʷšəblu and her family spent much of their lives away from these places, living in urban centers like Seattle, returning to these places during times of religious practice and purification took on the significance of holy pilgrimage.

Contemporary beliefs and practices surrounding syowen have changed since the nineteenth century.[96] One is far more likely to receive a spirit from inheritance rather than on a vision quest. And access to the landscape where such spirits live has become increasingly at risk. But the sense remains of syowen as an active agent, with the ability to empower and transform the individual. What we begin to see more clearly here is that a healthy self with a healthy working identity is defined in part by its relationship with spirit powers, which are tied to and part of a natural environment. Syowen empower individuals to take up their working identity: they fundamentally shape one's sense of self. And in the process, syowen create and reinforce relationships with the landscape from which syowen come. The "self" here is thus one that is interrelational with the natural world. Such relationships are earned by individual effort and personal practice. This is an individual, private spiritual life—but one expressed in public settings and dependent upon community support. To the extent that this remains the case for contemporary Coast Salish communities, then, successful healing practices must work to protect the natural environment and restore one's relationship with place.

9. "A Power Makes You Sick"

Illness and Healing in Coast Salish and Chinook Traditions

> The soul recovery ceremony is about healing, it's about recovery of the soul that was stolen. . . . We're going to bring it back. . . . We're not bringing it back for a theatrical production, we're bringing it back because our people need it.
>
> —CHIXAPKAID (D. Michael Pavel)

I have argued that the experience of illness is culturally specific, informed by local understandings of what it means to be a healthy self. Physical cures may be part of this process. But the more salient element within many healing systems is the renewal of the self, restoring the individual to a sense of self that *works*. Earlier chapters have described Coast Salish and Chinook perceptions of a healthy working identity, and this chapter addresses how illness and healing are understood within Coast Salish and Chinook worldviews. I discuss three kinds of illness and healing within Coast Salish and Chinook traditions: spirit sickness, disease-causing spirit powers, and soul loss. These various expressions all share a sense of health as a dynamic balance of personal autonomy and relational reciprocity. As such, they are spaces wherein traditional healing practices restore interpersonal relationships at the same time that they help sufferers gain a clearer sense of themselves as autonomous individuals.[1] Healing, therefore, occurs wherever this dynamic balance can be restored. It is important to note here that by interpersonal relationships I do not mean a merely human community but a community comprising spiritual beings as well: the plant and animal people within the surrounding landscape. Hence this is spiritual work. Healing requires ceremony, symbol, and ritual as a means of reconciling these complex and at times conflicting demands.

First, a caveat: in attempting to provide a synthesis of traditional Coast Salish and Chinook views of illness and approaches to healing, I emerge with a generalized overview: not everything here is true for every Coast Salish or Chinook community. Healing traditions differ from individual to individual, from family to family, from community to community. What I hope to offer in the pages that follow is an overall view of these traditions, tracing common themes and perspectives that are commonly held throughout the region.

"This Is What My Dream Tells Me": Healing and Spirit Sickness

If the healthy embodied self is in part defined by spiritual and human relationships, how might these relationships, once broken, be restored? Within Coast Salish and Chinook traditions of the nineteenth and early twentieth centuries, healers played an important role, gifted as they were with the ability to discern the initial cause of illness and provide a means for mending it. Through the use of herbal medicines, simple rituals, or complex ceremonies, healers sought to restore an individual to physical wellness. But they also worked to restore a healthy sense of self. This meant restoring a clear sense of individual identity and personal autonomy, while simultaneously affirming one's responsibilities toward one's kin and community.

HEALERS AND HEALING TECHNIQUES

Observers from the nineteenth century frequently attested to the remarkable skill of indigenous herbalists, most of whom were women. Alexander Ross, for example, described the "Keelalle," among the Chinook on the lower Columbia, "whose office it is to administer medicine and cure diseases." Even early Euroamerican observers, who generally discredited Native healing traditions, admired Coast Salish and Chinook herbalists, allowing that they were "a serviceable and skillful class of people. Their knowledge of roots and herbs enables them to meet the most difficult cases, and to perform cures, particularly in all external complaints."[2] The work of herbalists was accompanied by a complex spiritual tradition, including particular prayers and formulae to be recited when gathering plants, both to ensure their efficacy and to express gratitude to the plant and plant people. When herbs were administered, they were also often accompanied by prayer and song.

If herbal remedies were not effective, patients might seek out the services of a medicine man or woman, to discern the spiritual causes of illness.[3] Historical texts suggest that people of significant power who worked as healers within their communities were believed to have certain abilities: they could see things that were far away or things that were within a body; they could even see "a pain-power inside a person. That is why (they know) whatever sickness (it is) that has made him (a patient) ill"; and they could locate souls that had wandered far away.[4] A Clackamas Chinook narrative describes a female healer with a similar ability. The healer "saw that perhaps the sick person had been going somewhere at night in a bad place, perhaps by some cemetery somewhere. A shadow (a "dark thing" which is of dead persons or of their things) had covered him. Now then, she thought, 'That is what I shall do to this (sick) person.' They made pitch brands, sometimes they tied together five of them."[5] Following this prescribed ritual the patient was cured, and the "dark thing" was removed. Some healers also had the power to use the sgwədilič, a cedar divining board, still in use today. As Taqʷšəblu (Vi Hilbert) and Crisca Bierwert explain, the "sgwədilič was given to the Indian to heal the illness that would afflict people.'"[6] Sgwədilič is "a spirit power which some individuals earned by questing and occasionally by inheritance." It empowers owners to "see with the 'spiritual eye' to diagnose an illness or perform other tasks which the sgwədilič has the ability to perform."[7] Those who have the gift of the sgwədilič are able to examine a space, such as a dance house, and perceive the presence of disease powers.

Demonstrating the personalized nature of religious practice in this region, healers each had their own technique and method for treating patients.[8] Guided by their individual spirit powers, healers had their own dance and their own songs. Some might use a hands-on approach, touching or massaging the body. Others might only sit still and sing. Some used smudging, stones, or cedar divining boards such as the sgwədilič.[9] Some would take compensation, others not. As one individual explained: "This is what my dream tells me, 'you do not want to ask for compensation. If you take pay you will not have your power. That is why you are not to take pay when you try to cure a person, (you are to work) for nothing for a while. That is what my dream has told me. That is why I doctor for no pay."[10] Healers followed the directions of their individual spirit powers and, as a result, crafted individualized modes of healing, the goal of all being to honor their spirit power and maximize their strength and spirit for curing. Such healing techniques reflect the individualistic nature of Coast Salish religious life, dependent as it is upon an individual relationship with a spirit power that provides personal inspiration and guidance.[11] This can be compared with more formalized traditions that might be found among the Pueblo and Diné of the American Southwest, for instance, where healing rites are carefully prescribed, and each word and symbolic gesture is carefully recreated for each ceremony, without deviation. By contrast, Coast Salish traditions on the whole might be described as more variable, less centralized, charismatic rather than following prescribed structures.

Just as healing techniques were highly personalized, so was knowledge of particular spirits. Traditionally, each healer "knew" certain types of spirits and could make use of such personal knowledge to cure or injure. For instance, if rattlesnake power had caused an illness, a healer who had an established relationship with a rattlesnake spirit power could best effect a cure. Consider an account recorded by Melville Jacobs, in which a healer had to be found who "knew" the spirit power that caused an illness. Because of his knowledge of the particular power, this healer was able to remove the illness.[12] Disease power could also be lost control of, if the individual did not have a strong enough relationship with the spirit power that controlled it, and hence was extremely dangerous.[13] Healing ability was thus not a generalized power or ability but one premised on particular relations with specific spirit powers. Healing was both an expression of one's highly individualized spiritual life and at the same time completely dependent upon interrelationship with spiritual beings.

SPIRIT SICKNESS: BEING CALLED TO DANCE

Within Coast Salish and Chinook traditions, when first called to honor one's spirit power, an individual may suffer from what has been termed "spirit sickness." A Skokomish Twana elder described it this way to ethnographer William Elmendorf: "Any power makes you sick that way when it first comes to you. And you have to have a doctor, and he finds out what is wrong and opens a way so that power can come to you. When it comes to you, you know what is happening but can't help yourself, your power will sing from inside of you and work your jaws and make you talk and say things to people, whatever it wants to say: he is giving you sickness, your power."[14] An individual suffering from spirit sickness might be called to undergo initiation into a longhouse winter spirit dancing society. Honoring the spirit power publicly would cement a relationship with it and restore the individual to wellness.

The source of illness here appears to be the strain placed upon one's relationship with a spirit power when it is not being recognized and honored: health depends on that relationship staying healthy. As Smith notes, "Failure to meet the ceremonial requirements of one's power caused a friction which resulted in the illness or ultimate death of the human who was thus stubborn in refusal. Weakness of the body through fatigue or physical illness might cause the power to become detached or dislodged, a state, again, which involved illness and ultimate death if the power could not be recovered."[15] Jacobs observed this among the Coos as well. As one woman explained: "When her dream becomes too strong for her, if she (a healer) does not tie it together (dance publicly) she becomes ill. If the other watcher does not put it for her (help her) she may die. That is why she ties it together (dances) again. That is the reason why the shaman has the power increase dance again, because she is afraid (of becoming ill and dying)."[16] A Clackamas Chinook individual made a similar statement, telling Jacobs, "'That is why the people were fearful,' (of unhappy consequences if a new spirit-power was not sung and danced, at once, by its recipient). 'They would sing it at once; they would make him (sing and) dance (it at once). Then he would quit' (get through five nights of such singing and dancing)."[17] During such dances, all those present dance their own spirit dance, honoring the spirit power with whom they have a power relationship, adding strength to the healing of the initiate, and bringing the entire community's collective spirit powers together to assist in the healing process.[18] A milder form of such spirit sickness might recur annually, necessitating the individual's participation in winter spirit dances. According to one Skokomish Twana elder: "Your power calls by and sees you every winter. I don't know why, but tamanawis comes strong in the winter. Every winter your power will come to you and make you sick and you have to sing it and feed it and dance with it this way: your power has come into you now."[19]

When an individual suffers from spirit sickness the self is potentially overpowered by the spirit in question: the line between self and spirit has blurred, and the individual may be overwhelmed. Spirit dancing both affirms one's relationship with that spirit and distinguishes between one's self and the spirit. One's spirit power is "tied down," in a sense, allowing the individual to differentiate self from spirit power. Both historically and today, the process of initiation into the longhouse dance society and of dancing at annual gatherings serves to address this imbalance. The vitally important relationship between individual and *syowen* is thus recognized, reinforced, and ritually "fed." For those active in this tradition, such ceremonies are essential for one's continued health, wellness, and ability to function within community.[20] Winter spirit dances are powerful spaces of healing, reaffirming individuals' relationships with their own spirit powers, strengthening community and familial bonds, and providing a space to affirm publicly the working identity one is meant to embody within community.[21]

Winter spirit dancing provides a means by which the dynamic tension between personal autonomy and collective reciprocity is maintained. Bruce Granville Miller has argued that contemporary

Coast Salish society "is still fundamentally built around the idea of personal connections with spiritual entities or guardian spirits, which, once encountered, impart gifts or skills to humans. For this reason, Coast Salish people have been characterized as individualists par excellence."[22] At the same time that these traditions emphasize the importance of the personal and individual, participants in spirit dancing also depend upon the collective, particularly their extended family, to maintain these private spirit power relationships through ceremony. When one becomes ill with spirit sickness, it requires a *public* performance. Entering into the trance state necessary to perform one's spirit power requires the support of elders within the tradition as well as the spiritual presence of other dancers. The expense and ritual expertise necessary for sponsoring such an event require the support of one's family and community.[23]

Contemporary spirit dancing also creates relationships and social ties that extend beyond one's immediate family. A new dancer when first initiated into the longhouse is closely mentored by an elder for guidance through the first year as a spirit dancer. The initiate and initiator develop a close bond that "endures for life."[24] During this first year, the initiate is referred to as a "baby," and the mentor as "mother" or "father." Throughout their lives, whenever an initiate's "father" or "mother" hears the person preparing to sing, the mentor might come to provide support, walking alongside or joining the group of drummers and singers who surround the dancer. And when several individuals are initiated at the same time and undergo the period of supervision and care in the same longhouse, "a sibling-like bond is formed among them. . . . They know each other's songs and feel an obligation to help" fellow initiates when they dance.[25] Since most mentors and co-initiates are not blood relatives, the spirit dance longhouse provides an arena in which an individual's circle of kinship expands even further into these adoptive relatives. Such relationships have both spiritual and material consequences, as being part of the longhouse dance community binds individuals together within relationships of assistance and reciprocal exchange.[26]

Amoss has argued persuasively that both the Shaker Church and winter spirit dancing help resolve "the conflict between individual autonomy and kin solidarity," by providing dramatic space for individual spiritual fulfillment within a supportive group atmosphere.[27] Amoss goes on to identify three core values within Coast Salish society: "personal autonomy, kin solidarity and differential social status," and argues that "conflicts among them are resolved in the winter ceremonial complex."[28] Spirit dancing provides individuals with personal spiritual power, but it is expressed in a way that reinforces kinship ties and the exchange of resources. Spirit dancing is also preceded by "work," potlatch-like gatherings where personal status and rank are affirmed, but these occur within the community and are affirmed by the exchange of gifts. As she explains, being initiated into the spirit dancing tradition serves to resolve "the contradiction between the principles of rugged individualism and of mutual support, cooperation, and interdependence of kinsmen."[29] While spirit dancing appears to reinforce the Coast Salish value of personal autonomy and privacy, its very nature also embodies a profound sense of interdependency.[30]

Crisca Bierwert makes an important addition to Amoss's analysis, arguing that spirit power (syowen) triangulates the dynamic between individual and community. The relational dynamic here is not a dualism of self and collective but a triad of person-spirit-community. Syowen is experienced personally but is also inherited from and deeply interconnected with one's ancestors and place. Syowen provides a means for autonomous individuals to construct their own private means of relating to their ancestors, their place, and their community. The private nature of syowen provides a respite from a deeply kin-based community filled with reciprocal obligations, even while the fact that syowen comes from an ancestral landscape and lineage reminds one of one's place within that network of relations. When spirit dancing provides relief from spirit sickness, it does so not just by restoring a clear sense of identity and purpose but through the establishment and maintenance of a relationship with a living spiritual presence.

Within traditional Coast Salish and Chinook worldviews a different kind of spirit sickness can also result from offending one's spirit power. Offense might be caused by inappropriate actions, including traveling in dangerous places, having sexual intercourse at improper times, drinking too much water, walking near burial grounds, or hunting in a disrespectful manner.[31] Dreaming of something negative could also make one vulnerable to a disease power, particularly if one did not follow proper forms of behavior after such a dream. One Clackamas Chinook female healer, after doctoring a woman's eyes, suggested: "Possibly you dreamed of some bad thing (that is, a disease spirit-power came to you), and the following day you did not swim. Than you ate, you drank water (when you should have been fasting). It is this thing right here (a disease spirit-power) which is staying in your heart. It is swinging your head, although you may be supposing that your eyes are hurting you."[32] In this instance the ailment must be addressed both by restoring a fractured relationship with a powerful spirit and by carefully differentiating self from the spirit that may be "staying in your heart" and "swinging your head."

Failing to fulfill one's spirit-power-inspired role within one's community could also cause illness. If one was empowered to hunt or to heal, and failed to fulfill that task, one's spirit power might withdraw, and the individual would become ill. Elmendorf recorded one instance in which a Twana healer explained: "I've discovered that woman's tamanawis [spirit power] way up the mountain—dəxw'wa'kw' (Mt. Rainier). Now this woman's power has got mad at her because she never came to the mountain to pick berries. Her power was (a berry-picking power), it belongs to that mountain, and the purpose of that power is to pick berries. And that (power) got mad at that woman because she never went to the mountain to pick berries. That's the food of that power—berries. And now he had left that woman and made her sick."[33] Such traditions are significant for what they tell us about Coast Salish and Chinookan views of the self. A healthy self is one that is fulfilling one's working identity, embodying the role that it has been given. This is the identity of an autonomous individual, one who has been empowered with particular skills through a very private relationship with a particular spirit power. At the same time, individual identity is dependent upon relationships with nonhuman persons in the natural world, and individual status is earned not through self-interest but through demonstrations of responsible interactions with one's human community. The spirit power is a key part of this healthy working identity, an intimate bond between the self and the natural world. A breach in that relationship fundamentally compromises one's personal identity and vocation within one's community. Only restoring that relationship and embodying the identity it provides—fulfilling one's vocation—could cure such an ailment.

Healthy communities depend upon every individual properly honoring her or his obligations. If individuals honor their spirit powers and the gifts that those spirit powers offer, then the community will have healers, skilled hunters, basket weavers, fishermen, and herbalists. But if any of these obligations are not met, the health and well-being of the entire community is put at risk—important roles will not be fulfilled. As Amoss points out, because spirit dancing enables an individual to be a healthy, fully functioning member of the community, participation in the tradition is a source of general concern, even if the exact nature of one's participation is private.[34] Hence illness itself is a threat not merely to an individual, "but also to the others in the family who must take over his duties and finance the necessary curing ceremonies," and to the community who loses the gifts that person would otherwise bring.[35]

"The Poison Power of Some Person": Embodying Social Conflict, Restoring Relationships

A second spiritual cause of illness within traditional Coast Salish and Chinook worldviews are disease-causing objects or spirit powers thrown or shot into a person by an ill-intentioned individual. Reverend Myron Eells recorded in the 1880s that the Squaxin and

Skokomish blamed illness on a sickness power that had been sent out "in an invisible manner," by "wicked medicine men," which must then be removed.[36] In some instances the person who sent out the illness had to be identified, so that the individual could be cured and the social tensions removed. As one individual related to him: "It is the arrow (or bullet) poison-power of some person (which is in him)." When the individual was found, she was brought to and doctored the patient, removing the poison-power. The individual shortly thereafter fully recovered.[37] Jacobs recorded another instance in which a would-be rapist attacked a young woman. After successfully fending him off, she returned home but later grew ill and died. Her family soon discovered that her attacker had sent a poison power upon her, causing her death.[38] Such "hate magic" could also be used between entire communities, and according to Elmendorf was historically "commonly substituted for aggressive open warfare or raiding" among some groups.[39] In such instances, patients' bodies became the locus of social conflict, as medicine people and their spirit powers fought for dominance. Here illness signifies broken relationships, expressed through physical and mental disorders. Smith describes the Puyallup-Nisqually tradition in this way:

> A shaman could send his power, or it could wander without his volition, in search of powers weaker than itself which it might conquer. Having found such a power, the *tudáb* entered the man or woman to whom it belonged. "It just got into him." The conflict which ensued between his own and this foreign power made that individual sick. Another shaman had now to be called in to dislodge the foreign power from the man whom it had invaded and to restore his health. With the curing ceremony the conflict shifted, the patient became passive and the foreign power and that of the curing shaman continued the struggle. If the curing shaman was the stronger, he removed the invading or foreign *tudáb*, recognized it, once he had held it in his hands, and sent it back to 'its master.' If the foreign power was stronger, the patient died. . . . Struggles between powers were going on constantly. Every accident or misfortune was viewed in light of such attempts.[40]

Traditionally, because anyone who possessed a spirit power could potentially cause illness, individuals were encouraged to treat one another with care and caution. Indeed, fear of retaliation in the form of illness was a strong motivation for social solidarity. As Bruce Granville Miller has argued, the private nature of one's relationship with spirit powers, and their "emphasis on secrecy" regarding those relationships, served the vital purpose of "reinforcing the cultural emphasis on the individual" and balancing "obligations to the collectivity."[41] At the same time, as Alexandra Harmon explains, this secretive nature of spirit powers served to encourage individuals to treat one another with respect and courtesy, "in case he or she 'had something.'"[42] As Miller argues, it is this deeply personal nature of Coast Salish spiritual experience and personal commitment, reinforced by a "non-interference or privacy ethic," that grants a remarkable degree of privacy and freedom to the individual, thereby helping to eliminate those tensions that can arise within close-knit community living.[43]

Given the potentially lethal consequences of interpersonal animosity, social cohesion was an important deterrent to illness. When social networks broke down, or individuals fell through the cracks, the results could be dangerous.[44] This is reflected in a Kalapuya narrative involving a young orphan boy who had acquired the grouse guardian spirit while alone in the woods. The young boy, grieving over his loneliness and lack of family, and feeling unwelcome within his community, decided that he, along with his entire community, should die. "He stood to his dance" for five days, then returned home and slept for five days. "Now a sickness came (it was some type of diarrhea in which blood was passed), and all the people then became ill. They never got well; all who had become ill died. When they doctored them they never got well, a great many of them died." Healers determined that the boy and his grouse guardian spirit were to blame.[45] This narrative, told as a historical tale, happening "a long time ago," offers an ethical warning of the danger of broken human relationships. The community failed to welcome and support the orphaned child, and illness was the result.

Acting appropriately toward others, with kindness, generosity, and social decorum, was important to prevent such crises. Other stories attest to this as well, such as a Nehalem Tillamook story recorded by ethnographer Elizabeth Jacobs. Here, a young man brought an epidemic illness upon his community by breaking several important social rules: he had sexual relations with a "wild woman" who lived in the woods and then refused to marry her. The woman came to his village, lifted her walking stick toward the village, and immediately caused them all to become ill and die.[46] Or consider another Tillamook narrative of disease origin, providing a similar warning to individuals who might stray from traditional value systems. In this story, South Wind traveled to the area and placed his daughter "on the highest mountain near here." Before returning to his home in the south, he told her: "When our children become too mean, when too many of the people are being mean here, you will stand upon your mountain and raise your hand like this [palm outward], and you will say just one word. I will see you from the South, and I will answer you with one word. Our words will fly to meet each other and everywhere as they go there will be disease and people will die off.'"[47] This narrative reminds the people of their traditional obligations to their human, ancestral, and natural relations and their responsibility to maintain and honor their traditional heritage. The ethical violation in this story is "being mean," acting without generosity and kindness toward other living beings.[48] Hence inappropriate actions or offense to human or spiritual entities might bring about illness, even though the resulting symptoms may not manifest for some time. As one Clackamas Chinook individual pointed out: "One doesn't just become ill all of a sudden, it happens a long time ago. It is not a mere nothing. He is poisoned (by a lethal spirit-power). That is what is doing it to him."[49]

Disease and disease-causing spirit powers can manifest as semimaterial objects that a skilled healer can acquire, send out, clean, repair, set straight, call back, even steal. But unlike objects, these spirit powers are manifestations of dynamic relationships with sentient beings. Jacobs provides a Clackamas Chinook example of this:

"'Maybe some person did like that to her (put a poison power in her). The disease-power is right in here wriggling, just like a trout. This sickness is here just like a little fish (or small salmon). I have tried to catch it, but it slips by my fingers. It goes by and high up, it is swimming and wriggling around, and it is so large and slithery that I cannot reach it.' He did extract maybe two or three (other) disease-powers (which were smaller and were also in her); he killed them (one at a time). I gave him water in a pan, he blew on it (to weaken it after he had extracted it); he drowned the disease-power in it (in the water in the pan) there, before he killed it in his mouth. All done. Then he halted." The healer took no payment since he was a relative of the patient, and returned the next day to try again. Again he was unsuccessful, and, as he predicted, the patient died shortly thereafter.[50]

When successfully removed, the disease power might be cleaned, turned right, and restored to the individual as a spirit power, or it might be killed, discarded, or sent far away. Another Chinook narrative explains it this way:

> He is not doing this just for nothing. His spirit-power is doing like that (it has left him). You may say to me, what shall I do to him? Shall I remove the disease-power (which is inside him causing his illness)? Shall I throw it away? Or shall I replace it inside him? He sang, and when all done and following that, then he removed the disease cause. Sometimes he washed it (in order to cool and weaken it or merely clean it), and gave it back to him, he fixed it well. Now he sang. On the other hand sometimes he threw it (the disease power) away, he put inside some other (power). And then, that is the way he (the patient) would also sing.[51]

Such healing performances give flesh to social conflict as healers struggle against and seek to overcome a disease sent out from another individual or community. As such, they powerfully embody the tension between individualism and communalism. Removing invasive disease objects or helping individuals to "tie up" a spirit power that threatens to overwhelm them reaffirms Coast Salish values of autonomy. Healing rites that tangibly remove a disease-causing object help the individual to distinguish clearly between self and disease. The actions delineate a clear line between *you* and *not you*, helping to restore a patient to a clearer sense of self.[52] At the same time, restoring fractured relationships between those individuals, their spirit powers, and other members of their human community affirms the interrelational nature of Coast Salish identity. A medicine person was benefited by the presence of the patient's family and community: their physical presence and participation in song strengthened the healer, while the necessity of participation by community reinforced an awareness of interdependency with one's kin, and a sense of one's identity as a self-in-community.[53]

Respect for social relations as a source of health and well-being extended to plant and animal people as well: oral traditions described the importance of treating plants and animals with respect, lest individuals bring illness and death upon their communities. Many stories involved salmon in particular, such as those mentioned in the previous chapter, illustrating the significant interdependence of people and salmon, and the necessity of maintaining good relationships and careful respect for the salmon people. Jacobs, for instance, recorded one narrative in which young boys playing disrespectfully with some salmon caused a tidal wave that killed their entire community. "That is why it is not a good thing when children do all sorts of tricky things. You are not to do such things. You should not belittle food, because the people die (from that)," the storyteller explained.[54] Such modes of respect and obligation affirm the important interconnection between human and natural communities: respect and healthy relationships are foundational for survival. Traditional healing and spiritual practices in the Puget Sound and lower Columbia thus rely upon a notion of the embodied self as an autonomous individual embedded within a network of relationships and obligations: with spirit powers, with the natural world, and with human communities.[55]

Illness beliefs provide a means for negotiating and expressing fractured relationships, and because of this, social conflicts and tensions can be embodied and performed in healing ceremonies.[56] As George Guilmet and David Whited have pointed out, precolonial healers were not merely concerned with healing the individual but were also "responsible for dispute resolution, the integration of marginal individuals into society, and the establishment and interpretation of the meaning of existence." They were "necessary for the maintenance of daily social order."[57] If illness was caused by disrespect, improper behavior, or breaches in relationship, then healing and hope stemmed from the restoration of these relationships. And hence, when healers nearly vanished in the aftermath of epidemic diseases and colonial pressures of the nineteenth century, their loss was felt not just in terms of healthcare. Rather, their absence tore at the ethical and normative systems that had held communities together.[58]

"Fire and Sparks Falling Down": Soul Loss and a Working Identity

Even as some illnesses might be caused by a failure to recognize and protect the profoundly interrelational nature of the self, other ailments might indicate the loss of a clearly defined, distinct, autonomous self. An individual consumed by grief, overwhelmed by spirit power, or otherwise lacking a clear sense of identity is at risk for another kind of sickness: soul loss. Within both Chinook and Coast Salish traditional beliefs, individuals have a varying number of "souls," or different spiritual aspects of the self, one or more of which can wander or be stolen from the body, resulting in sickness or death.

According to both Suttles and Elmendorf, among the Skokomish Twana "a living and well human being contained a life soul (shəlé) and a heart soul (yədwás)." Elmendorf explains that "souls of the living were dual. Each individual possessed two souls, a life soul, and a heart soul. The life soul was a miniature image of its owner, about the length of a finger, and of fog-like consistency. It had its seat in the head and could leave or enter the body through the top of the head or breastbone. One informant stated that the life soul 'gathered together' in the head when it was about to leave the body in miniature form, but that normally it filled the entire body of its owner."[59] The life soul was immortal, while the heart soul died with the body. Life souls journeyed to the land of the dead by way of an underground trail. They remained in the land of the dead for a time, before journeying on to a second land of the dead, from which they might be reborn as an infant in the world of the living. Interestingly, Wayne Suttles and Barbara Lane note that "an infant dying in this world could leave this cycle of rebirth and become a parent's guardian spirit."[60]

For the Central Coast Salish, a living healthy person had "life" ("šxwhəlí"), "person" ("sməstə'yəxw"), "mind," and "shadow." Life and person were immortal, while mind and shadow tended to die along with the body. After death, one of these aspects of the self might become the "spəlqʷioaʔ" or "ghost." Ghosts might linger around one's grave or one's living family members, and periodically need to be "fed" food and clothing, which were offered at ceremonial burnings for the dead. Encounters with ghosts were (and are) considered dangerous and must be managed with ritual care. These ghostlike aspects of the self will eventually depart for the land of the dead, or might choose to be reborn with one of their descendents.

Any of these aspects of the self can leave the body during life, though it is usually the part of self described as one's "person." Such a departure can be temporary and benign, as in dreams and visions, or it can be more dangerous, as when it is "lured away by dangerous beings or the dead." It is the responsibility of medicine men and women to pursue such lost souls and return them to their bodies. Failure to do so can be lethal.[61] One nineteenth-century observer of Chinook communities put it thus: "They regard the spirit of man as distinct from the living principle, and hold that the spirit may be separated for a while from the body without causing death and without the individual being conscious of the loss. It is necessary, however, in order to prevent fatal consequences, that the lost spirit be found and restored as soon as possible."[62]

While particulars varied from group to group, there was a shared sense that contact with the dead, excessive grief or trauma, alienating one's spirit power, incurring the anger of a powerful person, or inappropriate thoughts or actions could cause soul loss.[63] Amoss explains that "souls could be lost by a sudden fright or by a strong attraction to a person, place, or thing. They could also be stolen by a hostile shaman or snatched away by a ghost or the dead in general."[64] One is particularly at risk if in a "weakened condition, physically, emotionally or ritually."[65]

If an individual's soul wanders too far from the body and becomes lost, the condition can be fatal.[66] One twentieth-century Chinook healer described a man whose spirit had wandered too far to be recovered: "Maybe he left us long ago now. We are just looking merely at his skin. Earlier perhaps we might have brought him back, but he has departed for too long a time."[67] Within Coast Salish Lushootseed traditions, the progression of the disease can be slow and gradual. First "the person began to wither, weaken, and languish, sleeping all the time and becoming colder and colder. Friends and family noticed a growing lethargy that soon became total unless desperate measures were taken and a specialist was consulted. Everyone knew that untreated soul loss was fatal."[68] According to Chinookan traditions, if the soul has drunk water in the land of the dead, has stayed away from the body for too long, or strayed too far, the patient will die. One reason given is that the soul has grown too small for the patient's body and will not be able to fill it anymore.[69]

RETRIEVING A LOST SOUL

Individual healers can restore a lost soul, if it has not been lost for too long or wandered too far.[70] As Eells notes regarding the southern Coast Salish: "Sometimes before a person dies, it may be months, it is supposed that a spirit comes from the spirit world and carries away the spirit of the person, after which the person wastes away or dies suddenly. If by any means it is discovered that this has been done, and there are those who profess to do it, then they attempt to get the spirit back by a tamanous, and if it is done the person will live."[71] Boas described one late nineteenth-century Chinook tradition in which "each person has two souls, a large one and a small one. When a person falls sick the lesser soul leaves his body. When the conjurers catch it again and return it to him he will recover." Boas described the Chinook soul as resembling "fire and sparks falling down," and explained that it departed toward the west, the direction in which healers and their spirit helpers went to retrieve it.[72] Sampson has likewise described Coast Salish views on the subject: "A man might walk on the earth, apparently in good health, yet his spirit might have been a long time with the dead, in which case he might die after a short illness, or just drop dead. . . . If the spirit of the living was taken to the Second Spirit World it could be brought back to the owner only by a trip to the spirit world by the medicine man."[73]

While singing their power song such healers travel the paths of the dead, gather up the lost soul, and return it to the patient. Elmendorf described one such event among the Skokomish Twana:

> And now (the doctor) came back with that sick man's shal˙ɛ́ (soul) and Tyee Charley stopped singing. And he told the people that his power had brought the man back all right. And he reached out in the air and took that man's shal˙ɛ́ from his power and held it in his cupped hands and then he put it on the man's head and stroked it in, without touching him. And he passed his hands up and down that man's body . . . and now that man stopped raving and talking wild, and he sat up and looked around him. And that man told the people, "I don't know what I was doing. Where was I?" And he was all well now.[74]

In particularly complicated cases, a more elaborate ceremony, the *spəłəʿdaq*, sometimes referred to as a soul retrieval ceremony or a spirit canoe ceremony, was held. This ceremony, described at length by Jay Miller, involved a team of healers who undertook a heroic journey to the land of the dead to recover the patient's lost soul.[75] Suttles describes a similar ceremony, writing that it was held at night, in front of large audience. Singers brought a spirit board painted with the image of their spirit power, a painted staff, and carvings of "earth dwarves" who would accompany them during their spiritual journey.[76] The spirit boards and other carvings were placed upright in the earth to outline a rectangle. The healers then stood within it, singing songs, and paddling as they pantomimed their spiritual journey to dead.[77] During a multinight ceremony the healers dramatized their journey, including encounters with ghosts, angry spirits, and various obstacles along the way. Eventually, they were able to outwit the spirits of the dead, outmaneuver the various obstacles, and retrieve the lost soul.[78] One Twana elder described a version of this ceremony to Elmendorf:

> When it comes on winter, if a number of people have been ailing, not looking good for some time, one of the relatives of an ailing person organizes a *sbəɬəda'q* to get the souls of those people back from the dead. All the families of the sick people pay to feed the crowd that gets together, and they pay to get doctors who bring the souls back. They have one doctor for each one who is sick, and each doctor brings back one soul. Some other people may go along just for the trip. . . . They only do the *sbəɬəda'q* in winter, and it takes four to six nights.[79]

If the healers are successful, when their "guardian spirits meet the soul, they turn it around, and the patient recovers at once."[80] While these elaborate ceremonies fell out of use in the early twentieth century, they are being revived among some contemporary communities. Consider for instance the art installation *Soul Recovery Ceremony*, by subiyay (Gerald Bruce Miller, Skokomish) and his nephew CHiXapkaid (D. Michael Pavel, Skokomish), included in the 2009 exhibit *S'abadeb—The Gifts: Pacific Coast Salish Art and Artists* at the Seattle Art Museum. The piece is a recreation of the ritual paraphernalia that would have been used in the ceremony, including the spirit boards and carvings of the earth dwarves who grant soul-recovering powers to healers. CHiXapkaid explains the significance of the piece:

> The ceremony is about healing, it's about being able to draw upon one's capacity to heal the people . . . clearly one of the purposes was to recover the soul that was stolen by one of the ghosts in the land of the dead. . . . The very purpose of this installation is to announce that we are bringing this ceremony back, that we have people in our community such as sm3tcoom, and other Indian doctors, who are quite familiar with all aspects of this ceremony, for they deal with it every time they're asked to heal. They know the songs, they know the procedure, they know the protocol, and we're going to bring it back. . . . We're not bringing it back for a theatrical production, we're bringing it back because our people need it.[81]

Soul loss is a powerful representation of how a compromised self can lead to illness. In a way that is indicative of Chinook and Coast Salish understandings of the healthy self, one is at risk of soul loss when one has lost a clear sense of who one is, when one's personal autonomy has been challenged. In such instances the boundaries of one's self have been breached, and one's identity as an individual has been severely undermined. A soul might begin the long journey to the land of the dead, for instance, "if someone hurt that person's feelings so badly that he or she wanted to die." Being away from home, or in a transitional state such as adolescence or old age, where one may lose a clear sense of self and purpose, also puts one at particular risk. "In other words, being out of place, in any sense, was a spiritual hazard."[82] One might also lose a clear sense of self through overattachment. For instance, being deeply in grief because of the loss of a loved one can put individuals at risk of losing themselves. If a mourner could not let go of the departed, the person's soul would be lured away by the ghost of the loved one, beginning the journey to the land of the dead before the mourner's time. Because of this, surviving spouses "and other close members of the family observed strict rules during the period of mourning." June Collins describes one such instance she observed during her time with the Upper Skagit in the 1970s: "I saw one young woman who was suffering soul loss after the death of her husband. She walked and sat with her head hanging down, did not appear to see others, and did not speak. She did not eat. In this case, her soul was returned to her; she lived for some years longer."[83] In all these instances it is the loss of a clear sense of personal identity, autonomy, and purpose that can put a person at risk.

At the same time one is also at risk of soul loss when interpersonal relationships are fractured. Rather than seeing the self as purely an independent isolated self, Chinook and Coast Salish worldviews insist that the self is defined by relationships. Because of this, offending others, whether one's spirit power or one's neighbor, could be potentially lethal. Offending a spiritual entity or another person might inspire that spirit power to seize one's soul. For instance, Franz Boas noted among late nineteenth-century and early twentieth-century Chinook that "when a person is angry at another, he engages a seer to watch for his enemy. If he finds him asleep he takes out his soul, which he hides in a graveyard, under the house, or in rotten wood. Then the person falls sick. His friends pay a conjurer to look for his soul. . . . If the soul is still unhurt the sick one will recover. If the conjurer's guardian spirit has eaten of it, he will die."[84] In this instance, social conflict translated, literally, to the dissolution of the self. The soul wandered and became lost, and the physical, mental, and spiritual self suffered as a result. Like the story of Lady Louse cited at the beginning of chapter 7, soul loss speaks to the danger of broken relationships and the importance of restoring them with care. Soul loss as a mode of diagnosis and cure reinforces values of social responsibility and the importance of maintaining a healthy balance of relationships. And it is a powerful metaphor for the loss of self that illness can bring and the vital necessity of restoring the person to a working identity.

A description and analysis of a contemporary soul recovery ceremony by Michael and Della Kew provides an example of the way in which such healing traditions are about restoring a sense of self. Kew and Kew describe a small family ceremony, performed informally in the patient's home. In contrast to the more elaborate soul retrieval ceremony, intimate healing ceremonies such as this are generally "held on short notice and are small in scale, being contained within the restricted social setting of the family and the private dwelling."[85] These events, geared toward the restoration of an individual's soul, are concerned with both self identity and the person's role within a family and community. Through song and drumming, the healer discerns the source of the patient's illness. He concludes that part of her has become lost, and in her weakened state bad things have settled upon her. He explains that one of her ancestors is calling her, and wanting to lead her soul away. The healer works over her body, removing those negative influences which are affecting her. To do so, he makes "upward sweeps culminating in a sudden pull from the region of the mouth and nose of the patient," which "are followed by wiping from the top of her head down to her neck, then forward to the mouth and free," or "from each shoulder to the hands and ending with a pull from the finger tips." His actions are accompanied by singing and drumming. Later, having retrieved the part of her soul that has become lost, the healer makes a "slow and deliberate gesture, picking something up in his cupped hands," and then releasing "them with a spreading motion before her face." Kew and Kew explain that "this is a motion which returns the shadow or part of Mary previously placed before her, into her actual body."[86] The effect of these songs, prayers, and ritual actions is to help the patient regain a sense of who she is and who she is not: to reclaim her true working identity within her family and community.

At the conclusion of the ceremony, the healer explains to the patient and her friends and family, "You know, people need help like that you folks gave this poor lady here today. People need friends, it makes their minds strong. Because, you know, the mind can weaken the body. The body can be strong all right, but something can hit that strong person's mind and his body will fail. . . . Something, some small thing even, could lift her mind and she would be strong. It's good to have friends like this, we all need them."[87]

Kew and Kew explain that while the healing ceremony focuses on one particular individual's need to reestablish a strong sense of personal identity and purpose, the rite is still "pre-eminently a social rather than a private ritual, despite the fact that the supernatural powers involved are private and personal." Rather than a "private therapy session behind closed doors," the healing ceremony includes patient, healer, spirit powers, and the patient's friends and family.[88] They observe that "we who are bit-players come away feeling supportive and supported," the healer "teaches about the importance of the context of friends and kinfolk in which all of us live. The patient as an individual is cleansed and made whole, and she and her family are brought into harmony. The day before the gathering she is disturbed and alienated, when we arrive she is ill in bed, and before we depart she is seated in her kitchen, restored and surrounded by her family."[89]

Illness is dangerous, but it is also an opportunity for spiritual recovery and growth. Through the journey of illness, individuals have the chance to regain a working identity, a sense of who they are meant to be and the role they are meant to play in their community. A moving illustration of this can be found in the life story of Taqʷšəblu (Vi Hilbert), Lushootseed elder and one of the most important figures within contemporary efforts to preserve Lushootseed language and culture. After suffering an aneurysm, Taqʷšəblu slowly recovered. As a friend recalled, she recovered from the ailment as a changed person with a renewed sense of purpose and calling. "She did regain her beauty, her quickness of speech and her amazing energy. But while she was sick she found, as according to her traditions her people do, a different vision of who she was to be. Out of the many threads of her former life, she selected those that were most important and laid the others aside. Preserving and perpetuating her people's language and culture, something she had only tentatively pursued before her illness, became a guiding principle for her."[90] Healing, then, does not simply end at the removal of an ailment or the elimination of pain. It is instead a re-forming of the person as a whole, a renewing, and perhaps a discovery, of one's working identity.

Conclusion

The Case of Ellen Gray, Reconsidered

In 1883 Reverend Myron Eells recorded the following account of a young girl's death:

> Ellen Gray was a school girl, about 16 years of age, and had been in the boarding school (at Skokomish) for several years, nearly ever since she had been old enough to attend, but her parents were quite superstitious. One Friday evening she went home, to remain until the Sabbath; but on Saturday, the first of January 1881, she was taken sick and the nature of her sickness was such that in a few days she became delirious (she suffered from the suppression of menses). Her parents and friends made her believe that a bad tamahnous had been put into her, and no one but an Indian doctor could cure her. They tamahnoused over her some. The Agency physician Dr. Givens, was not called until the sixth of January, when he left some medicine for her, but it is said that it was not given to her. Hence, she got no better, and her friends declared that the white doctor was killing her. The Agent and teacher did not like the way the affair was being maneuvered, took charge of her, moved her to a decent house near by, and placed white watchers with her, so that the proper medicines should be given and no Indian doctor brought in.
>
> The Indians were, however, determined if possible to tamahnous and declared that if it were not allowed, she would die, at three A.M. They kept talking about it, and she apparently believed it and said she would have tamahnous, but it was prevented, and before the time set for her death, she was cured of her real sickness. (Her menses returned.) But she was not well. Still, the next day she was in such a condition that it was thought safe to move her in a boat to the boarding house, where she could be more easily cared for. The Indians were enraged, and said

that she would die before landing, but she did not. Watchers were kept by her constantly, but the Indians were allowed to see her. They talked to her, however, so much about her having a bad tamahnous, that all except her parents were forbidden to see her. They also were forbidden to talk on that subject, and evidently obeyed. But the effect on her imagination had been so great that for a time she often acted strangely. She seldom said anything; she would often spurt out the medicine when given her as far as she could; said she saw the tamahnous; pulled her mother's hair; bit her mother's finger so that it bled; seemed peculiarly vexed at her; moaned most of the time, but sometimes screamed very loudly; and even bit a spoon off.

Sometimes she talked rationally and sometimes she did not. But by the fifteenth she was considerably better, walked around with help, and sat up when told to do so, but did not seem to take any interest in anything. Everything possible was done to interest her and occupy her attention and she continued to grow better for three or four days more, so that the watchers were dispensed with, except that her parents slept in the room with her. But one night she threw off the clothes, took cold, and would not make any effort to cough and clear her throat and on the twenty-second she died, actually choking to death. It was a tolerably clear case of death from imagination, easily accounted for on the principles of mental philosophy, but the Indians had never studied it, and still believe that a bad tamahnous killed her.[1]

Throughout researching and writing this book, I was haunted by the story of Ellen Gray. As this story makes clear, illness narratives *matter*, they have profoundly material and physiological repercussions. When conflicting narratives about health and the body are forced to confront each other, the experience is jarring, disruptive, and can even be violent. In such a confrontation each side can perceive the other as an extreme threat—and perhaps for good reason. This story describes a conflict between fundamental perceptions about the nature of the self, in which Native healers and Euroamerican missionaries competed for the lived-identity of the young Ellen Gray. To some degree, the mortal consequences each side feared were justifiable, on a cultural as well as physiological level. Eells wanted to change radically the personal and cultural identification of Miss Ellen Gray: he wanted to transform her sense of self, cutting her off from the spiritual relationships that would otherwise have defined who she was and who she was meant to be within her community. We may not even know her real name, being told only the English name she likely received at the boarding school. Her Coast Salish family and community were not ready to surrender the young woman to this cultural conversion, and nor, it appears, was she ready herself.

Eells and Ellen Gray's family understood her sickness in profoundly different ways. For Eells the disease was the girl's "suppression of menses." If forced to define her "illness" in Kleinman's terms, Eells would likely have said that it was the girl's refusal to abandon completely her old way of life. The "old superstitions," as he saw them, had instilled in the girl irrational fears, playing on her weakened physiological state, such that she refused to listen to "reason." The end result, he sadly concluded, was her death at her own hands, the self-imposed "death by imagination."

By contrast, Ellen's family and community had very different perspectives on her illness. As the last section of this book emphasizes, kinship and community were and remain central within Coast Salish and Chinook notions of the self. Salish and Chinook social relations, habitation, subsistence, wealth, status, religious traditions, and healing practices all depend upon healthy relationships with one's extended family and with the sentient beings abiding within the natural world. Coast Salish and Chinook healing traditions work to locate the individual within that network of relations, even as they craft a strong sense of individual identity and autonomy. This story presents us with a sense of how profoundly dangerous it could be to disrupt that dynamic balance. Ellen Gray's relationships with her family and community, as well as with the spiritual beings that inhabited her ancestral landscape, were intrinsic to her sense of self. When those were lost, the consequences were tragic.[2]

Eells was perhaps operating from the best of intentions: certain that her only option for survival lay in assimilation, Eells did everything in his power to remove Ellen Gray from her culture and community. He himself recognized that this separation was not easy, that it created sometimes irreparable damage to the interpersonal relationships of the children involved. He wrote elsewhere regarding the plight of his young Native students, noting that when they returned home, "the old folks say: 'your education and civilization are a splendid thing for you, when they make you so above your parents and relatives that you cannot treat them politely. Religion is a pretty thing, isn't it, when it leads you to treat us so.' So with all their honest efforts they are between two fires, and it is a hard place for them. Some get discouraged and fall back into the old ways."[3] Raised for years in this context, Ellen Gray had been alienated from her own family and community and the cultural traditions that defined them as a people.

It was this conflict, a spiritual battle of wills, that was now being played out within the body and spirit of Miss Gray. Forcibly removed from her community, imprisoned and guarded by "watchers," Ellen Gray was allowed to see her parents only when they had agreed to silence. They could not speak to her of their traditional beliefs. While they could be present to care for her physiologically, they were forbidden to address what may well have been the underlying cause of her illness: broken relationships, fractured identity. She was detached, isolated, her access to family regulated by Eells and guarded over by external authorities. For Ellen's family and community her illness would have been seen as a tangible expression of social conflict, and the "bad tamahnous" a manifestation of her inner discord. Her working identity was fractured, and the relationships that formed her as an embodied subject (relationships with human, fish, plant, and animal persons) had been strained to the point of breaking. Her soul needed restoring. The conflicted emotions inevitably arising out of such self-division became apparent as soon as she was allowed home. Her "hysteria" disrupts her physiologically, emotionally, spiritually. As far as her traditional family was concerned, the diagnosis appears to have been clear: soul loss, the result of disease-causing spirit powers. And from a Coast Salish perspective, the only cure would be spiritual intervention, the reweaving of the threads that tied her to kin, both living and deceased, and the spirits within her Native land base.

This is the story of a lost soul, a fractured identity. And what that identity *should* have been differed wildly, depending on whom one might ask: Eells, her parents, her community, or Ellen herself. For Eells, "death by imagination" was not an expression of the powerful forces underlying Ellen's beliefs, but of her "throwing off her clothes," and "refusing to cough or clear her throat." For Ellen Gray and her community, however, the healthy embodied self was one that existed in balanced reciprocal exchange with human, spiritual, and ecological relationships. These relationships had been disrupted, blocked, and perhaps irreparably damaged. For Ellen Gray, that was the true and dire illness, and her choking to death was the outward expression of a self that was offered no means of expression, reconciliation, or renewal. With no help given, Ellen Gray grew violent, lashed out at her mother, and embodied the broken sense of self that she felt internally. Finally, her choking to death, neither able nor allowed to speak, reflects with painful clarity the dire consequences that the destruction of one's working identity can have.

The words "death by imagination," if nothing else, demonstrate that illness narratives are not simply fairy tales. They have *real* implications, profound power, and they reflect even more powerful underlying lived-body experiences. Ellen Gray could not be easily divorced from her cultural surroundings, from the expectations and understandings she was given about the world. Our embodied experience *is intensely* affected by the ways we have been taught to see and interact with our world.[4] The working identity of this young woman was an inseparable combination of her physiology, her cultural and communal self, and her lived-body, and attempts to rend them apart had tragic consequences. The very foundations of Coast Salish and Chinook health and wellness were directly challenged by their experience with colonialism: epidemic disease, the loss of land and political autonomy, the suppression of Native cultures, religions, and languages, the removal of children to boarding schools, and the loss of commonly held land and extended family homes under the allotment system (among many other factors) worked to undermine Coast Salish and Chinook identities, families, and communities. This story and the many others told throughout this book help to illustrate an important point. When the foundations of a people's identity are undermined, regardless of intentions, the consequences are a form of cultural genocide. Symbols, philosophies, religious practices, social systems, political structures, subsistence activities: these form the basis for health and well-being when they inform the basis of the self. My point is that culture loss has material, physiological consequences for health and wellness. Concurrently, cultural and religious revival and the restoration of tribal sovereignty also have material implications for contemporary Coast Salish and Chinook healing and renewal.

Navigating Cultural Currents

Ellen's story is a tragic one, but it is not the place to end. Her story does not tell of the many ways Coast Salish and Chinook individuals found to negotiate and navigate the tricky currents of life in the colonial Northwest. Religious life underwent great changes in the nineteenth and twentieth centuries, as spirit power traditions inspired prophetic leaders, the Indian Shaker Church emerged as a new healing tradition, and winter spirit dancing saw a remarkable revival. The Shaker Church would soon flourish in Ellen's community, offering a means of healing and reconciliation—though not soon enough for Ellen herself. In the Shaker Church Native people from throughout the region would begin to rebuild a sense of a working identity that maintained their worldviews, ethos, and sensibilities, even as they incorporated Euroamerican symbols and practices.

In the contemporary context a wealth of new cultural and religious resources exist to assist young people in negotiating complex and sometimes competing identities. Coast Salish and Chinook communities are taking control of their healthcare, bringing together western biomedicine, holistic care, and traditional approaches to spirituality and wellness. While the approaches found in contemporary tribal wellness centers might appear very different from the guardian spirit healing traditions of the ancestors, they share in common a sense of what it means to be a healthy self, to have a working identity.

In 1989 the Paddle to Seattle revived an ancient tradition of summer intertribal canoe journeys along the Northwest Coast and Puget Sound. Since then the event has grown to include hundreds of canoes and their crews from throughout the Pacific Northwest. It has become a major event, inspiring thousands of Native people to reaffirm a sense of pride in their heritage and to lead healthy, sober lives. It is both profoundly modern and profoundly traditional. In 2006, for instance, the journey included a special canoe: the Pink Paddle Canoe, an intertribal effort "manned" by breast cancer survivors and their supporters. In a moving illustration of the union of traditional culture and contemporary healthcare, the team raised awareness of breast cancer prevention, even as they celebrated the renewal of canoe culture on the Northwest Coast. Such an event stands alongside the work of SPIPA's Women's Wellness Program and the Shoalwater Bay tribal community's Wellness Center as powerful illustrations of the ways in which contemporary communities are navigating a path between two cultures. As Charlene Krise (Squaxin Island) has suggested, the Canoe Journey can be seen as a modern soul recovery ceremony. As in the spirit retrieval ceremony of the nineteenth century, the people are pooling their physical and spiritual strength and undertaking an arduous journey to retrieve the soul of the people. What has been lost is being recovered, with great struggle, great effort, and the collaboration of all the people.[5]

If one were to look only at historical narratives such as the story of Ellen Gray, one might conclude that Coast Salish and Euroamerican views of what it means to be a healthy self are so fundamentally at odds that the imposition of one must imply the death of the other. Yet if this is the case, how can one make sense of neocolonial identities that are multiple, hybrid, fluid, flexible, and contingent? Can contemporary Coast Salish and Chinook identities be *both-and*, rather than *either-or*? To be more specific: can contemporary tribal communities integrate non-native approaches to health and wellness without doing damage to local Native understandings of what it means to be a healthy self?

The answer is a resounding yes.

As demonstrated here, by complicating the nature of subjectivity to envision a self of exchanges, obligations, and shared identities, the self is not lost but is seen within its intricate whole. The political possibilities of the self are maintained but not as a Cartesian master-subject. Rather, we can consider a notion of self that comprises community and a shared identity that makes political mobilization, survival, and healing possible. These are identities that are hybrid, adaptive, and vibrantly creative but that are built upon a continuous core of "tradition": a shared sense of what makes for a healthy self and a working identity.

Effective approaches to health and wellness within this contemporary context require some means of resituating the autonomous individual within a complex and extensive web of kinship relationships. These relationships include both close and distant relations, the living and the dead, and are symbolized by receiving inherited names, songs, spirit powers, or other rights and responsibilities. These relationships also include the ancestral landscape, as well as *syowen*, the animating spirits found within that landscape. Syowen help to shape one's identity, empowering one with particular gifts and abilities, as well as offering comfort, strength, and healing when needed. While syowen have an existence, personhood, and agency all their own (much as one's human relations do), they nonetheless play a key role in shaping one's individual identity and in effect can be considered to be a part of the self.

At the same time a healthy self is also one who is an autonomous individual demonstrating an ethic of hard work and self-sufficiency. Coast Salish religious life reinforces this value of the individual, centering on one's intimate, private relationship with a spirit power, expressed through a uniquely personal spirit song and spirit dance. While one's spirit power might enable one to succeed in life and achieve high status within one's community, the individual's success and status is expressed through an ethic of generosity, sharing, and interrelatedness with one's kin. Traditions surrounding illness and healing reflect this tension. Illness can stem from broken relationships or from a loss of a clearly defined self, and in such instances healing requires the restoration of balanced relationships and of a healthy working identity. The view of the healthy self that emerges here is that of an autonomous individual who is deeply rooted within a network of human and spiritual relationships and the responsibilities those entail.

It is through ceremony that the tension between individual autonomy and group solidarity is brought into flesh and blood performance. Private events like spirit dancing and public events like first salmon ceremonies and the Canoe Journey reveal core values and help to reconcile competing tensions within Coast Salish communities. Ceremonies work to articulate "ultimate existential concerns" as well as ongoing problems and conflicts within the community.[6] For the Coast Salish these ultimate concerns include communitarian values: the priority of kinship, of generosity, of interrelationship with the natural world. At the same time they also embody the cultural premium placed upon personal autonomy, privacy, and individual achievement and honor. Ceremonies work to reconcile these deeply individualist needs and concerns with those of one's community and extended kinship network. These ceremonies illustrate how such competing values are integrated and demonstrate the ways in which individual Coast Salish identity is strongly shaped by one's affiliation with a collective extended family and/or tribal group.

While individualism has often been seen as being intrinsically incompatible with "Indian communalism," the Coast Salish experience demonstrates that this is not the case. Quite the opposite: they are "ultimately inseparable."[7] As Bruce Granville Miller has argued, Coast Salish views of the individual, rather than reinforcing indifference and self-interest, "embed ideas of responsibility to the larger community, rather than primarily serving as a tool for the defense of the individual against the power of the collective."[8] A contemporary Nisqually woman, for instance, when asked about ceremonial activities within her community, explained: "We just have a lot of dinners . . . and a lot of get-togethers. That's a ceremony in itself. . . . We have got some four generations of living on Frank's Landing as a family . . . and I think that is a ceremony in itself."[9] From complex soul recovery ceremonies to a simple family meal, Chinook and Coast Salish ceremonial traditions help the individual navigate the currents of community, kin, and personal responsibility.

Understanding and considering indigenous views of wellness and the embodied self are absolutely vital for the creation of healthcare systems that will be truly effective in meeting the needs of Native people. Addressing health from a strictly biomedical point of view misses the issue entirely. If we are to move beyond *curing disease* to *healing illness*, practitioners must consider what it means to be healthy within the community in question. The greatest health risks faced by American Indian communities today are the results of fractured identities: broken communities, severed ecological relationships, soul loss. These can take the form of alcoholism, domestic violence, diabetes, heart disease, sexually transmitted diseases, violent and accidental deaths, and rising cancer rates, often due to environmental toxicity.[10] I hope the analysis presented here can join a broader ongoing conversation about Native healthcare, culture, and what it means to construct culturally relevant healthcare programs. If nothing else, I hope that this book has made a strong statement advocating for local tribal control of health and wellness services and in support of self-determination and sovereignty. Contemporary Native communities have the necessary tools and strategies for combating contemporary health risks, tools that they have maintained, though in continually modified forms, throughout the centuries.

Notes

Introduction

1. Myron Eells, missionary to the Skokomish, Squaxin, and Nisqually, in Castile, *Indians of Puget Sound*, 419–20.

2. See for example Csordas, *Sacred Self*; Law, *Religious Reflections on the Human Body*; Lewton and Bydone, "Identity Healing in Three Navajo Religious Traditions."

3. Geertz, *Interpretation of Culture*.

4. Tillich, *Theology of Culture*, 41–42.

5. Jaimes Guerrero, "Civil Rights vs. Sovereignty," 101.

6. This is a demand that many feminist researchers have taken into account as well. As Diane L. Wolf has written, "The most central dilemma for contemporary feminists in fieldwork, from which other contradictions have been derived, is power and the unequal hierarchies or levels of control that are often maintained, perpetuated, created, and recreated during and after field research. . . . Research demands that the researcher give up some of these controls and share them with others." See Wolf, *Feminist Dilemmas in Fieldwork*, 2–3.

7. Wolf, *Feminist Dilemmas in Fieldwork*, 27.

8. See Bruce Granville Miller, *Be of Good Mind*, 10.

9. Boxberger, "The Not So Common," 76.

10. Suttles, "Recognition of Coast Salish Art."

11. Harmon, *Indians in the Making*, 116–17.

12. Guilmet and Whited, *People Who Give More*, 73.

13. Dixon and Roubideaux, *Promises to Keep*, 71.

14. Swinomish Tribal Mental Health Project, *A Gathering of Wisdoms*, 34–38, 44.

15. Swinomish Tribal Mental Health Project, *A Gathering of Wisdoms*, 61.

16. Dixon and Roubideaux, *Promises to Keep*, 213.

17. Dixon and Roubideaux, *Promises to Keep*, 206.

18. Dixon and Roubideaux, *Promises to Keep*, 224. It is difficult to determine precolonial cancer rates, given the lack of medical treatment, biomedical diagnosticians, and Native terminology for cancer as we understand it. Still, epidemiologists appear to be in agreement that cancer rates are on the rise among indigenous communities.

19. Wilkinson, *Blood Struggle*.

20. Swinomish Tribal Mental Health Project, *A Gathering of Wisdoms*, 22–24.

21. See Wilkinson, *Blood Struggle*, 169, 202–3. In 1999 this was expanded to include the treaty right to half the shellfish harvest as well.

22. While the Wheeler-Howard Act of 1934 (the so-called Indian New Deal implemented under John Collier) marked the first formal shift toward religious freedom for American Indians, it is the American Indian Religious Freedom Act of 1978 that has been the foundation for Native-led court cases seeking to defend their access to free exercise of religion.

1. Theoretical Orientation

1. Levi, "Embodiment of a Working Identity."

2. Kleinman, *Illness Narratives*, 13, 27.

3. Hahn, *Sickness and Healing*, 5.

4. Hahn, *Sickness and Healing*, 5.

5. Hahn, *Sickness and Healing*, 39.

6. Lupton, *Imperative of Health*, 69.

7. Kleinman, *Illness Narratives*, 23.

8. Mauss, "Les Techniques du Corps."

9. Csordas, *Sacred Self*, 6.

10. Douglas, *Purity and Danger*; and Douglas, *Natural Symbols*.

11. Coakley, *Religion and the Body*, 8. The work of Paul Ricoeur and Clifford Geertz is also quite important here, in their conceptualization of culture as a system of symbols. As the vehicle of enacting such symbol systems, the body becomes, almost by default, a key element of symbol and ritual. See Geertz, *Interpretation of Culture*; and Ricoeur, *Figuring the Sacred*.

12. In the late twentieth century, cultural theorist Pierre Bourdieu looked beyond ritual studies to the way in which modes of embodiment were situated within the general social context as the lived expression of unconscious modes of being, or *dispositions*, defined by the *habitus*, society's unconscious set of organizing rules. For Bourdieu, cultural action is thus both social and embodied: it is through embodied practice that the unconscious rules of social conduct become manifest. Bourdieu referred to the meeting of the individual and social self within *hexis*, or deportment, which he saw as the result of the coming together of one's subjective reality and the cultural reality into which one was born. Bourdieu, *Outline of a Theory of Practice*; Bourdieu, *The Logic of Practice*; Spivak, *In Other Words*. Csordas's work with charismatic Catholic faith healing is an excellent example of Pierre Bourdieu's work applied to a religious setting, wherein he explores mystical phenomena and the mystical setting as examples of habitus and hexis.

13. Foucault, *Madness and Civilization*; Foucault, *Birth of the Clinic*; Foucault, *History of Sexuality*; and Foucault, *Discipline and Punish*. Thomas Kasulis has agreed, writing that Descartes' construction of mind/body dualism accompanied the rise of Protestantism and the need for a notion of the self that could be justified by faith, apart from works, a self that could be saved without a body. He concludes that Descartes himself was a product of culture.

14. Foucault argues: "Not only the names of diseases, not only the groupings of coding systems were not the same; but the fundamental perceptual codes that were applied to patient's bodies, the fields of objects to which observation addressed itself, the surfaces and depths traversed by the doctor's gaze, the whole system of orientation of his gaze also varied." Foucault, *Birth of the Clinic*, 54.

15. Kasulis et al., *Self as Body in Asian Theory*.

16. Several distinct schools of thought have been identified within feminist theory with regard to the female body. A group that might be called Egalitarian feminists, including such authors as Simone de Beauvoir, Shulamith Firestone, and Mary Wollstonecraft, criticized gender dualisms that disempowered women, arguing instead that any "natural" differences between the sexes could be overcome; women could be equal to men. Later theorists argued for a deconstruction of social and political narratives inscribed on the body, insisting that the body itself was not the cause of social inequalities but that the discourses created about the body were the cause. Psychoanalytic feminist theorists could be found among these scholars. Marxist materialist feminists took a similar route but emphasized instead a focus on changing not the discursive expressions about bodies but the economic and material conditions that produced those narratives.

17. Denise Riley, *Am I That Name?*, 101.

18. Denise Riley, *Am I That Name?*, 102–3.

19. Denise Riley, *Am I That Name?*, 106. Italics hers.

20. Butler, *Bodies That Matter*, 10.

21. Butler, *Bodies That Matter*, 33. See for example Lindsey French, "The Political Economy of Injury and Compassion: Amputees on the Thai-Cambodia Border," in Csordas, *Embodiment and Experience*, 77.

22. Judith Butler writes, "Paradoxically, it may be that only through releasing the category of women from a fixed referent that something like 'agency' becomes possible." Butler, "Contingent Foundations," 16.

23. Butler, "Contingent Foundations," 13.

24. Jana Sawicki argues that power is defined by "relations that are flexible, mutable, fluid, and even reversible," while domination is "a situation in which the subject is unable to overturn or reverse the domination relation." Sawicki, "Feminism, Foucault, and 'Subjects,'" 170. See also David Hoy, "Critical Resistance: Foucault and Bourdieu," in Weiss and Haber, *Perspectives on Embodiment*, 19. Hoy argues that "power implies having more than one option open. . . . One could not speak of power unless one could also speak of freedom."

25. Foucault, *History of Sexuality*, 99.

26. Sawicki, "Feminism, Foucault, and 'Subjects,'" 161.

27. Foucault, *History of Sexuality*, 96.

28. Turner, "Bodies and Anti-Bodies," 30, 36.

29. Turner, "Bodies and Anti-Bodies," 44.

30. Ebert, *Ludic Feminism and After*, 77.

31. See Weiss, *Body Images*, 2.

32. See for example Elizabeth Grosz's discussion of Deleuze and Guattari, in *Volatile Bodies*, 164. See also David Abram's analysis of Merleau-Ponty's work in Abram, *Spell of the Sensuous*.

33. Glass, "Intention of Tradition," 300. Even the use of the word *colonialism* can raise questions here. On the one hand, one should not reduce to a single monolithic entity the enormously complex and diverse historical experience of more than five hundred years of history involving vastly different peoples with different motivations and agendas, operating in different times and places. Nor should the term be used to occlude the complex power relations that exist between people. At the same time the term can be necessary to call attention to the historical experience of "colonized" people, both for scholarly causes and for political mobilization.

34. For Marxist materialists, postmodern discursive analysis and Foucauldian power relations strip communities of the possibilities of genuine resistance or social change. Postmodern theorists counter that real change can only happen when a priori categories have been disrupted. Regardless, an important contrast exists between a notion of bodies as belonging to active individuals—individuals with agency and the ability to impact, react to, and modify their world—and a notion of bodies as objects, passively inscribed by cultural classifications, norms, and modes of being. See Lyon and Barbalet, "Society's Body," 56–57.

35. Judith Butler, quoted in Sawicki, "Feminism, Foucault, and 'Subjects,'" 166.

36. Deveaux, "Feminism and Empowerment," 216.

37. Bordo, "'Material Girl,'" 53.

38. Grosz, *Space, Time and Perversion*; and Grosz, *Volatile Bodies*; and Bordo, *Unbearable Weight*.

39. Grosz, *Volatile Bodies*, 19.

40. See Griggers, *Becoming-Woman*. For instance, Griggers argues, the sign systems of late capitalism have constructed a subject that is both constrained and productive, and by means of which contemporary inequalities are held in place. Paula Cooey's work on the role of religion and the body likewise presents a working solution. Religious ideas about the body and day-to-day body practices may not always appear identical. However, it is the space between the ideal and the lived that is useful. Cooey proposes that "we think of the body lived in relation to the body imagined as a testing ground or crucible, indeed in some cases a battleground, for mapping human values, as these are informed by relations of and struggles for power." Cooey, *Religious Imagination*, 9; Jagger and Bordo, *Gender/Body/Knowledge*.

41. Jenkins and Valiente, "Bodily Transactions," 176–77.

42. Maher, "Body Counts."

43. Crosby, *Columbian Exchange*; Cronon, *Changes in the Land*; Merchant, *Ecological Revolutions;* Valencius, *Health of the Country*.

44. White, *Organic Machine*.

45. Nash, *Inescapable Ecologies*.

46. Mittman, "Geographies of Hope"; Mittman, *Breathing Space*.

47. As David Arnold has observed in his work on the history of disease in British India, illness can play a significant role in the colonial process. As he argued, "Colonialism used, or attempted to use, the body as a site for the construction of its own authority, legitimacy, and control. In part, therefore, the history of colonial medicine, and of the epidemic diseases with which it was so closely entwined, serves to illustrate the more general nature of colonial power and knowledge and to illuminate its hegemonic as well as coercive processes." Arnold, *Colonizing the Body*, 8.

48. Bordo, "Bringing Body to Theory," 96.

49. Bigwood, "Renaturalizing the Body," 101.

50. Descartes, *Meditations on the First Philosophy*.

51. Welton, *The Body*, 3. See also Charles Taylor, *Sources of the Self*.

52. Haraway, "Situated Knowledges."

53. Scheper-Hughes and Lock, "The Mindful Body," 9. And indeed, Descartes himself was deeply committed to the development of what would become biomedical practice and devoted himself to the dissection and study of animal and human anatomy. See Leder, "A Tale of Two Bodies."

54. A telling testimony to the resiliency of Descartes' dualism can be found in a recent article in the *New England Journal of Medicine*, Sloan et al., "Should Physicians Prescribe Religious Activities?" In the article, a group of hospital chaplains and biomedical physicians and researchers conclude that religion and science should be kept separate. To mix the two will merely produce weakened versions of both. The authors conclude: "Religion and science, and religion and medicine, exist in different domains and are qualitatively different."

55. Haraway, "Situated Knowledges," 586.

56. Haraway, "Situated Knowledges," 581.

57. Haraway, "Situated Knowledges," 582, 589.

58. Haraway, "Situated Knowledges," 577.

59. Mohanty, "Under Western Eyes," 65. See for instance Spivak, *In Other Words*. Feminist women of color have issued strong critiques against white feminist theorists who have not written from an embodied location or recognized their own views as partial and limited. Chandra Mohanty has critiqued feminist theorists who, in writing about women of the third world, recolonize them through creating discourses that attempt to speak on behalf of women, creating totalizing images of women, ignoring heterogeneity, and denying them the ability to speak for themselves. Mohanty critiques authors who "discursively colonize the material and historical heterogeneities of the lives of women in the third world, thereby producing/re-presenting a composite, singular 'third world woman,' an image which appears arbitrarily constructed, but nevertheless carries with it the authorizing signature of western humanist discourse." Mohanty, "Under Western Eyes," 53.

60. See also Hartsock, "Postmodernism and Political Change," 48.

61. Hartsock, "Postmodernism and Political Change," 44.

62. Merleau-Ponty, "The Lived Body," 156.

63. Merleau-Ponty, *Primacy of Perception*; Merleau-Ponty, *Phenomenology of Perception*. Carol Bigwood describes Merleau-Ponty's work as "his attempt to recover a noncultural, nonlinguistic body that accompanies and is intertwined with our cultural existence, and thereby [he is] arguing for what I call the body's fleshy presencing in the world-earth-home." Bigwood, "Renaturalizing the Body," 101.

64. Csordas, *Embodiment and Experience*; Merleau-Ponty, *Primacy of Perception* and *Phenomenology of Perception*.

65. Csordas, *Embodiment and Experience*, 8.

66. Welton, *Body and Flesh*, 11–23, 95–121, 150–77.

67. See Abram, *Spell of the Sensuous*.

68. Merleau-Ponty, "The Lived Body," 168–69. He goes on to discuss his notion of "natural perception." This is "not a science, it does not posit the things with which science deals, it does not hold them at arm's length in order to observe them, but lives with them; it is the 'opinion' or 'primary faith' which binds us to a world as to our native land, and the being of what is perceived is the antepredicative being toward which our whole existence is polarized." Merleau-Ponty, "The Lived Body," 170.

69. Drawing from the work of Merleau-Ponty, Csordas has argued for a similar foundation of knowledge in embodiment rather than culture. The body, he argues, acts as a source of culture. Csordas challenges his readers to consider how individuals experience being-in-the-world, rather than the ways in which culture inscribes the abstract body. As he insists, scholars are less likely to move beyond the limits of Cartesian dualism "by writing *about the body* in its individual, social, or political aspects, than *from embodiment* as the preobjective condition of social life" (*Sacred Self*, 278). Csordas suggests we locate our inquiries in embodied experience, recognizing the importance of representation and language, but seeing it as distinct from being-in-the-world, "for it is the difference between understanding culture in terms of objectified abstraction, and existential immediacy." As he explains, there is a great deal of difference between a discussion of religious experience and the religious experience itself (*Embodiment and Experience*, 9–10, quote on 10).

70. Csordas, *Sacred Self*, 5.

71. Csordas, *Sacred Self*, 276.

72. As Christine Battersby suggests, "not all talk of identity involves thinking of the self as unitary or contained; nor need boundaries be conceived in ways that make the identity closed, autonomous or impermeable. We need to think about individuality differently, allowing the potentiality for otherness to exist within it, as well as alongside it. We need to theorize agency in terms of patterns of potentiality and flow. Our body-boundaries do not *contain* the self, they *are* the embodied self." Battersby, "Her Body/Her Boundaries," 355.

73. Or consider McKim Marriot's analysis of Ayurvedic medicine wherein he describes the *dividual body*. In contrast to the *in*dividual subject of the enlightenment, the body he presents is "a constellation of substances and processes that is connected to other bodies through a complex network of transactions." Holdrege, "Body Connections," 11. Or consider Dorinne Kondo's work on Japanese culture and embodi-

ment, which she contrasts with Cartesian dualism, and its assumption of a "division between the inner space of selfhood and outer world," and a "Transcendental Signified, a substance which can be distilled out from the specificities of the situations in which people enact themselves." She argues that in Japan the embodied subject is "constituted in and through social relations and obligations to others. Selves and society did not seem to be separate entities; rather the boundaries were blurred." Kondo, *Crafting Selves*, 33, 35, 22. Kondo cites as an example the use of multiple "I's" in Japanese. Different words for "I" are used, depending on the context and distinct social relationships existing in the present social moment. As she argues: "In short, proper use of Japanese teaches one that a human being is always and inevitably involved in a multiplicity of social relationships. Boundaries between self and other are constantly changing depending on context and on the social positioning people adopt in particular situations." It is "this accommodation to others that makes them fully mature human beings, that creates their personality." Kondo, *Crafting Selves*, 33.

74. Sawicki argues the self is a "process of signification within an open system of discursive possibilities." Sawicki, "Feminism, Foucault, and 'Subjects,'" 166. Because of this, one can employ "creativity in the production of one's identity." Lloyd, "Feminist Mapping," 247. As Grosz puts it, the self is a space of "linkages" and "transformations" and "becomings," not a finished object. See Grosz, *Volatile Bodies*, 165.

75. Csordas's discussion of the self may be influenced by his own work with Navajo healing systems. See Csordas, *Ritual Healing in Navajo Society*.

76. See Grounds et al., *Native Voices*.

77. Schwarz, *Molded in the Image of Changing Woman*, xix.

78. O'Nell, *Disciplined Hearts*, 46–47.

79. O'Nell, *Disciplined Hearts*, 64.

80. O'Nell, *Disciplined Hearts*, 56.

81. O'Nell, *Disciplined Hearts*, 77–78, 110, 143.

82. O'Nell, *Disciplined Hearts*, 43.

83. O'Nell, *Disciplined Hearts*, 77.

84. Blackfeather, "Cultural Beliefs and Understanding Cancer," 140.

85. See Jaimes Guerrero, "Feminism and Tribalism."

86. Voss et al., "Tribal and Shamanic-Based Social Work Practice," 231.

87. Voss et al., "Tribal and Shamanic-Based Social Work Practice," 234. Leenhardt, in a 1947 study of Melanesian medicine (cited by Csordas), similarly argues that "in the indigenous worldview the person was not individuated, but was diffused with other persons, and things in a unitary sociomythic domain." Csordas, *Sacred Self*, 7.

88. See Farella, *Main Stalk*; Schwarz, *Molded in the Image of Changing Woman*, Csordas, *Ritual Healing in Navajo Society*; and McNeley, *Holy Wind in Navajo Philosophy*.

89. See Basso, *Wisdom Sits in Places*; Bierwert, *Brushed by Cedar*; Nelson, *Make Prayers to the Raven*; Thornton, *Being and Place among the Tlingit*.

90. O'Nell, *Disciplined Hearts*, 206–7.

91. O'Nell, *Disciplined Hearts*, 10.

92. O'Nell, *Disciplined Hearts*, 12.

93. "An individual will perceive pathology, as an alteration of the normal, according to value-laden qualities that have been constructed as important in his or her culture. Thus a teenage girl from mainstream American society in the 1980s or 1990s who is confined to a back brace because of a curvature of the spine might well experience her pathology in terms of a diminished sense of attractiveness—at a time in her life when personal attractiveness is emphasized for young women within her culture. For a Flathead person, pathology is apprehended, is felt at the phenomenal level, when he or she no longer feels connected to family and friends. And it is in those culturally emphasized terms that depressed affect may or may not be perceived as an alteration of the normal." O'Nell, *Disciplined Hearts*, 204.

94. Garroute and Westcott, "'The Stories Are Very Powerful,'" 164.

95. See Jacob, "This Path Will Heal Our People," and Frey, "If All These Stories Were Told," both in Crawford O'Brien, *Religion and Healing*.

96. Numerous works mention local traditions that distinguish between "white ways" and "white illnesses" and "Native illnesses." Within these particular Native communities there is the generally accepted assumption that many illnesses and diseases are culturally specific, and the treatments for them should be as well. For instance, see Basso, *Wisdom Sits in Places*; Bierwert, *Brushed by Cedar*; and Schwarz, "Lightning Followed Me."

97. See Vine Deloria, *Custer Died for Your Sins*; Jaimes, *The State of Native America*; Sale, *Conquest of Paradise*; Charney, *Encyclopedia of Genocide*.

98. Morsink, "Cultural Genocide."

99. See for instance Thornton, *American Indian Holocaust*.

100. Tinker, *Missionary Conquest*, 4.

101. Tinker, *Missionary Conquest*, 5.

102. Tinker, *Missionary Conquest*, 6.

103. Numerous other scholars have viewed colonial history through this lens of cultural genocide. See for instance Churchill, *A Little Matter of Genocide*; Fenelon, *Culturicide*; Van Krieken, "Stolen Generations"; Smith, *Conquest: Sexual Violence and American Indian Genocide*.

2. "The Fact Is They Cannot Live"

1. Meeker, *Pioneer Reminiscences of Puget Sound*, 511.

2. This chapter takes as its focus Euroamerican responses and actions. This is not to suggest that Native people were passive victims who did not in their own turn respond and act. Indeed, Coast Salish and Chinook people took an active role in shaping their responses to changing situations, and I focus on those responses in later chapters.

3. Jay Miller, *Lushootseed Culture*, 40. Suttles and Lane, "Southern Coast Salish," 500.

4. Suttles and Lane, "Southern Coast Salish," 499. The word "regularize" appears in quotes because I am citing Suttles and because the word is clearly problematic. From Native people's perspectives their marriages were likely already "regular"! From missionaries' perspectives, their unions did not fulfill Christian expectations

and needed to be reformed to follow Euroamerican standards. These included formalizing the rite of marriage and limiting men to one wife.

5. Harmon, *Indians in the Making*, 47.

6. Collins, *Valley of the Spirits*, 33; Collins, "Religious Change," 146; and Bagley, *Early Catholic Missions in Old Oregon*, 1:69.

7. Harmon, *Indians in the Making*, 47.

8. Jay Miller, *Lushootseed Culture*, 40.

9. Suttles and Lane, "Southern Coast Salish," 500.

10. Suttles and Lane, "Southern Coast Salish," 500. See also Collins, *Valley of the Spirits*.

11. See for example Boyd, *Coming of the Spirit of Pestilence*; Ruby and Brown, *Chinook Indians*; Todorov, *Conquest of America*; Trafzer, *Death Stalks the Yakama*; and Scott, "Indian Diseases as Aids."

12. Guilmet et al., "Legacy of Introduced Disease," 4–5.

13. Guilmet et al., "Legacy of Introduced Disease," 7.

14. Boyd, *Coming of the Spirit of Pestilence*, 34.

15. Harris, "Voices of Disaster," 591. Swinomish Tribal Mental Health Project, A *Gathering of Wisdoms*, 18.

16. See Boyd, *Coming of the Spirit of Pestilence*; Ruby and Brown, *Chinook Indians*. It is significant that the spread of disease was in large part reflective of the new emerging economy: trade systems surrounding cattle and oysters facilitated the spread of measles and smallpox in the mid-nineteenth century. It is no small irony that many contemporary illnesses among Native communities are also due to economic demands: from oyster farming on Willapa Bay to uranium mining on the Navajo Reservation.

17. The Reverend Samuel Parker noted in 1835 that "since the year 1829, probably 7/8, if not as doctor McLoughlin believes 9/10, have been swept away by disease, principally by fever and ague." Parker, *Journal of an Exploring Tour*, 188. William Fraser Tolmie noted much the same devastation on the Columbia in the late 1830s: "On its lower bank, just opposite to Coffin Island, is the site of an Indian village, which a few years ago contained two or three hundred inhabitants, but at present only its superior verdure distinguished the spot from the surrounding country. Intermittent fever which has almost depopulated the Columbia River of its aborigines, committed its fullest ravages and nearly exterminated the villagers, the few survivors deserting a spot where the pestilence seemed most terribly to wreck its vengeance." Large, *Journals of William Fraser Tolmie*, 183.

18. Indian Claims Commission, "The Quileute Indians of Puget Sound," 209.

19. Gary, "Diary," 275.

20. Lee and Frost, *Ten Years in Oregon*, 308, 314.

21. Ruby and Brown, *Chinook Indians*, 188.

22. *Wapato*, sometimes referred to as wild potato or water potato, is a bulb root and staple food that grew throughout the Pacific Northwest.

23. Wyeth, "Correspondence and Journals," 149.

24. Lupton, *Imperative of Health*, 8.

25. Scheper-Hughes and Lock, "The Mindful Body," 8–10. Although dealing with a very different religious community, Thomas Csordas's examination of Catholic faith healing is also useful in this discussion of Euroamerican embodied subjectivity. Within Csordas's study, he found a view of the embodiment (the "sacred self") that suggested a distinctly independent self. As Csordas argues, the goal of such healing was ultimately to separate oneself from the influences of others: "The sacred self is thus created by a performance act that powerfully enacts the cultural ideal of ego integrity and psychological differentiation, in vivid contrast to ritual healing societies where boundary lines between selves are not so definitively drawn." Csordas, *Sacred Self*, 44–45. Csordas observes that for Christian believers, illness and unease were often attributed to demonic influences: demons violated the sanctity of the independent self, entering without consent. This violation is placed in contrast with the presence of God, to whom believers surrender control. Control, however, is never forcefully taken: the healthy individual is always in control; the person's ego remains intact and unthreatened. As Csordas observes, "Behind this contradiction lies a fundamental uneasiness about a cherished western value—integrity of the ego—in the face of an unsettling prospect raised by the ritual practice—dissolution of the self." Csordas, *Sacred Self*, 238. The goal of such healing, Csordas argues, is not the loss of self but the solidification of self, within "person to person" interaction with the divine. Csordas, *Sacred Self*, 243. The contrast is seen most clearly in "the space between an absolute wholeness of divine healing, and an absolute nihilation of demonic self destruction." Csordas, *Sacred Self*, 271. This sacralization of the individual self, the sacred-self, is a central tenet not only of Christianity but of Enlightenment philosophy, which has informed western biomedicine, politico-economic practice, and social norms. And it can be seen as informing nineteenth-century Euroamerican narratives of and approaches to illness and healing in encounters with Northwest Native communities. Euroamerican missionaries saw within indigenous healing practices an attack upon the individuated self and reacted with fear and alarm. The necessity of protecting what Thomas Csordas calls the "integrity of the ego" was inevitably accompanied by the constraint, control, and careful definition of the embodied experience. As Brian Turner explains, "We can consequently approach the history of western culture as [one that] starts with the control of the flesh and ends with the control of the self." See Brian Turner in Coakley, *Religion and the Body*, 38. This ideal of the carefully controlled self, the constrained body, is seen in the narratives that Euroamericans told about themselves and about the people they encountered.

26. See Said, *Orientalism*; Pearce, *Savagism and Civilization*; Berkhofer, *The White Man's Indian*; and Parkhill, *Weaving Ourselves into the Land*.

27. This view is by no means the norm within the Christian tradition, which maintains a wide range of beliefs and interpretations regarding the causes of illness. See Amundson and Numbers, *Caring and Curing*, for a comparative look at how different Christian traditions approach illness and healing.

28. Merk, *Fur Trade and Empire*, 94–104.

29. Ruby and Brown, *Chinook Indians*.

30. Jackson, *Letters of the Lewis and Clark Expedition*, 506.

31. Ogden, *Traits of American Indian Life*, 68–70.

32. Boyd, *Coming of the Spirit of Pestilence*, 154. Such language is reminiscent of current discourse over HIV and AIDS, especially among cultural and sexual minority groups.

33. Dunn, *History of the Oregon Territory*, 116.

34. Bolduc, *Mission of the Columbia*, 118.

35. Parrish (1855), in Boyd, *Coming of the Spirit of Pestilence*, 133–34.

36. Thwaites, *Original Journals of the Lewis and Clark Expedition*, 43.

37. O. Larsell, *The Doctor in Oregon, A Medical History* (Portland, 1947): 221.

38. Cox, *Adventures on the Columbia River*, 167.

39. See Coues, *New Light*, 836.

40. Boyd, *Coming of the Spirit of Pestilence*, 72.

41. Henry, 1856–58 *Monthly Medical Reports*, 185, cited in Boyd, *Coming of the Spirit of Pestilence*, 76.

42. Boyd, *Coming of the Spirit of Pestilence*, 76; Gibbs et al., "Tribes of Western Washington and Northwest Oregon," 198–99, 208.

43. See Gibbs et al., "Tribes of Western Washington and Northwest Oregon," 198–99, 208.

44. See for example Lupton, *Imperative of Health*, 8. She writes: "The civilized body is controlled, rationalized, and individualized, subject to conscious restraint of impulses, bodily processes, urges and desires." The uncivilized body, by default, is none of these things. Margrit Shildrick and Janet Price likewise discuss this trend within western philosophical thought, when they describe the female body, which is marked "as out of control, beyond and set against the force of reason . . . the female body demands attention and invites regulation." Price and Shildrick, *Feminist Theory and the Body*, 3–4. In the Northwest, Native bodies were feminized by Euroamerican observers, reduced to the carnal, the out-of-control, the bleeding, the transgressive, the dangerous, in need of control and restraint. Elizabeth Spelman has argued that this association of women with the irrational body and men with rational spirit can be traced to Plato, where "the body is seen as the source of all the undesirable traits a human being could have, and women's lives are spent manifesting those traits." Spelman, in Price and Shildrick, *Feminist Theory and the Body*, 39. As this chapter demonstrates, Euroamerican observers associated Native cultures with fleshly experience, with embodied existence, with irrationality and all the unpleasantness that carnality could imply.

45. Bagley, *Early Catholic Missions in Old Oregon*, 49–50.

46. Bagley, *Early Catholic Missions in Old Oregon*, 50–51.

47. See Pearce, *Savagism and Civilization*; Berkhofer, *Salvation and the Savage*; Berkhofer, *The White Man's Indian*; Vine Deloria, *Custer Died for Your Sins*; and Vine Deloria, *God Is Red*.

48. Dunn, *History of the Oregon Territory*, 293. As David Thompson argued, their illnesses were "on account of their filthy manner of living, their bad food, and the incessant rain for six months in the year." Coues, *New Light*, 820.

49. Collins, "Religious Change," 64.

50. Bagley, *Early Catholic Missions in Old Oregon*, 1:84.

51. Bagley, *Early Catholic Missions in Old Oregon*, 2:35.

52. Thwaites, *Oregon Missions and Travels: De Smet*, 27.

53. Lee and Frost, *Ten Years in Oregon*, 164.

54. Bolduc, *Mission of the Columbia*, 119.

55. Cox, *The Columbia River*, 178.

56. Dunn, *History of the Oregon Territory*, 127.

57. Bagley, *Early Catholic Missions in Old Oregon*, 1:83–4.

58. Gary, "Diary," December 18, 1844.

59. Landerholm, *Notices and Voyages of the Famed Quebec Mission*, 89.

60. Ruby and Brown, *Chinook Indians*, 93.

61. Harmon, *Indians in the Making*, 24.

62. Guilmet and Whited, *People Who Give More*, 116.

63. Guilmet et al., "Legacy of Introduced Disease," 14.

64. Ruby and Brown, *Chinook Indians*, 196. "This great mortality among the Indians has been attributed to the manner in which the disease has been treated, or rather to their superstitious practices. Their medicine men are no better than jugglers, and use no medicine except some deleterious roots, while from the character of these Indians, and their treatment of an unsuccessful practitioner, the whites decline administering any remedies, for fear of consequences later those to which I have alluded." Wilkes, *Narrative of the U.S. Exploring Expedition*, 369–70.

65. Irving, *Astoria*, 117–18. See also Cox, *The Columbia River*, 314–15. See also Ruben Thwaites, *Oregon Missions and Travels: De Smet*, 23.

66. Ruby and Brown, *Chinook Indians*, 186; Boyd, *Coming of the Spirit of Pestilence*, 112–13.

67. Lee, "Letter of 22 May, 1840," *Christian Advocate*, August 25, 1841, Oregon Historical Society Archives. See also Ruby and Brown, *Chinook Indians*, 186.

68. Swan, *The Northwest Coast*, 65.

69. Swan, *The Northwest Coast*, 150.

70. Collins, "Religious Change," 158.

71. Boyd, *Coming of the Spirit of Pestilence*, 189. While priests had been driven away when they first attempted to convert Native communities, many of these same communities welcomed them following their struggles with epidemics. Farther north, up the coast, the Se'shalt are one such example, who first rejected conversion but in 1862, following a devastating epidemic, welcomed a mission and the rapid acculturation that followed. By 1868 the Se'shalt lived at the mission under the guidance of Oblate Father Pierre-Paul Durieu, who introduced his strict 'systeme' under which dancing and potlatching were outlawed, and the community adapted a Euroamerican style of governance, homes, and cultivation. See Lemert, "Life and Death of an Indian State."

72. Harmon, *Indians in the Making*, 39.

73. Harmon, *Indians in the Making*, 69.

74. Harmon, *Indians in the Making*, 39.

75. Boyd, *People of the Dalles*, 172–73.

76. Chirouse, *Letters*, Oblates of Marie Immaculate (1862), Oregon Historical Society, MSS 1581.

77. Guilmet et al., "Legacy of Introduced Disease," 14.

78. Boyd, *Coming of the Spirit of Pestilence*, 156.

79. Chirouse, *Letters*.

80. Guilmet et al., "Legacy of Introduced Disease," 14; quoting Boyd, "The Introduction of Infectious Diseases" (unpubl.), 168–70.

81. By denying healthcare and vaccines to all but the most acculturated, Euroamerican settlers and missionaries demonstrate what Judith Butler argued in her 1993 work, that only those individuals who subject themselves to regulatory norms within a society are granted subjectivity, are *allowed to matter*.

82. Cox, *The Columbia River*, 169.

83. Ruby and Brown, *Chinook Indians*, 80.

84. Large, *Journals of William Fraser Tolmie*. These views persisted well into the twentieth century, as attested by Melville Jacobs. His research among the Clackamas Chinook in the 1940s demonstrates this. As one woman recounted, "Long ago the people did not know this illness [measles]. Soon after the myth [white] people had come to this land, they brought with them all sorts of illnesses such as these. At first they [merely] announced it, they said that a disease was coming. A person will cough, forthwith his breath will be shortened [and he will not be able to breathe as well as usual], and then he will die [of tuberculosis]." Jacobs, *Content and Style of an Oral Literature*, 545.

85. Boyd, *Coming of the Spirit of Pestilence*, 135.

86. Merk, *Fur Trade and Empire*, 106.

87. Frost, "Journal, 1840–43," 360.

88. Lee and Frost, *Ten Years in Oregon*, 252, 261.

89. Lee, "Diary," 17.

90. Frost, "Journal, 1840–43," 359.

91. Davenport, "Recollections of an Indian Agent," 234.

92. Frost, "Journal, 1840–1843," 364, 359. George Gary reflected that "the prevailing opinion was that all or nearly all the good that resulted from it [the missions] was that quite a number had experienced religion here, and died when in school and hopefully gone to heaven. All agreed the Indian community had not been benefited by anyone who had left the school and returned to various walks of life." He further concluded that the mission school had done as much "as could be expected all things taken into account. These children receive no check or restraint on their animal propensities from their parents and friends any more than the pigs in the street, and, as far as I am able to learn, as is the child, so is the parent and the grave is opening to receive them all. A most appalling scene, but so it is." Gary, "Diary," 84.

93. Hines, *Missionary History of the Pacific Northwest*, 176–77. Charles Wilkes noted this shift in priorities in his critique of the Oregon missions. Their emphasis had shifted to white parishioners (he noted only twenty pupils and four servants in the mission schools and doubted they were having any lasting impact on local Native communities). He noted their almost total lack of interest in reaching Indians and found it incongruous with their talk of increased funding for developing mission buildings and business. Wilkes, *Narrative of the U.S. Exploring Expedition*, 354–45.

94. Hines, *Missionary History of the Pacific Northwest*, 345.

95. Hines, *Missionary History of the Pacific Northwest*, 367.

96. Kasulis et al., *Self as Body in Asian Theory*.

97. This is of course an oversimplification of Protestant and Catholic theologies. Both contain a diversity of opinion on the question of the relationship between body and soul. Both carry traditions of the bodily resurrection, for instance, which would suggest an eternal, spiritual body. But the prevailing tradition throughout both Catholic and Protestant history has been a sense of the dual nature of body and spirit, largely inherited from Greek philosophy.

98. Bosse, *Memoirs d'un Grand Brainois*, 65.

99. Catholic belief does allow for the possibility that baptism and last rites could offer miraculous healing, but such cures were unusual.

100. Bolduc, *Mission of the Columbia*, 100–1.

101. Bolduc, *Mission of the Columbia*, 115, 126.

102. Bolduc, *Mission of the Columbia*, 119.

103. Bolduc, *Mission of the Columbia*, 113.

104. Bolduc, *Mission of the Columbia*, 108–9. Father J. Nobili described similar activities at Fort Vancouver on June 1, 1846: "While I remained at Ft. Vancouver, I baptized upwards of 60 persons, during a dangerous sickness which raged in the country. The majority of those who received baptism died with all the marks of sincere conversion." Thwaites, *Oregon Missions and Travels: De Smet*, 223. Blanchet described baptizing 122 children on May 31, 1840, at Whidbey Island. He noted: "The children were scared and crying, and soon all retired." Schoenberg, *History of the Catholic Church in the Pacific Northwest*, 56. Such an image is not necessarily that of a joyous conversion but rather acts of desperation in the midst of illness.

105. Ruby and Brown, *John Slocum and the Indian Shaker Church*, 20; see also Schoenberg, *History of the Catholic Church in the Pacific Northwest*, 129, 153.

106. As Hare and Barman have argued in their study of the Methodist mission to the Tsimshian at Fort Rupert, Natives who cooperated with missions did so for their own reasons, often pursuing their own interests. They were not passive but active participants within mission settings, enabling the missions to succeed and negotiating the degree to which they accommodated missionaries' expectations. Missionaries and their Native parishioners were engaged in a mutual "reciprocal relationship," each dependent upon the other, in different ways. See Hare and Barman, *Good Intentions Gone Awry*, xxii, xix.

107. Bolduc, *Mission of the Columbia*, 89.

108. Bolduc, *Mission of the Columbia*, 102–3.

109. Bolduc, *Mission of the Columbia*, 95.

110. Collins, *Valley of the Spirits*, 33.

3. "Civilization Is Poison to the Indian"

1. Berkhofer, *The White Man's Indian*; Pearce, *Savagism and Civilization*; Mihesuah, *American Indians*.

2. Spencer, *Principles of Biology*.

3. Evans-Pritchard, *History of Anthropological Thought*; Kuklick, *The Savage Within*; Stocking, *Race, Culture and Evolution*; Gould, *Mismeasure of Man*.

4. Suttles, *Coast Salish Essays*, 222. However, in most cases, band membership was then based on patrilineal descent, in direct contrast to Coast Salish traditions of ambilateral descent and ambilocal residence.

5. Harris, *Making Native Space*, xxix.

6. Harris, *Making Native Space*, 67.

7. Harris, *Making Native Space*, 265.

8. One man is reported to have objected to the notion of removal to a single reservation, arguing that "that little creek was the only place he cared for, as he always got his salmon there and he liked the place." American Friends Service Committee, *Uncommon Controversy*, 21.

9. American Friends Service Committee, *Uncommon Controversy*, 19.

10. Typically acquired through raids on other Native groups, slaves occupied a lower-class status among Coast Salish communities. Though it was not hereditary, the taint of slavery on one's lineage tended to prevent people from entering higher-class status.

11. American Friends Service Committee, *Uncommon Controversy*, 26.

12. Marino, "History of Western Washington since 1846," 169.

13. Marino, "History of Western Washington since 1846," 171.

14. Suttles, *Coast Salish Essays*, 222.

15. American Friends Service Committee, *Uncommon Controversy*, 16.

16. American Friends Service Committee, *Uncommon Controversy*, 17. For a history of the genocidal violence waged against Native people in southern Oregon by settlers and gold miners, seek Beckham's *Requiem for a People*.

17. Zenk, "Kalapuyans," 551.

18. Zenk, "Kalapuyans," 551.

19. Recognition of the Chinook Nation has been resisted by some recognized tribes, fearful of losing federal funds.

20. American Friends Service Committee, *Uncommon Controversy*, 17.

21. Thrush, *Native Seattle*, 42.

22. Thrush, *Native Seattle*, 59. The 1855 Color Act voided marriages between Indians and whites in Washington State and was amended in 1858 to nullify all future marriages as well. The 1866 Marriage Act denied "even common-law legitimacy to indigenous-white relationships." And the 1866 Legitimacy Act "barred mixed-race

children from inheriting their father's estate if children existed from a previous marriage to a white woman." Thrush, *Native Seattle*, 58–59.

23. Thrush, *Native Seattle*, 89.

24. Thrush, *Native Seattle*, 99.

25. Guilmet et al., "Legacy of Introduced Disease," 17.

26. Guilmet et al., "Legacy of Introduced Disease," 18.

27. Guilmet et al., "Legacy of Introduced Disease," 20.

28. In an 1885 census: 527 Puyallup reservation; 162 Skokomish; 167 at Nisqually reservation; 112 at Squaxin Island; 467 at Tulalip; 222 at Swinomish; 234 at Lummi; 142 at Port Madison. Two-fifths of these chose to live off-reservation where there were more opportunities. Harmon, *Indians in the Making*, 119. Alternatively, some Natives like the Jamestown Klallams or the Upper Skagit accommodated to white lifestyles so that they could stay on aboriginal land and not go to a reservation. Harmon, *Indians in the Making*, 120.

29. Thrush, *Native Seattle*, 108.

30. Elmendorf and Kroeber, *Structure of Twana Culture*, 276.

31. Jacobs, *Clackamas Chinook Texts*, 563.

32. See for example Kan, *Memory Eternal*.

33. Marino, "History of Western Washington since 1846."

34. Harmon, *Indians in the Making*, 108.

35. Furtwangler, *Bringing Indians to the Book*.

36. Neilson, "Focus on the Chehalis Indians" (unpubl.), 77–78; and Castile, *Indians of Puget Sound*, 29.

37. Kew, "Central and Southern Coast Salish," 476.

38. Jay Miller, *Lushootseed Culture*, 40–41. Carlson writes that early Sto:lo alliances with missionaries in the nineteenth century centered on temperance and a shared goal of freeing their communities of whiskey traders. Carlson, *You Are Asked to Witness*, 96. But missions also divided communities: "communities were pulled apart by interdenominational feuding between the different missionaries. . . . Competition for the loyalty and allegiance of Sto:lo leaders remained a characterizing feature of Catholic-Protestant and interdenominational Protestant relations in the Fraser Valley throughout the nineteenth century." Carlson, *You Are Asked to Witness*, 96. Missionaries appointed their own community leaders. According to Oblate priest Father Edward Peytavin (1886): "There are now three (chiefs) in this little village, it is the Catholic Chief who has the most subjects, the Methodist Chief is in Control of thirteen, and the Episcopalian has only his wife to govern." Carlson, *You Are Asked to Witness*, 97.

39. Eells, *Indians of Washington Territory*, 674.

40. For instance, in the 1930s Marian Smith interviewed traditional healers who explained that it was common for healers never to request payment and only to receive gifts after their first two years in practice. After that people might receive gifts, though some refused any payment if directed to do so by their spirit power. See Smith, *Puyallup-Nisqually*, 76.

41. Eells, *Indians of Washington Territory*, 677.

42. Quoted in Castile, *Indians of Puget Sound*, 409.

43. Guilmet et al., "Legacy of Introduced Disease," 21.

44. Guilmet et al., "Legacy of Introduced Disease," 19–20.

45. Eells, *Indians of Washington Territory*, 414.

46. The first missionaries to the area were Methodists, led by Jason Lee, who founded the Willamette Mission in 1834 and later outposts at the Dalles and Oregon City. He was followed shortly thereafter by Presbyterians and Catholic missionaries, arriving in the latter half of the 1830s. Presbyterian missions were established at Puyallup, Nisqually, and among the upper Chehalis on the Chehalis River. Congregationalist missions were founded among the Twanas, Klallams, and Squaxins, and Catholic missionaries worked among the Snohomish, Port Madison communities, Muckleshoot, Lummi, Swinomish, Clatsop, and Cowlitz. Often reservation agents shared the roles of legal authority, missionary, and physician. As physicians, their work was limited to dispensing purgatives and painkillers; see Holt, *Saddlebag Medicine*; and Boyd, *Coming of the Spirit of Pestilence*.

47. Guilmet et al., "Legacy of Introduced Disease," 20. Eells himself was determined to bring the Coast Salish within the territory under his authority. Miller writes that Eells went so far as to have "Klallam houses on the Port Townsend beach burned in a vain attempt to force a move to his reservation." Jay Miller, *Lushootseed Culture*, 43.

48. Castile, *Indians of Puget Sound*, 426.

49. Guilmet and Whited, *People Who Give More*, 29. As is discussed in the next chapter, such experiences may not have "unwound" the entire religious structure as much as sparking new religious responses, such as the revitalization movements and prophetic leadership like that within the Shaker Church. See Wallace, *Revitalizations and Mazeways*.

50. Elmendorf and Kroeber, *Structure of Twana Culture*, 274.

51. See Child, *Boarding School Seasons*.

52. Adams, *Education for Extinction*; Hoxie, *A Final Promise*.

53. Mauro, *Art of Americanization*.

54. Similar promotional images from the Tulalip Indian School show young Native women being taught how to bake bread and young men learning agriculture or logging. Carey C. Collins, "Through the Lens of Assimilation"; Carey C. Collins, "Oregon's Carlisle"; Marr, "Assimilation through Education," University of Washington Digital Collections, http://content.lib.washington.edu/aipnw/marr.html, accessed June 10, 2011.

55. Reyes, *White Grizzly Bear's Legacy*, 112–18. See also Adams, *Education for Extinction*, and Hoxie, *A Final Promise*.

56. Bonney, "Puyallup Indian Reservation." History of Cushman School (typescript), Special Collections Division, Washington State Historical Society, n.d.

57. See Vecsey, "The Lord's Prayer."

58. Sullivan, "Eugene Casimir Chirouse" (unpubl.), 46–62.

59. See Hoxie, *A Final Promise*; Adams, *Education for Extinction*; and Bonney, "Puyallup Indian Reservation."

60. See Child, *Boarding School Seasons*.

61. Jay Miller, *Mourning Dove*.

62. Szasz, *Education and the American Indian*.

63. By the 1930s most Native children in the country attended public schools, and those residential schools that remained began to soften their policies toward Native cultures and languages. The Wheeler-Howard Act of 1934 changed policies toward Native cultures, encouraging schools to be more tolerant of Native languages and cultures and to include them in curricula where appropriate. Substantial changes occurred in the 1970s as well. In Alaska, the 1976 Molly Hooch decision paved the way for local schooling by declaring that the state was obligated to make local or home schooling possible for Alaskan Native high school students, who had previously been required to travel great distances to attend residential schools. The Indian Child Welfare Act of 1978 transformed federal policies once again, contracting with local tribes to direct their own local reservation schools.

64. As Harvey Hines wrote, regarding Jason Lee, "He saw what was near, the speedy extinction of the Indian tribes; the sure and swift coming of an American population to occupy the splendid country from which the Indians were disappearing." Hines, *Missionary History of the Pacific Northwest*, 345.

65. Davenport, "Recollections of an Indian Agent," 246.

66. Bagley, *Early Catholic Missions in Old Oregon*, 2:142.

67. Castile, *Indians of Puget Sound*, 31–32.

68. Castile, *Indians of Puget Sound*, 294.

69. Strong, *Cathlamet on the Columbia*, 56–57.

70. As Margrit Shildrick and Janet Price have argued, the creation of a narrative of victimization could be used in various ways to justify colonization. By imaging indigenous peoples as victims of primitive culture, in need of civilization, or by seeing them as the victims of that civilization, the end result is the same: an image of a people in need of an outside savior, outside control, outside regulation. Price and Shildrick, *Feminist Theory and the Body*, 389, 394.

71. Davenport, "Recollections of an Indian Agent," 247.

72. Davenport, "Recollections of an Indian Agent," 233.

73. See also Beckham, *Requiem for a People*.

74. Thrush, *Native Seattle*, 79.

75. Thrush, *Native Seattle*, 159.

76. Thrush, *Native Seattle*, 159.

77. Thrush, *Native Seattle*, 92, 69, 139.

78. Thrush, *Native Seattle*, 92–93.

79. Thrush, *Native Seattle*, 130, 128.

80. Raibmon, *Authentic Indians*, 7–9.

81. Raibmon, *Authentic Indians*, 201.

82. See Philip Deloria, *Playing Indian*.

83. Raibmon, *Authentic Indians*, 11, 16.

84. Raibmon, *Authentic Indians*, 10.

85. Raibmon, *Authentic Indians*, 134.

86. Despite this, in her study of the Puyallup community in the 1930s, Marion Wesley Smith argued that "Native people on Puget Sound . . . had 'come through remarkably well,'" demonstrating a "successful adaptation." Cited in Thrush, *Native Seattle*, 151. In many ways they had, becoming a part of the new economy and navigating the complex sea of cultural changes.

87. Of four hundred treaties made between 1778 and 1871 only twenty-four provided for medical service. The Treaty of Medicine Creek was one of them. As such Puyallup consider medical care a treaty right. Guilmet and Whited, *People Who Give More*, 19.

88. Harmon, *Indians in the Making*, 194.

89. Until 1955 the Bureau of Indian Affairs sought to administer healthcare for Native people, generally through assigning physicians to reservations. After 1955, with the creation of the Indian Health Service, healthcare shifted to a network of centralized facilities, which often required an individual to travel some distance from home.

90. Jacobs, *Clackamas Chinook Texts*, 549–50.

91. Jacobs, *Coos Myth Texts*, 92–93. A lengthy collection of successful curing stories can also be found in Smith, *Puyallup-Nisqually*, 78–99.

92. Jacobs, *Clackamas Chinook Texts*, 545–48.

93. Foucault, *Discipline and Punish*, 138. As I argue later, it is important to note that these bodies were *not* docile by any means. Euroamerican narratives constructed an image of them as such, and in so doing obscured the ways in which Native people subverted such colonial efforts.

94. One might consider the work of scholars such as Sandra Lee Bartky, on the social construction of the female body and femininity, in which she argues that cultural expectations create docile women, forced to conform to preapproved roles and bodily performativity. Bartky's work, while insightful, has also been widely criticized and reinterpreted by feminist scholars of the body, who argue that women are not simply docile dupes, easily blown about by the winds of culture. Women can and do make choices, resist, and reinterpret the cultural narratives with which they are faced. See for example Bartky, "Foucault, Feminism, and the Modernization of Patriarchal Power," 143.

4. "A Good Christian Is a Good Medicine Man"

1. Material from this and the following chapter was included in my essay "Healing Generations in the South Puget Sound," in Crawford O'Brien, *Religion and Healing*, 135–59. Reproduced with permission of ABC-CLIO, LLC.

2. Sampson, *Indians of Skagit County*, 11.

3. Sickness here is understood as *spirit-sickness*, the result of strained relationships with one's spirit power. The cure is to dance at the winter spirit dances, to

honor and affirm the relationship. The *xewsa'kwtl*, or new dreamer, who is made ill by this spirit song, relies upon a ritualist to assist in controlling the song and "to *mi'tle*, to dance with it in a state of possession." See Suttles, *Coast Salish Essays*, 200, 201, 203–4. Spirit songs might also come to persons suffering from grief, or they might be "induced to possess persons by means of a ritual abduction and isolation resembling the Wakashan Sacred Society initiation. Each winter persons with songs acquired in these various ways danced possessed at public gatherings held for the purpose." Suttles, *Coast Salish Essays*, 204.

4. See Amoss, *Coast Salish Spirit Dancing*; Bierwert, *Brushed By Cedar*; and Suttles, *Coast Salish Essays*.

5. Sampson, *Indians of Skagit County*, 57–58; Vibert, "'The Native Peoples Were Strong to Live'"; Cline, "Religion and Worldview," 172; Christopher Miller, *Prophetic Worlds*; Hunn et al., *N'ch'i-Wana, "The Big River"*; Boyd, *People of the Dalles*; and Bierwert, *Brushed by Cedar*.

6. *Tamanawas* is the Chinook *wawa* term for such activity and the one used most often in historical sources. Anthropologists and many white observers have used the term *tamanawas* to describe the experience of meeting a spirit power, the spirit power itself, the ability to heal, and as a generic term for all indigenous modes of religious practice and "magic." Scholars have concluded that belief in such guardian spirits is widespread throughout Native North America and virtually universal on the Columbia River and Northwest Coast. See Spier, *Ghost Dance of 1870*; Spier, *Prophet Dance*, 25–29; Benedict, *Concept of the Guardian Spirit*; Suttles, *Coast Salish Essays*; Boyd, *Coming of the Spirit of Pestilence*; and Boyd, *People of the Dalles*.

7. On cold destroying the power see Boas, "Doctrine of Souls and Disease," 41.

8. Spier, *The Prophet Dance*, 13.

9. A Snohomish narrative describes a healer who died as a young boy, visited the dead, and returned with spirit power to heal. See Haeberlin and Gunther, *Indians of Puget Sound*, 81. Narratives of Kwakwak'wakw, Tlingit, and Bella Coola shamans visiting the land of the dead can be found in Dawson, *Notes and Observations on the Kwakiool*, 16; Boas, *Mythology of the Bella Coola Indians*, 37, 42; Boas *First General Report on the Indians of British Columbia*, 843–45.

10. Throughout the Northwest Coast the traditional manner in which one becomes a healer follows a relatively standard form that reflects this notion of identity re-creation. In many recorded oral traditions, an individual experiences a severe illness and death or a near-death experience. In this state the individual is met and healed by a spirit helper, who gives a spirit song, and perhaps also a new name, or a healing ritual. The individual thereafter maintains a lifelong relationship with that spirit helper. In many contexts, upon recovery the healer-initiate performs a healing ceremony or takes part in a longhouse spirit dance to demonstrate having a new role in the community, demonstrating restored identity through dance, ritual performance, and healing of others. For more information, see Amoss, *Coast Salish Spirit Dancing*.

11. Aberle, "The Prophet Dance and Reactions to White Contact"; Walker, "New Light on the Prophet Dance Controversy"; Christopher Miller, *Prophetic Worlds*;

Vibert, "'The Native Peoples Were Strong to Live'"; Spier, *Prophet Dance*; Suttles, *Coast Salish Essays*.

12. Vibert, "'The Native Peoples Were Strong to Live,'" 217; see also Hunn et al., *N'ch'i-Wana, "The Big River,"* 242.

13. Vibert, "'The Native Peoples Were Strong to Live,'" 218. See also Ray, *Cultural Relations in the Plateau*, 95–99.

14. By 1802, prior to the arrival of non-native settlers to the area (although some European ships had already traveled the coast), smallpox epidemics had reduced populations on the Columbia Plateau by 45 percent, and around 1800 a volcanic eruption showered the area with ash.

15. Ross, *Adventures of the First Settlers*, 289.

16. Spier, *Klamath Ethnography*, 229.

17. Sampson, *Indians of Skagit County*, 28, 60.

18. Collins, *Valley of the Spirits*, 34.

19. DuBois, *Feather Cult*, 9.

20. DuBois, *Feather Cult*, 27; Tyrell, *David Thompson's Narrative*, 437, 512–13; Ross, *Adventures of the First Settlers*, 92, 111. Wáášhat, the Longhouse, or Seven Drums are the names used interchangeably for the contemporary religious tradition arising from these prophetic movements. Wáášhat, or what Hunn has called "the Indian religion of the Plateau," emerged during the nineteenth century, drawing from these older prophetic movements, to craft a religious tradition that met the contemporary needs of Indian people. Rooted in indigenous tradition, this movement also adapted certain features of Christianity, features that enabled the tradition and Indian people to survive the radical social upheaval with which these communities were faced during the nineteenth and early twentieth centuries. Consider as well the case of Kau-xuma-nupika (also Kokomenepeca), an individual whom DuBois credits as one of the original founders of the Wáášhat. Alexander Ross was one Euroamerican who met Kau-xuma-nupika in person. As he recalled: "Among the visitors who every now and then presented themselves were two strange Indians, in the character of man and wife, from the vicinity of the Rocky Mountains, and who may probably figure in our narrative hereafter. The husband, named Kocomenepeca was a very shrewd and intelligent Indian, who addressed us in the Algonquin language, and gave us much information respecting the interior of the country." A page later, Ross notes, as if as an afterthought, "they were both females." Ross, *Adventures of the First Settlers*, 92–93. A Kutenai woman married to a white trader, Kau-xuma-nupika left her husband, declaring that she was at heart a man, and intended to live as such. She joined and led several war parties among her people, gaining status as a leader, warrior, and prophet. Spier has written that "at length she became the principal leader of her tribe, under the designation of 'Manlike Woman.' Being young, and of delicate frame, her followers attributed her exploits to the possession of supernatural power, and therefore received whatever she said with implicit faith." Spier, *Prophet Dance*, 26–27. In 1811 David Thompson recorded her return to the lower Columbia River valley, bringing with her "a young wife, of

whom she pretended to be very jealous; when with the Chinook, as a prophetess, she predicted diseases to them which made some of them threaten her life, and she found it necessary for her safety to return to her own country at the head of this River." David Thompson, "July 28, 1811," in Tyrell, *David Thompson's Narrative*, 512–13, 920. He later described a group of Chinook men who questioned him, in the presence of the prophetess, asking if "it is true [what she says] that the white men have brought with them the smallpox to destroy us ... is this true, and are we all soon to die?" Vibert, "'The Native Peoples Were Strong to Live,'" 214. Kau-xuma-nupika predicted epidemics brought by white immigrants, the imminent end of Indian lands, the destruction of the world, and the subsequent arrival of a golden age in which Indian peoples would be restored to their former strength and the dead would return to life. As a prophet and religious leader she sought to encourage Native resistance to white settlement, and the restoration of Native control of the Columbia River. The movement also incorporated certain Christian elements, however, elements that enabled it to stand up against the incursions of Christian missionaries. Such Christian features included the incorporation of Sunday meetings, organized to resemble slightly a Christian prayer meeting in style, with prayer on one's knees, the observance of some Christian holidays, and the recognition of a Supreme Deity. Spier, *Prophet Dance*, 31. See Barry, "Ko-Come-Ne-Pa-Ca, the Letter Carrier," and Sperlin, "Two Kootenay Women Masquerading as Men?"

21. For more on Transformer ("Dokibatl"), see Eells, *Indians of Washington Territory*, 680; Castile, *Indians of Puget Sound*, 362; and Elmendorf and Kroeber, *Twana Culture*, 535–36.

22. Beckham et al., *Native American Religious Practices*.

23. Suttles, *Coast Salish Essays*, 185.

24. Suttles, *Coast Salish Essays*, 185–86.

25. Suttles, *Coast Salish Essays*, 155.

26. *Trafzer, Death Stalks the Yakama*. See also Hunn et al., *N'ch'i-Wana, "The Big River."*

27. Vecsey, "The Lord's Prayer," 50.

28. Vecsey, "The Lord's Prayer," 51.

29. Vecsey, "The Lord's Prayer," 51.

30. Vecsey, "The Lord's Prayer," 52.

31. Bagley, "Historical Sketches of the Catholic Church in Oregon 1838–1878," in *Early Catholic Missions in Old Oregon* 1:69. Historians have argued that the likely introduction of such Christian elements came not from white missionaries but from a band of Iroquois men, who traveled west to join the Flathead communities in Montana and northern Idaho in 1820. These Iroquois became a part of the Flathead nation, intermarrying with the community. As Catholic converts, the Iroquois brought with them elements of Catholic tradition, such as the gospel, the Lord's prayer, the sign of the cross, the Sabbath, baptism, and, of course, the notion of a supreme deity. While the Iroquois arrived in the Northwest in the 1820s, the first Christian missionaries did not arrive until 1834. See Spier, *Prophet Dance*.

32. DuBois, *The 1870 Ghost Dance*, 184.

33. Large, *Journals of William Fraser Tolmie*, 172. He also describes an instance where the Native community reacted to a converted Native, known as "the Frenchman," as they would to prophets, adapting these new voices into their already understood worldview: the Frenchman "took the opportunity of haranguing them on the miserable and wretched condition and the numberless advantages which would accrue to them, from being at peace with each other, and obeying the dictates of our blessed religion which he at the same time explained as simply as possible, and was listened to with breathless attention by old and young. The Indians afterwards formed a large semi circle round a fire at the North end of the store, and an animated dialogue was kept up for more than an hour between the Frenchman and Chiatsasa, and a simultaneous hum of approbation followed every pause. Just as we were going to bed, perhaps 10½, the religious dance was performed in nearly the same manner as at Fort Vancouver—the Frenchman being master of ceremonies, after dancing in a circle, all dropped except him and Chiatsasa, and they repeated a short chaunt when the latter also squatted down and the Frenchman kneeing uttered a prayer which terminated the affair," (Wednesday July, 1833). Large, *Journals of William Fraser Tolmie*, 214.

34. Consider for instance the narrative of Dr. Tolmie when visiting the "Klalums": "H & I explained to them the creation of the world, the reason why Christians and Jews abstained from work on Sunday [*sic*], and had got as far as the Deluge in the Sacred History when we were requested to stop, and the Indians could not comprehend this clearly. The Chinook [jargon] is such a miserable medium of communication, that very few ideas can be expressed in it. The savages seem anxious for instruction and with good interpreters, could be induced to alter for the better their conduct. They afterwards danced the Samanowash, in a large circle, the women and boys keeping together." Large, *Journals of William Fraser Tolmie*, 221–22.

35. Hunn et al., *Nch'i-Wana, "The Big River,"* 241. The prophet dance spread from the Plateau along Puget Sound and Georgia Strait, taking a different form, one that was referred to as "religious dance," or "praying dance," centered around worship of the Transformer. Prophet Dances could be found all along the Northwest coast, as far south as northern California, and inland as far south as northern Nevada. See Suttles, *Coast Salish Essays*, for more on this. Prophetic movements provided communities with a means of resisting Euroamerican cultural aggression, accommodating certain aspects of Christianity while maintaining distinctly indigenous approaches to healing, subsistence, kinship, and community. Mythologies and oral traditions also gave voice to Native resistance to Euroamerican coercion and control. These mythic narratives emphasized several key themes: outsmarting disease and death; a reaffirmation of traditional values as a means of avoiding illness and devastation; and a stubborn insistence on survival. Jacobs and colleagues recorded an illuminating Kalapuya narrative, in which Coyote is presented as a culture-hero capable of outsmarting death.

> A sickness came toward here. All those who were persons (Native people) were frightened. Now then they talked to one another, "What shall we do now? Now

a sickness is coming toward here. Wonder where we may go to now? Oh it is well if we go up above. Ready then let us go." So then they all went. The birds bore them aloft, they carried them on their backs. Coyote accompanied the people, riding on the back of a turkey buzzard as they flew to higher ground. The buzzard, annoyed by Coyote who persisted in nibbling him on the back of the neck, eventually dropped him to the ground below. Left behind, Coyote returned to the (Willamette) Valley, where he indeed met with Disease, who was searching for persons to make sick. Coyote decided to outsmart Disease. "I am a Disease too!" he announced. To prove this, he had secretly filled his mouth with grasshoppers. "Where have you come from?" He asked. "Have not they all died where you have come from?" "Here from above I come, they have all died. I am a disease too. I eat up people. Look at my mouth!" So saying, Coyote showed Disease his open mouth, filled with grasshoppers that appeared to be tiny people. The two camped together for the night. But while Disease slept, Coyote sent mice to steal the disease-power from Disease. Coyote then fled, carrying away Disease's disease-causing-spirit-power. "It was not strong (after that). He had stolen (some of) what was his disease."

Coyote was able to steal the spirit power from Disease, taking away his ability to harm future communities. Jacobs et al., *Kalapuya Texts*, 90. In much the same way, Native communities who had survived disease could see themselves as having outsmarted death. Frederica De Laguna recorded similar narratives among the Yakutat Tlingit, whose stories described individuals who had been taken away in the Disease Boat to the land of the dead. These men and women returned and brought with them special abilities to outsmart disease and protect their villages. De Laguna, *Under Mount Elias*, 710, 713–14.

36. Silas Heck, Chehalis, in Barnett, *Indian Shakers*, 25.

37. Slocum, recorded by Wickersham, in James Mooney, *Ghost Dance Religion*, 753.

38. Amoss, "Indian Shaker Church."

39. Amoss, "Indian Shaker Church"; Amoss, "Resurrection, Healing, and 'the Shake'"; Gunther, "The Shaker Religion," 37–77. Sacket, "The Siletz Indian Shaker Church."

40. Amoss, "Symbolic Substitution in the Indian Shaker Church," 230.

41. Harmon, *Indians in the Making*, 127.

42. Castile argues that the severity with which Edwin suppressed traditional religions worked against his brother Myron's more tolerant efforts and resulted in driving South Puget Natives away from Myron's mission and toward the Shaker Church. Castile, "The Half-Catholic Movement."

43. Neilson, "Focus on the Chehalis Indians," 83.

44. Quoted in Mooney, *Ghost Dance Religion*, 749.

45. Ruby and Brown, *John Slocum and the Indian Shaker Church*, 36.

46. Gunther, "The Shaker Religion." Gunther reports that those guilty of "Indian doctoring" received thirty to forty-five days imprisonment on the Tulalip reservation.

47. Collins, "Religious Change," 13.

48. Collins, *Valley of the Spirits*, 205.

49. Barnett, *Indian Shakers*, 151.

50. Amoss, *Coast Salish Spirit Dancing*, 81.

51. Collins, "Religious Change," 83–84.

52. Spier, *Prophet Dance*, 52. See also Haeberlin and Gunther, *Indians of Puget Sound*, 77; Gunther, "Klallam Folk Tales," 292; Boas, *Chinook Texts*, 208; Spier and Sapir, *Wishram Ethnography*, 243, 246.

53. "Acting through the hands of one who is possessed, power cures by 'drawing' and 'brushing' sin or some evil force from the patient's body, or it finds and helps to restore the soul of a sick person. Since it guides the search for such disembodied souls and leads the hands to sickness, power, therefore, has preternatural insight and volition." Barnett, *Indian Shakers*, 150. See also Castile, *Indians of Puget Sound*, 416.

54. Gunther "The Shaker Religion," 50.

55. Collins, "Religious Change," 87.

56. Collins, "Religious Change," 88.

57. Collins, "Religious Change," 106.

58. Collins, "Religious Change," 80.

59. Barnett, *Indian Shakers*, 149–50.

60. Collins, "Religious Change," 88.

61. Collins, "Religious Change," 82.

62. Collins, "Religious Change," 81.

63. Mooney, *Ghost Dance Religion*, 749.

64. Smith, *Puyallup-Nisqually*, 86.

65. As Amoss has noted, while pre- and early colonial diagnosticians were limited to religious specialists who could see into other realms, since the 1880s this role has been filled by Shaker Church members, who are able to see introduced spirit powers, or lost souls, and discern in what way a soul had been threatened. Amoss, *Coast Salish Spirit Dancing*, 44.

66. See for example Trafzer, *Death Stalks the Yakama*.

67. Harmon, *Indians in the Making*, 125.

68. Harmon, *Indians in the Making*, 129.

69. Harmon, *Indians in the Making*, 225.

70. Harmon, *Indians in the Making*, 128, 231.

71. Harmon, *Indians in the Making*, 128.

72. Eells notes as well that "parental and filial love are quite strong, and the poor are generally cared for by their relatives and friends." Eells, *Indians of Washington Territory*, 615.

73. Within this new context Shakers took up many of the intertribal public duties that might once have been filled by intervillage networks of shamanic healers and ceremonial leaders. See Jay Miller, *Lushootseed Culture*, 8.

74. Harmon, *Indians in the Making*, 128.

75. Pike Ben, quoted in Neilson, "Focus on the Chehalis Indians," 90

76. Collins, "Religious Change," 89.

77. Collins, "Religious Change," 86.

78. Amoss, "Indian Shaker Church," 638.

79. Jay Miller, *Lushootseed Culture*, 144–45.

80. Mooney, *Ghost Dance Religion*, 754.

81. Barnett, *Indian Shakers*, 29. Neilson quotes Pike Ben, an early member of the church who saw a clear distinction between the Shakers and the old way. As he says: "I now see that the Indian Tah-nah-nous doctor is a real devil. I am afraid of him now. That shake comes to me now if I am sick, and sends the sickness away, and God is angry if the Shaker charges anything, because He gives the Shaker power to send the sickness away. All people, young and old, can cure sickness if they are Shakers. To do this, they must catch the sickness in their hands. We call the Shake a medicine sent from God." Neilson, "Focus on the Chehalis Indians," 90.

82. Smith, *Puyallup-Nisqually*, 85.

83. Collins, "Religious Change," 104.

84. Castile, *Indians of Puget Sound*, 430.

85. Spier, *Prophet Dance*, 49.

86. Sampson, *Indians of Skagit County*, 17. See also Ruby and Brown, *John Slocum and the Indian Shaker Church*, 173–95.

87. Quoted in Mooney, *Ghost Dance Religion*, 748. Castile and Gunther, among others, have argued that the Shaker Church thrived where Catholic missions were absent.

88. Wickersham, letter of December 5, 1892, cited in Mooney, *Ghost Dance Religion*, 750. During the 1940s the Shaker Church split over the role that the Bible was to play in the Church, forming the Indian Shaker Church and the Full Gospel Church. Led by Lans Kalapa from Neah Bay (Makah), the FGC advocated the use of the Bible in church services and a closer adhesion to evangelical theology. Barnett estimates that about one quarter of Shakers agreed with the Bible-centered church and went with the FGC; the remaining three quarters continued with the Shaker Church.

89. This direct experience reflects a clear continuity with previous prophetic traditions, in which the leader was able to travel to and return from the spirit world with messages for followers. Early adherents to the Shaker Church reported similar phenomena themselves, as they were able to visit with the dead and report these words back to their congregations. As Reverend Eells noted in his journals, individuals in the church claimed to have visions: "Among other things, he saw an old friend of his, named Sandyalla, who had died many years previous, and his friend taught him four songs. They were mainly about Heaven, and there was not much objection to them except that this species of spiritualism was mixed up in them. He taught them to his friends." Eells also notes that following the death of a church leader, the congregation "must get together and talk about what he had said, and sing his songs." Castile, *Indians of Puget Sound*, 428. Such actions demonstrate an engaging continuity with previous prophetic traditions.

90. In some ways the beliefs of the Shakers mirror other charismatic and Pen-

tecostal traditions that argue for direct interaction with the Holy Spirit. This similarity was not lost on Reverend Eells, who argued that the Shaker tradition "is evidently based upon the same principles of the mind as the jerks and shouting at camp meetings among the whites of the southern and western states fifty years ago, when they were more ignorant and less acquainted with *real religion* than they are now." Mooney, *Ghost Dance Religion*, 747 (italics mine). Such emphasis upon individual experiential interaction with the divine has helped to structure the organization of the church as well, leaving it with "spontaneous individual leadership, with lack of direction by, and absence of responsibility to, officially constituted officers." Barnett, *Indian Shakers*, 124. Any such structure or attempts at organization, Barnett argues, had been made to please Euroamerican bureaucracies, in order to gain a guarantee of religious freedom for Church members.

91. Harmon, *Indians in the Making*, 127.

92. Ruby and Brown, *Dreamer Prophets*, 44. Reverend Mann argued that the healing ritual of the Shakers "closely resembled Indian Ta-nah-nous which was expressly forbidden by Rule 6 of the official 'Rules Governing Indian Offences.'" Neilson, "Focus on the Chehalis Indians," 83.

93. Agent Evan Estep observed in 1924: "The Yakamas are cursed not only with medicine men, but with medicine women." Trafzer, *Death Stalks the Yakama*, 35, 38.

94. Barnett, *Indian Shakers*, 104.

95. It seems significant that Slocum, Louis, and Sam were working so closely with Walker, who was *both* a Shaker and a traditional healer. It implies that the relationship between the Shaker Church and traditional *tamanawas* healers was not exclusive, but cooperative, and thus indicates similar philosophical understandings regarding the embodied self and approaches to healing. Collins observed that Shakers were willing to work with Indian doctors, or against them, depending on the nature of the illness and the particular doctor in question. Collins, *Valley of the Spirits*, 105.

96. Barnett, *Indian Shakers*, 92–93. Neilson also notes an instance when "John Smith, assisted by Peter Yo-kim, Thomas Heck, and George Walker were in charge of the doctoring. As a result of the trial, these four along with Puyallup Bill, were sentenced to ten days at hard labor and were also confined to the 'skukum house' (jail)." Neilson, "Focus on the Chehalis Indians," 89.

97. As one observer reported of the church at White Swan, "There is dancing and singing. Everyone has a chance to get into the act. . . . This idea of everyone participating is really prevalent among the Indians." Harmon, *Indians in the Making*, 155.

98. Waterman, "The Shake Religion of Puget Sound," 146; Amoss, "Symbolic Substitution," 234.

99. Barnett, *Indian Shakers*, 156.

100. Ruby and Brown, *John Slocum and the Indian Shaker Church*, 34.

101. Quoted in Mooney, *Ghost Dance Religion*, 749. In addition to healing, Shaker power has been reported to be effective in providing the clairvoyant ability to locate lost objects, to predict the future, or predict someone's death.

102. Mooney, *Ghost Dance Religion*, 748.

103. Neilson, "Focus on the Chehalis Indians," 84–88.

104. Shaker churches can be found all over the Northwest, as far north as British Columbia and south into northern California. Spier recorded churches found among the Squaxin, Skokomish, Nisqually, Chehalis, Lower Columbia tribes, Klallam, Quinalt, Tulalip, Squamish, Yakama, Warm Springs, Klamath, Modoc, Oregon coastal tribes (Siletz and Grand Ronde reservations), the Yurok, and the Hupa. Spier, *Prophet Dance.*

105. Barnett, *Indian Shakers*, 147.

106. Eells, "S'kokomish Agency, Washington," 167.

107. Castile, *Indians of Puget Sound*, xix.

108. Castile, "The Half Catholic Movement," notes the irony of the historical record, in which Judge Wickersham is praised for his benevolence toward the Indian Shaker Church and his efforts to secure them legal protections. However, Castile notes, Wickersham was a proponent of allotment and citizenship for Native peoples so as to free up reservation land for white settlement. His interests were far from purely benevolent.

109. Quoted in Castile, *Indians of Puget Sound*, 426.

110. Long, *Significations*, 118.

111. Amoss, "Symbolic Substitution," 246.

112. Neilson, "Focus on the Chehalis Indians," 91; Johnson, *Report to United States Commissioner of Indian Affairs*, 276.

113. Buckley, "The Shaker Church and the Indian Way," 1.

114. Long, *Significations*, 119.

115. McNally, "Uses of Ojibwe Hymn Singing," 141, 148. Thomas Buckley's work with the Yurok and Pamela Amoss's work with the Coast Salish provide intriguing evidence of the role of the Shaker Church in the contemporary revival of indigenous "precolonial" religious practices. As Buckley points out, "If the Shake was a 'continuation of the Indian Way,' as the most respected members of the Church have always claimed, then, too, the resurgent local Indian Way must be viewed as a 'continuation' of the Shake." See Thomas Buckley, *Standing Ground*, 267. See also Buckley, "The Shaker Church and the Indian Way," 1–14. This can be seen too in the ways in which some Shaker leaders are entering into or blessing the revival of Native traditional practices. For instance, a Shaker Church elder at Squaxin Island recently offered the opening prayer and blessing at the community's First Salmon ceremony, welcoming the arrival of king salmon at the beginning of the salmon season.

116. Elmendorf and Kroeber, *Structure of Twana Culture*, 276.

117. Suttles, "Central Coast Salish," 472.

118. Bierwert, *Brushed by Cedar*, 165. See also Cole and Chaikin, *An Iron Hand.*

119. Kew, "Central and Southern Coast Salish," 476.

120. Bierwert, *Brushed by Cedar*, 166.

121. Kew, "Central and Southern Coast Salish," 476, 479.

122. Bierwert, *Brushed by Cedar*, 167. At the same time, spirit dancing has become more acceptable by local Catholic congregations. In the 1970s, for instance, one non-Indian member of a religious order was initiated as a spirit dancer and later ordained as a priest, and Catholic clergy on Vancouver Island and at Squamish have "sponsored memorial services for Christ as the focal event of invitational gatherings in smokehouses at Easter, which usually coincides with the end of the winter dance season." Kew, "Central and Southern Coast Salish," 480.

123. Collins, *Valley of the Spirits*, 237, 239–40; Collins, "Religious Change," 13.

124. Collins, *Valley of the Spirits*, 241–42.

125. Collins, *Valley of the Spirits*, 243; Harmon, *Indians in the Making*, 224.

126. Collins, "Religious Change," 65.

127. Kew, "Central and Southern Coast Salish," 479.

128. Kew, "Central and Southern Coast Salish," 479.

129. Amoss, *Coast Salish Spirit Dancing*, 54.

130. Vi went out one winter morning, fetching a bucket of water, and undressed and bathed in the stream, praying to the four directions. When nothing happened, she went in. "Mom came in all wet and blue from her bathing. Grandpa asked her what she had been doing. She told him. Grandpa just laughed and laughed and put her in his lap. He told her again that when the time was right, this would happen. Her spirit power would come to her." Coy, "My Mom's Spirit Power," 20.

131. Kew, "Central and Southern Coast Salish," 477. See also Barnett, *Coast Salish of British Columbia*, 29–33.

132. Collins, "Religious Change," 94.

133. Collins, "Religious Change," 94.

134. Collins, "Religious Change," 84, 96.

135. Collins, "Religious Change," 95.

136. Collins, "Religious Change," 93.

137. Collins, "Religious Change," 103–4.

138. Amoss, "Symbolic Substitution," 82.

139. Kew and Kew, "People Need Friends," 33.

140. Amoss, "Symbolic Substitution," 244.

141. Amoss, "Symbolic Substitution," 245; and Amoss, "Indian Shaker Church," 637.

142. Amoss, "Symbolic Substitution," 245. Since 1947 Pentecostals have also made inroads into Coast Salish communities, though their growth has been slower than that seen among spirit dancers. Pentecostals' "emphasis on healing with supernatural power and on speaking in tongues provides some counterpart with the guardian spirit religion." Collins, *Valley of the Spirits*, 44.

143. Collins, "Religious Change," 82.

144. Collins, "Religious Change," 82.

145. Collins, "Religious Change," 90.

146. Collins, *Valley of the Spirits*, 43. As she notes, while possession of a guardian spirit was nearly universal among Upper Skagit in 1942, a majority of Upper Skagit also belonged to the Indian Shaker church. Those who joined the church

"believed that their guardian spirit was transformed into their Shaker spirit or 'power.'" Collins, *Valley of the Spirits*, 172. See also Collins, "Religious Change," 122.

147. Jay Miller, *Lushootseed Culture*, 32. Collins noted a particular example wherein one woman's hummingbird spirit helped her to heal others as a member of the Shaker Church. Collins, *Valley of the Spirits*, 150.

148. Yoder, *Dxwʔdal taq*^{w}*šəblu*, 16–17.

149. Collins, "Religious Change," 90–92.

150. Amoss, "Symbolic Substitution," 243.

151. Bierwert, *Brushed by Cedar*, 12.

152. Collins, "Religious Change," 70.

153. Amoss, "Symbolic Substitution," 245.

154. Amoss, "Symbolic Substitution," 246.

155. Amoss, "Symbolic Substitution," 227.

156. Amoss, "Symbolic Substitution," 235.

157. Suttles, *Coast Salish Essays*, 208.

158. Bierwert, *Brushed by Cedar*, 167.

159. Harmon, *Indians in the Making*, 224.

160. Harmon, *Indians in the Making*, 224.

161. See Bucko, *Lakota Ritual of the Sweat Lodge*, for a discussion of tradition and its evolution among Plains tribes.

162. Glass, "Intention of Tradition," 280.

163. Glass, "Intention of Tradition," 280.

164. Glass, "Intention of Tradition," 281.

165. Glass, "Intention of Tradition," 281.

166. Adelman, "A Drink From Miriam's Cup," 109.

167. Adelman, "A Drink From Miriam's Cup," 110–12.

168. Raibmon, *Authentic Indians*, 199. As she wrestled with this same question, Crisca Bierwert distinguished between "emergent cultural systems," which "comply with dominant, hegemonic, controlling forms," and "residual" cultural forms, "that is, those that are like 'vestiges,' not articulating well with the dominant cultural forms." Bierwert, "I Can Lift Her Up," 184.

169. Glass, "Intention of Tradition," 296.

170. Bruce Granville Miller, *Be of Good Mind*, 19.

171. Sider, "The Walls Came Tumbling Up," 286–87.

172. American Friends Service Committee, *Uncommon Controversy*, 67.

173. Guilmet et al., "Legacy of Introduced Disease," 24.

174. Jay Miller, *Lushootseed Culture*, 79.

175. Jay Miller, *Lushootseed Culture*, 80. As the American Friends Service Committee has argued, traditional Coast Salish culture has survived but out of sight. Feasting, dancing, entertaining guests, the giving of names at potlatches, the carving and use of cedar canoes, arts and crafts, seasonal mobility, and a reliance on salmon all remain strong within Coast Salish communities. And more than anything, they argue, attitudes have survived, in particular, their view of time "which is

for living" and their "sense of continuity with those who have gone before." American Friends Service Committee, *Uncommon Controversy*, 69.

176. Jay Miller, *Lushootseed Culture*, 1.

177. Jay Miller, *Lushootseed Culture*, 1.

5. Both Traditional and Contemporary

1. Material from this and the previous chapter was included in my essay "Healing Generations in the South Puget Sound," in Crawford O'Brien, *Religion and Healing*. Reproduced with permission of ABC-CLIO, LLC.

2. Long, *Significations*, 119.

3. As Susan Friedman has argued, scholars need to go beyond narratives of 'how we colonized them,' to discussions of how they *reacted to* those colonial efforts, how Native peoples made use of their creative and resilient agency to respond to colonization through modes of cultural exchange and adaptation. Haraway and Friedman insist that by refusing to fetishize difference, we can achieve a more complex understanding of identity, one which is, in Friedman's words, a "historically embedded site, a positionality, a location, a standpoint, a terrain, an intersection, a network, a crossroads of multiply situated knowledges." There is here a need to affirm difference, without an essentialist notion of identity that fails to recognize its permeable borders and the realities of ongoing cultural navigation and hybridity. See Friedman, *Mappings*, 19, 5. See also Anzaldua, *Borderlands*; and Clifford *Routes*.

4. As is discussed later in this chapter, the definition of *traditional* is a complex one and not readily apparent. Communities and generations continually redefine what it means to be traditional, reflecting their views on history, culture, the body, and what it means to be a healthy person in community.

5. Rhoades, *American Indian Health*, 89.

6. See for example Nebelkopf and Phillips, *Healing and Mental Health for Native Americans*, which discusses a wide array of community-directed programs. These include the Friendship House Healing Center in San Francisco; the Healthy Nations Initiative, which is funding a variety of tribal programs; Yup'ik and Cup'ik community-centered substance abuse programs; and Native Circle, a holistic HIV/AIDS mental health program. The Diné Nation has, in many ways, been at the forefront of this effort. For an excellent history of contemporary efforts, see Davies, *Healing Ways*.

7. Dixon in Dixon and Roubideaux, *Promises to Keep*, 74–75.

8. Guilmet and Whited, *People Who Give More*, 21.

9. Guilmet and Whited, *People Who Give More*, 22.

10. Thrush, *Native Seattle*, 166–67.

11. As discussed in the previous chapter, Seattle's urban Indian population is very diverse. In fact, as Coll Thrush notes in *Native Seattle*, the majority of Native people in the Seattle area are not indigenous to this region but rather come from other parts of North America, including Alaska, California, and the Midwest. This diverse population presents unique challenges when it comes to addressing con-

cerns such as health services, community cohesion, and the celebration of Native cultures and identities.

12. Thrush, *Native Seattle*, 167–68, 162, 171. Activism among Canada's First Nations communities likewise increased at this time, inspired in part by a new 1969 governmental policy, known as the "White Paper," which proposed eliminating Indian status, and in turn "prompted a nationwide resurgence in Aboriginal peoples' activity in defining and asserting themselves at broader levels of collective identity and governance." Schaepe, "Sto:lo Identity and the Cultural Landscape," 235.

13. Guilmet and Whited, *People Who Give More*, 23.

14. Guilmet and Whited, *People Who Give More*, 96.

15. "There are two basic choices available to federally recognized tribes: 1) they can receive their health care through the Indian Health Service, a federal agency in the U.S. Department of Health and Human Services; or 2) they can receive money from the IHS to operate their own health care delivery system," or various combinations of the above. Tribes can either contract to provide specific services or contract to provide a full range. Neither the Indian Health Service nor tribes can provide everything, and so must contract out for specialized care. Dixon, "Unique Role of Tribes," 39, 40. Tribes that fully manage care have more options when determining whether to contract out or provide their own.

16. "The Tribal Leaders' Summit," quoted in Dixon and Roubideaux, *Promises to Keep*, 53–54.

17. Dixon and Roubideaux, *Promises to Keep*, 98.

18. Dixon and Roubideaux, *Promises to Keep*, 98.

19. Dixon and Roubideaux, *Promises to Keep*, 101.

20. Baldridge, "The Elder Indian Population and Long Term Care," 150–51. Elder care is also a conundrum for many tribes, for whom care for elders is an important familial prerogative. Placing elders in nursing homes can feel like a break with tradition, unless done carefully and with full community engagement.

21. Forquera, "Challenges," 121.

22. Forquera, "Challenges," 133.

23. Forquera, "Challenges," 126.

24. Thrush, *Native Seattle*, 181.

25. Swinomish Tribal Mental Health Project, *A Gathering of Wisdoms*, 96.

26. Forquera, "Challenges," 126.

27. Thrush, *Native Seattle*, 69.

28. Guilmet and Whited, *People Who Give More*, 38.

29. Guilmet and Whited, *People Who Give More*, 69.

30. Harmon, *Indians in the Making*, 119.

31. Harmon, *Indians in the Making*, 121.

32. Harmon, *Indians in the Making*, 190–91.

33. Bruce Granville Miller, *Be of Good Mind*, 17.

34. Jay Miller, *Lushootseed Culture*, 32.

35. Killen, *Religion and Public Life*.

36. Swinomish Tribal Mental Health Project, *A Gathering of Wisdoms*, 33.

37. According to Guilmet and Whited, sweat lodges were only rarely used among Coast Salish communities prior to the mid-twentieth century, and many scholars argue that they did not serve a spiritual purpose, as they did among cultures of the Plateau and Plains. Guilmet and Whited, 75.

38. Guilmet and Whited, *People Who Give More*, 82.

39. I would point out that in many ways this religious diversity is reflective of Coast Salish and Chinook approaches to religion. Religion was (and often still is) an individual, private affair. Respect for the individual autonomy of others and the need for each person to establish individual spiritual practice runs deep in this part of the world.

40. Harmon, *Indians in the Making*, 156.

41. Harmon, *Indians in the Making*, 236–37.

42. Guilmet and Whited, *People Who Give More*, 78.

43. In considering those spaces where cultures meet, spaces of integration and hybridity, Donna Haraway describes an emerging postmodern subject, what she calls the *cyborg*. Haraway defines cyborgs as hybrids, people with no easy origin stories. Their lives and stories are locations of "transgressed boundaries, potent fusions, and dangerous possibilities." Such individuals, existing in the space between cultures, inhabiting both-worlds-in-part is a theme to which many women of color have turned as an affirmation of the complexity and heterogeneity of contemporary ethnic identities. Such discursive efforts, as Haraway describes them, are not simply "literary deconstructions, but liminal transformations." In this context, where meanings, identities, and experiences encompass multiple histories and meanings, one finds spaces of cultural continuity, survival, complexity, and affirmation of identities that reflect the real experiences of Native people, not the ideal "Indians" of non-native construction. Haraway's "cyborgs are the people who refuse to disappear on cue, no matter how many times a 'Western' commentator remarks on the sad passing of another primitive, another organic group done in by 'western' technology. . . . Survival is the stakes in this play of readings." Recognizing spaces of cultural hybridity as legitimate and authentic locales of identity challenges universal and totalizing notions of American Indian identity. This is not to suggest that American Indian culture has been lost to the dominating forces of so-called civilization and modernity but quite the opposite. It is to argue for the inherent strength, adaptability, and agency of American Indian cultures and the complexity of contemporary American Indian experience. See Haraway, "Manifesto for Cyborgs," 154, 176–77, 181.

44. *South Puget Intertribal News* 15, no. 7 (October–November 2005): 11.

45. SPIPA, *Planning Agency Annual Report*, 1999, 13.

46. Jay Miller, *Lushootseed Culture*, 1.

47. Waters, "Native American Food Production Systems," 6–7. In 2002 an article in *Intertribal News* reported that the Nisqually Community Garden was planting a crop of camas, "an important historical crop . . . second only to salmon." In

addition to acting as a source of healthy traditional foods, the community garden also had an "intergenerational" focus, which encouraged "both elders and youth to work on the garden." The garden is part of a series of Traditional Food and Food Systems Workshops that took place at Skokomish, Nisqually, Chehalis, and Squaxin Island in 2001 and 2002.

48. Collins records nineteenth-century Upper Skagit dietary practices that in many ways support this representation. "The Upper Skagit ate two meals a day; one in the morning after everyone had gone bathing in the river and had dried out by the fire, and one in the evening. At each meal they ate a dish of fish or meat followed by camas, wild carrots or other roots if these were available. Water was their only beverage. The diet was rich in protein and low in starch and sugar. For this reason the Upper Skagit have a tradition that sugar and flour were very welcome items when they were introduced at the nearby trading posts." Collins, *Valley of the Spirits*, 57.

49. *South Puget Intertribal News*, February–March 2006, 6. A comparative example can be found at the Porcupine Clinic, founded by Lorelei DeCora on the Lakota Pine Ridge reservation in 1981. In 1997 DeCora instituted a grassroots effort to combat diabetes. Because of traditional diets and modes of subsistence, diabetes was virtually unknown in precontact days but became epidemic on many reservations following the high-fat, high-sugar rations provided by the Bureau of Indian Affairs. DeCora's program recruited elders to teach community members about traditional foods, preparation, and preservation techniques. One tribal elder's comments were revealing: "This approach to diabetes isn't just about food. When you bring back the knowledge and skills about preparing food, you bring back the ceremonies that go with them. Maybe this is a message from the Creator that we have to hang on to those traditions to survive in the next century." Sandrick, "The Wisdom of the Old Ways," 42. Such a message is a call for a return to traditional foods drawn from the traditional landscape. What such programs illustrate is a notion of healing that insists upon the interaction of community, extended family, and the natural environment.

50. *South Puget Intertribal News*, February–March, 2006, 11.

51. Field notes, August 2001. This is reflected in the comments made by David Ramon (Morongo Tribal Health Services) to a Bridge the Gap Luncheon sponsored by SPIPA's social services: "It's not the Native way to harm a woman, mentally or physically. Historically, Indian men weren't abusers, but treated women with respect and understanding." *South Puget Intertribal News*, July–August–September 2002, 7.

52. When I was first told this story, we were seated at a community dinner on the Shoalwater Reservation. Excited by what I had just learned (and perhaps not exercising the best judgment), I turned to the other woman at the table, blurting out what I had just been told. "Condom carriers!" I gleefully announced, to a woman I was later to learn was the oldest member of the Shoalwater community. I paused for a moment, realizing I might have spoken a bit too quickly. But the elder woman smiled, nodding her head and sitting back in her chair as she crossed her arms over her chest. "Well, whatever works!" she said, much to my relief.

53. "Celebration Dinners Planned: The Nisqually Native Women's Wellness Program Is Planning Two Dinners to Celebrate Womanhood," *Native Women's Wellness*, Winter 2002–3, 5.

54. Consider, for example, comments given at the opening of the Squaxin Island Health Center. Physician's Assistant Tiff Barret described the facility to the Women's Wellness Program's staff: "Center. That's different than a clinic. Center implies more than just medical." The Squaxin Island center provides family practice and other preventative medical care as well as "alternative medicine such as acupuncture, acupressure, and alpha stimulation for pain management. . . . There are also dental, mental health and family violence counseling services. In addition, the clinic has an Indian Child Welfare caseworker and a community health coordinator." See SPIPA, "Tribal Clinic Profiles," 21–22.

55. Swinomish Tribal Mental Health Project, *A Gathering of Wisdoms*, 79.

56. Swinomish Tribal Mental Health Project, *A Gathering of Wisdoms*, 212.

57. Jay Miller, *Lushootseed Culture*, 129.

58. Amoss, *Coast Salish Spirit Dancing*, 83.

59. Guilmet and Whited, *People Who Give More*, 39–40.

60. Guilmet and Whited, *People Who Give More*, 40.

61. Swinomish Tribal Mental Health Project, *A Gathering of Wisdoms*, 215, 228–29. Another example of this is the Native American Women's Wellness through Awareness (NAWA) program based in Denver and Los Angeles, which provides Native Sisters to support women undergoing cancer treatments. For instance, one woman had her Sister accompany her through a sweat lodge prior to screening, while another helped arrange for a traditional medicine woman to smudge and bless women following screening and detection. Burhansstipanov, "Cancer: A Growing Problem," 245.

62. Swinomish Tribal Mental Health Project, *A Gathering of Wisdoms*, 48, 55.

63. Guilmet and Whited, *People Who Give More*, 66.

64. Guilmet and Whited, *People Who Give More*, 66.

65. Chandler et al., *Personal Persistence, Identity Development*, vii–viii.

66. Chandler et al., *Personal Persistence, Identity Development*, 2.

67. Chandler et al., *Personal Persistence, Identity Development*, 75.

68. Chandler et al., *Personal Persistence, Identity Development*, 3.

69. Chandler et al., *Personal Persistence, Identity Development*, 73. Those with none of these "cultural markers" had the highest suicide rates, while no suicides were reported among those with the strongest evidence of cultural strength. Chandler et al., *Personal Persistence, Identity Development*, 74.

70. Field notes, Nisqually Tribal Center, May 2004.

71. Megan MacDonald, field notes, summer 2004.

72. SPIPA, "Women and Girls' Gathering, Annual Report," 2004.

73. Whitener, "Language Program," *Klah'Che'Min*, August 2001, 9.

74. Foster, "Cultural Resources Management," *Klah'Che'Min*, August 2001, 11.

75. The reverence and care for one's ancestors is reflected in Coast Salish burn-

ings for the dead: "The other way we take care of our ancestors occurs when we have our spiritual burnings, each spring and each fall." McHalsie, "We Have to Take Care," 118. For a description of a burning for the dead see Rudine, "Center of the World," 43. Recognizing the presence of one's ancestors and seeking to honor them is entirely different from contact with ghosts, however. Historically, most avoided contact with ghosts at all costs, as contact with ghosts could result in soul loss and perhaps death. Amoss, *Coast Salish Spirit Dancing*, 18.

76. Swinomish Tribal Mental Health Project, *A Gathering of Wisdoms*, 214.

77. Swinomish Tribal Mental Health Project, *A Gathering of Wisdoms*, 210.

78. Swinomish Tribal Mental Health Project, *A Gathering of Wisdoms*, 292.

79. Swinomish Tribal Mental Health Project, *A Gathering of Wisdoms*, 138.

80. Miller states that in his experience Shaker healers are more often called to address ailments stemming from community disharmony, while shamans may be called to address "instances of cosmic disharmony and spiritual disaffection." Jay Miller, *Lushootseed Culture*, 34.

81. Swinomish Tribal Mental Health Project, *A Gathering of Wisdoms*, 227.

82. Megan MacDonald, field notes, summer 2004.

83. Cecilia Firethunder, keynote address, Women and Girls' Gathering, Panhandle Lake, Washington, August 18, 2001.

84. *Native Women's Wellness Newsletter*, Winter 2000–2001, 8.

85. A small news item in the Squaxin Island tribe's monthly newspaper illustrated this well. The staff from the Fitness Center reported that the stereo had gone missing from the exercise room. "We would like the person or persons responsible to know that acts like this don't affect only one person, but the whole community. The clients that utilize the Fitness Center really enjoy listening to music while they do their workout. Some even brought their own CDs. This is their time to enjoy what makes them happy and healthy. Now all they have to listen to until we can find money to replace the radio is the sound of the fitness equipment and their own breathing. . . . So the next time you decide to take something that is not yours, think about how many other people you would be affecting." *Klah'Che'Min*, August 2001, 3.

86. SPIPA, "Women and Girls' Gathering, Annual Report," 2004.

87. Rogers, "Sharing the Message at Home," 5.

88. Field notes, July 30, 2004.

89. Field notes, August 1, 2004.

90. SPIPA, "Women and Girls' Gathering, Annual Report," 2004.

91. Field notes, August 17, 2001. "After this presentation I took a walk around the lake, following a nature trail that the owners of the camp have built. Along the path, the camp owners have placed markers next to certain plants, describing the plant, how it grows, and the ways in which Native Americans *used to* use the plants. The use of past-tense on the signs seems strikingly incongruous. 'Red Elderberry used to be an important source of food for Native Americans.' 'Some Northwest Tribes thought the shrub (Black Gooseberry) had powers to ward off

evil influences.' 'Oregon Grape was used for medical purposes.' Tall Oregon Grape: 'Native Americans used the bark to make a bright yellow dye for basket materials.' As I walked, I thought of the women inside, teaching each other the art of basketry even at this moment. Osoberry, or Indian Plum: 'Native Americans used many parts of the plants medicinally.' I again think of the women inside, still discussing the plants their grandmothers taught them to use. 'Big Leaf Maple: Native Americans used the wood for bowls, utensils, and canoe paddles, and the bark for making rope.' I am remembering a woman I met recently whose husband has built a traditional canoe, traditional paddles. 'Cascara: Native Americans used the bark for laxatives, washing sores, and treating heart strain.' Cedar: 'Native Americans used this tree for many religious and medical purposes . . . as remedy for toothache, sore throats, cuts and poisoning. Bark was used to make clothing and baskets.' Hemlock: 'bark was used to tanning hides and making dyes.' Salal: 'the dark juicy berries were the most plentiful and important fruit for Native Americans.'' Red Huckleberry: 'used for fish bait.' All these 'used to's' are maddening—the women inside are *still* doing these things!"

92. Krise, "Memories of Gathering."

93. These tribal communities continue to hold First Salmon ceremonies, including some that are open to the public, such as the Squaxin Island's First Salmon Ceremony at the Arcadia Boat Launch Beach during the first or second weekend of August.

94. Field notes, "Talent Show, Women and Girls' Gathering, Panhandle Lake, August 18, 2001."

95. *South Puget Intertribal News*, February–March, 2006, 2.

6. Coming Full Circle

1. SBIN, *Shoalwater Bay Indian Nation FY2001 Congressional Appropriations Request* (hereafted cited as SBIN 2001 *Appropriations Request*).

2. SBIN 2001 *Appropriations Request*. Throughout this chapter I prefer to use the term "child loss" or "pregnancy loss" as opposed to "miscarriage." There are several reasons for this. First, as Linda Layne and other child-loss scholars have noted, the term miscarriage implies a fault on the part of the mother, that she did not *carry* this child properly. It is a misnomer, for in most instances the mother's actions are not responsible for the loss of the pregnancy at all. I also prefer the term "child loss" because it provides a link between mothers who lost infants prior to birth and those women in the community who have lost children later in life. This is not to suggest that these losses are the same; they are quite different. But many women in the Shoalwater Bay community, in reflecting upon these losses, also reflected upon the deaths of their children who died later in life. See Layne, *Motherhood Lost*.

3. SBIN, "The Pregnancy and Infant Mortality Emergency . . . Joint Report," in SBIN 2001 *Appropriations Request*, sec. 6: 7.

4. Kim Zillyet, March 6, 2000, quoted in the *Seattle Post-Intelligencer*.

5. Personal communication, October 6, 2000. This brings to mind Linda Layne's work on the silences surrounding pregnancy losses, in which she discusses the reluctance of contemporary women, their families, and their care providers to discuss the experience of pregnancy loss. See Layne, "Breaking the Silence."

6. *Seattle Post-Intelligencer*, February 2, 1999.

7. CDC to NCCDPHP, October 14, 1999, in SBIN 2001 *Appropriations Request*, sec. 2: 17.

8. Statement to the CDC, printed in the CDC report to the NCCDPHP, October 14, 1999, in SBIN 2001 *Appropriations Request*.

9. Carolyn St. James, "Shoalwater Bay Looks Forward to New Learning Resources Center, Clinic," *South Puget Intertribal News* 3, no.1, January–March 2003, 8.

10. See SBIN references for additional agencies.

11. When discussing the spiritual presence of ancestors in this chapter I am referring to the actual spiritual presence of their deceased ancestors, not guardian spirit powers (*syowen*), which are almost never the spirits of departed human beings. This is complicated by the fact that syowen can be inherited from one's ancestors, however.

12. For George Engel, this intersection of culture, religion, subjectivity, and physicality is expressed within a "biopsychosocial" model of medicine, which views the individual as a complex combination of biological, psychological, and social factors. Western biomedicine, he argues, is undergirded by two fundamental worldviews: reductionism, "the philosophic view that complex phenomena are ultimately derived from a single primary principle," and mind-body dualism, "the doctrine that separates the mental from the somatic" and "assumes that the language of chemistry and physics will ultimately suffice to explain biological phenomena." Challenging these principles of reductionism and mind-body dualism inherent in a focus on biomedical "disease," Arthur Kleinman argues for a focus on "illness," one that requires an understanding of how the community defines health, and how that definition of health relates to their sense of self and embodied subjectivity. Understanding health in relation to illness, rather than disease, is to see "health as a condition in which the great number of elements in a complex system are being sufficiently well managed in relation to each other." See Kleinman, *Illness Narratives*, 3–4. See also Engel, "The Need for a New Medical Model."

13. This is what Emily Martin refers to as a shift toward a "complex systems model." Martin, *Flexible Bodies*, 89–90. In many ways this also parallels medical anthropologist Thomas Csordas's argument that healing is essentially about restoring the self. As described in chapter 2, for Csordas, the self is "an indeterminate capacity to engage or become oriented in the world, characterized by effort and reflexivity." Achieving health, for the members of the Shoalwater community, has to do with orienting themselves within the cosmos, within their communal, spiritual, and natural worlds. Csordas, *Sacred Self*, 5. And as Deborah Lupton has suggested in her work on community perceptions of cancer, "Health has become a way of defining the boundaries between Self and Other, constructing moral and social categories and binary oppositions around gender, social class, sexuality, race, and ethnicity."

These boundaries and definitions emerge within the ways in which the Shoalwater community responded to the crisis, drawing from their own Coast Salish and Chinook traditions and community strengths. Lupton, *Imperative of Health*, 69.

14. Nancy Scheper-Hughes and Margaret Lock have identified what they see as three distinct bodies present in anthropological literature: the individual body, the social body, and the body politic. The individual body is the lived body-self, the experience of the individual of his or her bodily life, as described in phenomenology and autobiography. The social body is the body as symbol, used to represent social, natural, or supernatural orders. Discussions of the social body point out how the body is used, symbolically, as a microcosm of phenomena, such as political or social structures. Discussions of the body politic argue that relationships between individual and social bodies are not merely metaphors; they carry the ability to impact those systems, and as such, narratives of the body are about power and control. I argue that it is important to keep all three of these bodies in mind: the lived experience of individual Shoalwater women and men, the ways they represent their bodies through symbolic representation, verbal and otherwise, and the way those narratives of the body take part in religious, political, and economic discourses of power and resistance. Scheper-Hughes and Lock, "The Mindful Body."

15. An ectopic pregnancy is one in which the fertilized egg does not make it to the uterus and instead begins to develop in the fallopian tube. Typically, by the sixth to eighth week of gestation, ectopic pregnancies cause severe abdominal pain, cramping, and bleeding. If undetected, ectopic pregnancies can be life-threatening and might cause severe internal bleeding.

16. SBIN, "The Pregnancy and Infant Mortality Emergency . . . Joint Report," October 27, 1994, in SBIN 2001 *Appropriations Request*, sec. 6: 4.

17. Minutes, Shoalwater Bay Indian Tribal Health Advisory Committee Meeting, February 5, 1999; SBIN, EPA, "Shoalwater Bay Reservation, A Limited Environmental Assessment," January 17, 1997, in SBIN 2001 *Appropriations Request*.

18. Appendix to the NCCDPHP Report, in SBIN 2001 *Appropriations Request*, sec. 2: 32. During a visit in 2000, I was informed that some environmental scientists consider the bay to be "dead," exceeding contamination levels that allow for the sustainability of native plant and animal species. Personal communication, October 6, 2000.

19. SBIN, Tom Anderson, "Cultural Assessment Report: A Brief History of the Shoalwater Bay Reservation to Clarify the Issues; Cultural, Environmental, and Otherwise," in SBIN 2001 *Appropriations Request*, sec. 10: 1–10. See also Hajda, "Southwestern Coast Salish," 514.

20. Upper Chehalis are found in the interior on the upper Chehalis River, near the present-day Chehalis reservation in Washington. Lower Chehalis lived along the lower Chehalis River, on the Pacific Coast near Gray's Harbor, and on the Columbia River.

21. Personal Communication, November 8, 2000.

22. Personal communication, November 29, 2000.

23. SBIN, Tom Anderson, "Cultural Assessment Report," in SBIN 2001 *Appropriations Request*, sec. 10: 3.

24. Personal communication, November 8, 2000.

25. Personal communication, November 29, 2000.

26. SBIN, "The Pregnancy and Infant Mortality Emergency . . . Joint Report," October 27, 1994, in SBIN 2001 *Appropriations Request*, sec. 6: 7. The joint report issued by the tribal council, Indian Health Service, and state Department of Health attested: "Since declaration of the health emergency, the SBIT [Shoalwater Bay Indian Tribe] itself took several steps to deal with the situation. It helped arrange for mental health counseling on-site. It called in traditional healers and religious leaders to help individuals and the community cope with their grief. It made all tribal offices smoke-free. This joint report is another step of the SBIT taking control over events which individuals, the community, and health care appeared impotent to prevent."

27. *Seattle Post-Intelligencer*, March 6, 2000. For a similar discussion among African-American communities, see Roberts, *Killing the Black Body*. Iris Young, in her discussion of the phenomenological experience of pregnancy, points out its unique position as "a bodily experience in which transparent unity of self dissolves and the body attends positively to itself at the same time that it enacts its projects." As she goes on to argue, "this move to situate subjectivity in the lived body jeopardizes dualistic metaphysics altogether. There remains no basis for preserving the mutual exclusivity of the categories subject and object, inner and outer, I and world." See Young, "Pregnant Embodiment." Her point seems particularly important here, where Coast Salish and Chinook notions of health and wellness already challenge an essentialist and individualist notion of the self, suggesting instead a porous and community-based notion of subjectivity. Pregnancy, as an inherently liminal state existing between self and nonself, highlights this notion all the more clearly.

28. *New York Times*, March 26, 2000.

29. *Seattle Post-Intelligencer*, May 26, 2000.

30. Minutes, Shoalwater Bay Indian Tribe Health Advisory Committee Meeting, February 5, 1999.

31. A 2002 study confirmed that miscarriage rates in the surrounding counties remained at national averages and that a scourge of failed pregnancies in the late 1990s was limited to the Shoalwater Bay tribe. Paul Shukovsky, "Failed Pregnancies Isolated to Shoalwaters, Health Study Finds," *Seattle Post-Intelligencer*, April 18, 2002, http://www.seattlepi.com/default/article/Failed-pregnancies-isolated-to-Shoalwaters-1085541.php (accessed June 25, 2012).

32. See Layne, *Motherhood Lost*.

33. Personal communication, November 8, 2000.

34. Judith Altruda Anderson, "Foreword," *Summertime*, 15.

35. Joan Shipman, "Separation," in Anderson, *Summertime*, 63.

36. Midge Porter, "Marie Riddel," in Anderson, *Summertime*, 80.

37. Midge Porter, "Marie Riddel," in Anderson, *Summertime*, 80.

38. Recall from chapter 4 that traditionally Chinook and Salish youth would spend five days in isolation on the island in the bay as they sought spirit powers at puberty.

39. See chapter 5 for a discussion of such traditional, community-based approaches to healing as they are being put into practice with the South Puget Intertribal Planning Association's Women's Wellness Program.

40. Personal communication, November 29, 2000.

41. Personal communication, November 8, 2000.

42. Economic concerns are an important part of well-being in coastal tribal communities. Hajda noted that in 1985 unemployment rates in this region ranged from 30 percent on the Quinault reservation to 33 percent at Shoalwater and 39 percent at the Chehalis reservation. Hajda, "Southwestern Coast Salish," 515.

43. SBIN, EPA, "Shoalwater Bay Reservation, A Limited Environmental Assessment," January 17, 1997, in SBIN 2001 *Appropriations Request*, iii.

44. Personal communication, November 8, 2000.

45. For a similar analysis of the way in which key subsistence species can become a central symbol of a people's identity, see Nesper, *The Walleye War*.

46. "Shoalwater Reservation Centennial: From Carcowan through the Charleys—100 Years," *Sou'Wester* 1, no. 3 (Autumn 1966).

47. Because many Shoalwater tribal families received allotments on the Quinault reservation, they can legally act under the Quinault treaty. Here the judge ruled based on traditional salmon fishing for the Quinault, who live farther north up the Pacific coast, ignoring that many Native communities covered under the Quinault treaty were not Quinault but Columbia River tribes. SBIN, Tom Anderson, "Cultural Assessment Report," in SBIN 2001 *Appropriations Request*, sec. 10: 4.

48. SBIN, Tom Anderson, "Cultural Assessment Report," in SBIN 2001 *Appropriations Request*, sec. 10: 4.

49. *Seattle Post-Intelligencer*, March 6, 2000.

50. Personal communication, November 8, 2000.

51. Guilmet and Whited, *People Who Give More*, 14.

52. *New York Times*, March 20, 2000.

53. Midge Porter, "Uncle Dave," in Anderson, *Summertime*, 75–76. The product name is Sevin; cabaryl is the active ingredient.

54. Minutes, Shoalwater Bay Indian Tribe Health Advisory Committee Meeting, February 5, 1999.

55. Personal communication, October 6, November 8 and 29, 2000.

56. Personal communication, November 1, 2000.

57. Tom-Orme, "Native American Women's Health Concerns."

58. Personal communication, November 29, 2000.

59. In 2001 the community had already raised more than seven thousand dollars toward construction costs from the sale of baked goods, arts, crafts, and books.

60. Personal communication, November 29, 2000. The visiting healer, from the Tulalip reservation, brought "spirit boards, a divining device phonetical-

ly pronounced squi-day-lich." Upon reading the cedar boards, "'the spirits revealed to him that death was coming down in the form of rain,' Teresa Whitish said" (*Seattle Post-Intelligencer*, February 2, 1999). The *squi-day-lich* is described by Sampson as a "manifestation of the spirit" of Big Lake, or the Skagit River, which "took the form of a piece of vine maple formed in a circle about six inches in diameter with the two ends crossed, leaving handholds. The vine maple circle was wrapped with buckskin and adorned with tassels of mountain goat hair. Down the river it was made of cedar and cedar bark." See Sampson, *Indians of Skagit County*, 58–60.

61. See Hilbert and Bierwert, "Naming Ceremonies," in *Ways of the Lushootseed People*.

62. Personal communication, November 29, 2000.

63. See Linda Layne's work on pregnancy loss and the need for rituals to address these losses. Layne, "Breaking the Silence"; Layne, *Motherhood Lost*, 69–99.

64. Joan Shipman, "Separation," in Anderson, *Summertime*, 70.

65. Rosalita Shipman, "Memories," in Anderson, *Summertime*, 73

66. Anita Couture, "Agnes James, A Beautiful Woman," in Anderson, *Summertime*, 94–95.

67. For a study of community ethics and their influence on community understandings of health and wellness, see Balshem's *Cancer in the Community*.

68. Lynn Clark, "Irene Shale," in Anderson, *Summertime*, 85.

69. Lynn Clark, "Irene Shale," in Anderson, *Summertime*, 98–100.

70. Personal communication, November 8, 2000.

71. Midge Porter, "My Name Is Chinook," in Anderson, *Summertime*, 96.

7. "Rich in Relations"

1. Hilbert and Miller, "Storied Arts," 12.

2. Chandler et al., *Personal Persistence, Identity Development*, 111.

3. Jay Miller, *Lushootseed Culture*, 89.

4. Chandler et al., *Personal Persistence, Identity Development*, 14.

5. Chandler et al., *Personal Persistence, Identity Development*, 95.

6. Chandler et al., *Personal Persistence, Identity Development*, 13.

7. Chandler et al., *Personal Persistence, Identity Development*, 14.

8. Jay Miller, *Lushootseed Culture*, 89.

9. American Friends Service Committee, *Uncommon Controversy*, 69.

10. Swinomish Tribal Mental Health Project, *A Gathering of Wisdoms*, 179.

11. Swinomish Tribal Mental Health Project, *A Gathering of Wisdoms*, 178–79.

12. Swinomish Tribal Mental Health Project, *A Gathering of Wisdoms*, 69.

13. Palmer, "Taqʷšəblu and Indian Time," 32.

14. Bruce Granville Miller, "The Individual, the Collective," 113.

15. Collins, *Valley of the Spirits*, 3.

16. Collins, "The Influence of White Contact," 106.

17. Amoss, *Coast Salish Spirit Dancing*, 35–36.

18. Hilbert and Bierwert, *Ways of the Lushootseed People*, 38. There are two Lushootseed words for people: "The first, 'ʔaciłtalbixw' is a more general term, meaning any group of Indian people. The second word for people, 'ʔi(h)išəd' refers only to those people who are one's relations."

19. Bierwert, *Brushed by Cedar*, 18, 203. See also Bierwert, "I Can Lift Her Up," 191, and Swinomish Tribal Mental Health Project, *A Gathering of Wisdoms*, 155. Coast Salish groups in Washington and southwest British Columbia have been portrayed as relatively decentralized, with an egalitarian social structure where hierarchies were based on cultural knowledge rather than inheritance (though the two often went together), and access to subsistence resources was gained through kinship relations.

20. Charles Hill-Tout, in Maud, *The Salish People*, 33.

21. Suttles, *Coast Salish Essays*, 226.

22. Collins, "The Influence of White Contact," 116.

23. Hajda, "Southwestern Coast Salish," 511. See also Collins, *Valley of the Spirits*, 86–87.

24. Collins, *Valley of the Spirits*, 86–87.

25. Swinomish Tribal Mental Health Project, *A Gathering of Wisdoms*, 146.

26. Guilmet and Whited, *People Who Give More*, 70.

27. Bierwert, *Brushed by Cedar*, 210–11. See also Swinomish Tribal Mental Health Project, *A Gathering of Wisdoms*, 155.

28. Swinomish Tribal Mental Health Project, *A Gathering of Wisdoms*, 211.

29. McHalsie, "We Have to Take Care," 100.

30. Harmon, "Coast Salish History," in Bruce Granville Miller, *Be of Good Mind*, 34.

31. Harmon, "Coast Salish History," 36.

32. Swinomish Tribal Mental Health Project, *A Gathering of Wisdoms*, 147.

33. Swinomish Tribal Mental Health Project, *A Gathering of Wisdoms*, 148.

34. Carroll L. Riley, "Ethnological Field Investigation," 75.

35. Swinomish Tribal Mental Health Project, *A Gathering of Wisdoms*, 175.

36. Carroll L. Riley, "Ethnological Field Investigation," 43.

37. Suttles has noted that among the southern Coast Salish (the group with which this book is primarily concerned), villages were not only one's primary permanent site of residence but were also relatively closed to outsiders. See Suttles and Lane, "The Southern Coast Salish," 493.

38. "Their territorial unit was the village although they did recognize special ties among those who lived on the same drainage system." Collins, *Valley of the Spirits*, 4. The independent political nature of the Coast Salish village reflected the value placed upon kinship. In a culture where the "highest unit of common allegiance was the extended family," one's allegiance was to one's village rather than to any higher collective or abstract political identity. Barnett, *Coast Salish of British Columbia*, 241.

39. Bruce Granville Miller, *Be of Good Mind*, 82–84.

40. Bruce Granville Miller, *Be of Good Mind*, 81. See also Bierwert, *Brushed by Cedar*, 18, 203.

41. Riley reports that such longhouses reached "100 feet or more," Riley, "Ethnological Field Investigation," 50. Pavel, Miller, and Pavel write that longhouses in the southern Puget Sound more typically ranged from 100 to 200 feet long, and 60 to 140 feet wide. Pavel et al., "Too Long, Too Silent," 61.

42. Maud, *The Salish People*, 44.

43. Carlson, *You Are Asked to Witness*, 89; see also Keith Thor Carlson in Bruce Granville Miller, *Be of Good Mind*, 152.

44. Riley, "Ethnological Field Investigation," 58.

45. Pavel et al., "Too Long, Too Silent," 61.

46. Quoted in Jay Miller, *Lushootseed Culture*, 81.

47. Carlson, *You Are Asked to Witness*, 89.

48. Carlson in Bruce Granville Miller, *Be of Good Mind*, 152.

49. Collins, *Valley of the Spirits*, 62.

50. See Collins, *Valley of the Spirits*, 62; Maud, *The Salish People*, 44; Jay Miller, *Lushootseed Culture*, 84.

51. Bruce Granville Miller, *Be of Good Mind*, 152. See also Collins, *Valley of the Spirits*, 64, and Jay Miller, *Lushootseed Culture*, 83.

52. Jay Miller takes a more esoteric approach in his description of the metaphorical significance of longhouses, noting that "the shape of the house mirrored that of the universe, as did the body. . . . The house frame was imagined to be a body on its hands and knees, with the face at the front. Therefore, the outer skin . . . house walls, and rim of the world were equated, as were the inner heart, hearth, and helios. In regions with gabled roofs, moreover, the ridge pole was equated with a spine, river, and the Milky Way, as were the four support posts with human limbs and sky pillars." Jay Miller, *Lushootseed Culture*, 36.

53. Bruce Granville Miller, "The Individual, the Collective," 114.

54. On children's autonomy see Guilmet and Whited, *People Who Give More*, 70.

55. Elmendorf and Kroeber, *Twana Culture*, 397.

56. Amoss, *Coast Salish Spirit Dancing*, 37. See also Jay Miller, *Lushootseed Culture*, 96.

57. Jay Miller, *Lushootseed Culture*, 94. While individual judgment is highly valued, however, it is also the case that failure to comply with group consensus can mean shunning. See Jay Miller, *Lushootseed Culture*, 93. Further, Coast Salish communities appear historically to have valued personal achievement and rank rather than collective class or status. June McCormick Collins has argued that this emphasis on personal status and rank changed after the arrival of Euroamericans in the mid-nineteenth century, with the resultant centralization of wealth in fewer hands. As individuals increased in wealth, it often put them in conflict with kinship loyalties. Collins, "Religious Change," 106. For example, Harmon argues that Coast Salish views of interpersonal conflict differed from nineteenth-century Euroamerican views. During the 1855 Seattle war, Euroamerican Seattleites saw Native aggression as a sign of political uprising and an attack on white culture and society. For its Native participants, Harmon argues, the conflict had much more to do with avenging "personal injuries or to seize slaves and property" rather than

an abstract political statement. In a similar manner, murders "were not crimes that imperiled an abstract public order; they were injuries to and by individuals and their families, who had responsibility for rectifying the social consequences. Personal losses and relationships were likewise the motivations for acts of war and arrangements to end war." See Harmon, *Indians in the Making*, 89, 93. Among contemporary communities, Bruce Granville Miller has argued, it remains a serious offence to fail "to recognize individual achievement, status or distinctiveness." See Bruce Granville Miller, "The Individual, the Collective," 114.

58. Jay Miller, *Lushootseed Culture*, 15.

59. American Friends Service Committee, *Uncommon Controversy*, 5.

60. Harmon, *Indians in the Making*, 30, 37.

61. Elmendorf and Kroeber, *The Structure of Twana Culture*, 402.

62. Suttles, *Coast Salish Essays*, 219.

63. Harmon, *Indians in the Making*, 8.

64. Harmon, "Coast Salish History," 37–38.

65. Elmendorf and Kroeber, *The Structure of Twana Culture*, 306–8.

66. Harmon, "Coast Salish History," 33; and Suttles, *Handbook of North American Indians*, 15.

67. Kew, "Central and Southern Coast Salish," 46. See also Kew, "Salmon Availability."

68. Suttles, *Coast Salish Essays*, 210, 220.

69. Suttles, *Coast Salish Essays*, 22.

70. Carlson, *You Are Asked to Witness*, 112.

71. Jay Miller, *Lushootseed Culture*, 26.

72. Collins, *Valley of the Spirits*, 187.

73. Raibmon, *Authentic Indians*, 109.

74. Suttles, *Coast Salish Essays*, 210, 222.

75. Suttles, *Coast Salish Essays*, 223. Elmendorf described various other aboriginal "intercommunity culture complexes," such as "upper-class marriage, the s'i'wad give-away feast, the secret-society initiation ritual (sXä˙dəb), intervillage disk-game gambling (swák'xac'), and intervillage eating contests. . . . In all of these intercommunity relations the village community or the extended-village community was the social unit involved." Elmendorf and Kroeber, *The Structure of Twana Culture*, 298–99. Particular activities were limited to the wealthy. These included "exercising of wealth powers (s'iya'lt guardian spirits), sponsorship of or ceremonial recognition by sponsor at the s'i'wad give-away feast and the secret-society initiation, and the reciprocal wealth-exchange type of marriage. All these institutions operated intertribally, that is, cooperation of more than one village community was necessary for their occurrence." Elmendorf and Kroeber, *The Structure of Twana Culture*, 404.

76. "The Shaker religion generated new institutional identities among its followers at the same time as it perpetuated intervillage ties among the Coast Salish. . . . The doctrine of the Shaker church is an additional example of information—

this time religious, rather than political—exchanged at the hop fields." Raibmon, *Authentic Indians*, 111, 113.

77. Amoss, *Coast Salish Spirit Dancing*, 38.

78. At such a gathering, Pamela Amoss tells us, the first action one undertakes is to locate one's relatives. As Amoss describes it, "he may then initiate exchange of small friendly services, such as bringing food when his relatives are putting up a party, or sending his son along to help with the wood cutting or other work. Then gradually, if the overtures are successful, the frequency and weight of the reciprocal exchanges are intensified." Amoss, *Coast Salish Spirit Dancing*, 36.

79. Two canoes, from Lower Elwha and from La Push, Washington, made the round trip. It took two months and covered thirteen hundred miles.

80. Suttles, *Coast Salish Essays*, 228.

81. Bruce Granville Miller, *Be of Good Mind*, 21.

82. Hajda, "Southwestern Coast Salish," 511.

83. Riley, "Ethnological Field Investigation," 53–54.

84. Harmon, "Coast Salish History," 34.

85. Amoss, "Symbolic Substitution," 228–29.

86. Harmon, "Coast Salish History," 48. "This flux of peoples, coupled with marriages that were almost always between people from different house groups (often from different population clusters) and with property rights held by house groups and conjugal families, created intricate webs of socio-economic relationships that spread well beyond the region. Social space had few clear boundaries. Individuals could belong by right of birth and marriage to several different house groups. People from different winter population clusters would have rights, therefore, to many of the same resources. Ties of kin crossed dialect and language boundaries that, in any case, were not sharp. The obligations incurred by gift-giving at the feasts added another layer to the web." Harris, *Resettlement of British Columbia*, 73–74.

87. Riley, "Ethnological Field Investigation," 46.

88. Harmon, *Indians in the Making*, 143.

89. Harmon, *Indians in the Making*, 138.

90. Harmon, *Indians in the Making*, 181.

91. Harmon, *Indians in the Making*, 202. I would argue this is another reason why the South Puget Intertribal Planning Agency works: it simultaneously recognizes the independence and autonomy of local tribal communities and maintains and makes use of long-standing intertribal relationships.

92. Harmon, *Indians in the Making*, 216, 247.

93. Sider, "The Walls Came Tumbling Up," 276.

94. Jay Miller, *Lushootseed Culture*, 126.

95. Jay Miller, *Lushootseed Culture*, 127.

96. Swinomish Tribal Mental Health Project, *A Gathering of Wisdoms*, 162.

97. Bierwert, *Brushed by Cedar*, 112.

98. Jay Miller, *Lushootseed Culture*, 111. Bruce Granville Miller put it well: "The human being is made up of several components, these being the body; the soul,

which only some can see, which continues after death, and which can be lost; the breath/vitality/life, which is not a condition, which can be disassociated from the body, thereby creating a state of illness, and which can be returned; and the shadow/reflection, which can also be lost or stolen. Although everyone has all four components, they are not well integrated in the young, the feeble, the ill, and others who are consequently vulnerable to spiritual dangers. There is another part of the self that not all acquire: Sil'ye, the guardian spirit power. This power is gained in various ways, coming to some unbidden and to others through the rigorous process of fasting, training, and purification necessary to become acceptable prior to undergoing a quest for the spirit power. Once a relationship is established a human becomes a different kind of human being. This relationship is invoked in the complex known as Spirit Dancing, or *Syowen*, a term that refers to the visible aspects of the nonhuman world given to humans. The initiate into Spirit Dancing draws closer to the nonhuman sphere and, eventually, gains new powers and abilities once the relationship becomes properly managed. The private relationship with the spirit power becomes dangerous if spoken of, and if the spirit is offended, an upset in the relationship can cause the death of the human partner. A healthy person, then, knows who they are (their self) and maintains a proper spirit relationship." Bruce Granville Miller, "Rereading the Ethnographic Record," 313–14.

99. Sergei Kan identifies parts of the "complete social persona": the Ghost, which settles in the cemetery; the Spirit which finds a permanent home in village of the dead; the Reincarnated Spirit which is reborn as a baby of a matrilineal relative; and names, regalia (ritually passed on to matrikin), social position (title, wealth, spouse). Personhood was tied to names. If you were sick, you might be renamed in an attempt to give you a new life. Shagoon was likewise a part of one's social persona. It was one's "origin/destiny," "the root concept in Tlingit culture . . . an individual's or matrilineal group's ancestors, heritage, origin, and destiny . . . The clan's totemic animal(s) as well as the crest(s) representing it were also called Shagoon." Kan, *Symbolic Immortality*, 42–44 (parts of persona), 68–69 (destiny), 72 (renaming).

100. Swinomish Tribal Mental Health Project, *A Gathering of Wisdoms*, 162.

101. Such notions are reminiscent of property holdings by some aristocratic families in England, for instance. Great manor houses were only stewarded by each generation, who were responsible for caring for the house and passing it on to the next generation. With the privilege of living in the home came crests, titles, lands, and resources but also a great sense of responsibility and, in many instances, a sense that one did not actually *own* the estate, at least not as an individual, but was merely one in a long line temporarily holding it.

102. Hilbert and Miller, "Storied Arts," 36.

103. Harmon, "Coast Salish History," 49.

104. Amoss, *Coast Salish Spirit Dancing*, 17.

105. Hilbert and Bierwert, *Ways of the Lushootseed People*, 18–19.

106. Hilbert and Miller, "Storied Arts," 36.

107. Carlson, *You Are Asked to Witness*, 112.

108. Swinomish Tribal Mental Health Project, *A Gathering of Wisdoms*, 153.

109. For a description of contemporary initiation into winter spirit dances, see Jay Miller, *Lushootseed Culture*, 103–4.

110. Elmendorf and Kroeber, *The Structure of Twana Culture*, 498.

111. Amoss, *Coast Salish Spirit Dancing*, 72.

112. Collins, "Religious Change," 23. In another publication Collins also argued that "people usually, if not exclusively, acquired spirits which had belonged to one of their ancestors." Collins, *Valley of the Spirits*, 180.

113. Collins, *Valley of the Spirits*, 180.

114. Collins, "Religious Change," 23.

115. Jay Miller, *Lushootseed Culture*, 57.

116. Elmendorf, *Twana Narratives*, 191. Elmendorf also notes, "When a power that belonged to a dead ancestor comes to a person or wants to come to him that makes the person sick. Then a doctor comes and diagnoses the case and brings the power to that person, so he can show it and use it and then he gets well." Elmendorf, *Twana Narratives*, 190. Smith shares this view that powers could be inherited from deceased relatives: "But the power said, 'Don't kill me. I used to belong to your uncle . . . I belong to you." Smith, *Puyallup-Nisqually*, 84.

117. Bierwert, *Brushed by Cedar*, 162–63.

118. Holm, "Art," 613.

119. Suttles, *Coast Salish Essays*, 105–32.

120. An intermediate display could be located among northern Coast Salish groups, particularly those who have adopted the sxwexwey masking tradition, which includes an inherited right to perform the mask as well as a more developed and shared graphic artistic expression of it. See Barnett, *Coast Salish of British Columbia*, 310.

121. Barnett, *The Coast Salish of British Columbia*, 309.

122. Swinomish Tribal Mental Health Project, *A Gathering of Wisdoms*, 135. Hill-Tout described such an instance when he witnessed a woman singing and dancing her deceased mother's song at a winter spirit dance. Maud, *The Salish People*, 48.

123. Bruce Granville Miller, *Be of Good Mind*, 19.

124. Elmendorf and Kroeber, *The Structure of Twana Culture*, 248.

125. Jay Miller, *Lushootseed Culture*, 26–27.

126. Carlson, *You Are Asked to Witness*, 112.

127. McHalsie, "We Have to Take Care," 95–97.

128. In Halkomelem, the individual responsible for stewarding a site is referred to as the *Sia:teleq*. See McHalsie, "We Have to Take Care," 98.

129. One "could fish where there were people who regarded him as kith or kin." Harmon, "Coast Salish History," 39.

130. Carlson, *You Are Asked to Witness*, 113.

131. Suttles, *Coast Salish Essays*, 4. See also Jay Miller, *Lushootseed Culture*, 89–90.

132. Suttles, *Coast Salish Essays*, 6.

133. Suttles, *Coast Salish Essays*, 91.

134. Carlson, *You are Asked to Witness*, 89.

135. Jay Miller, *Lushootseed Culture*, 21–23. See also Bierwert, *Lushootseed Texts*.

136. Suttles, *Coast Salish Essays*, 20.

137. Suttles, *Coast Salish Essays*, 20.

138. Amoss, *Coast Salish Spirit Dancing*, 36.

139. Jay Miller, *Lushootseed Culture*, 25.

140. Swinomish Tribal Mental Health Project, *A Gathering of Wisdoms*, 170.

141. Suttles, *Coast Salish Essays*, 8.

142. Carlson, *You Are Asked to Witness*, 12.

143. Bruce Granville Miller, *Be of Good Mind*, 159.

144. Harmon, *Indians in the Making*, 27.

145. Riley, "Ethnological Field Investigation," 47.

146. Riley, "Ethnological Field Investigation," 47; Elmendorf and Kroeber, *The Structure of Twana Culture*, 334; Harmon, *Indians in the Making*, 27.

147. Riley, "Ethnological Field Investigation," 73.

148. Amoss likewise concludes that when the economic system was undermined, it "inevitably undermined the credibility of native beliefs and rituals as well." See Amoss, "Symbolic Substitution," 226.

149. See Collins, *Valley of the Spirits*, 82, 123, 172, 179.

150. Jay Miller, *Lushootseed Culture*, 92.

151. Snyder, "Quest for the Sacred," 150.

152. Elmendorf and Kroeber, *The Structure of Twana Culture*, 330.

153. Suttles, *Coast Salish Essays*, 21.

154. Harmon, *Indians in the Making*, 50.

155. Snyder, "Quest for the Sacred," 151. See also Collins, *Valley of the Spirits*, 142. Jay Miller identifies three reasons for potlatches: to cement relationships, to celebrate the end of winter spirit dances, and to honor the dead at the memorial potlatch. See Jay Miller, *Lushootseed Culture*, 99.

156. Kathleen Mooney, "Social Distance and Exchange," 326.

157. Kathleen Mooney, "Effects of Rank and Wealth."

158. Mooney, "Effects of Rank and Wealth," 393.

159. Mooney, "Effects of Rank and Wealth," 402.

160. Mooney, "Effects of Rank and Wealth," 401, 342.

161. Mooney, "Social Distance and Exchange," 344.

162. Mooney, "Social Distance and Exchange," 326.

163. Mooney, "Social Distance and Exchange," 326–27.

164. Mooney, "Social Distance and Exchange," 345.

165. Bierwert, *Brushed by Cedar*, 32.

166. Mooney, "Social Distance and Exchange," 330.

167. Taqʷšəblu (Vi Hilbert), in Yoder, *Dxwʔdal taqʷšəblu tulʔal ti syeyaʔyaʔs*, 18. Carlson quotes one Sto:lo man explaining that after he caught a first spring salm-

on and did not share any, "the rest of the season I only got two more. That's all I got that season—three Springs. I told my wife Mary, 'See, I didn't give that first Spring away and I only got two more all season—bad luck.'" See Carlson, *You Are Asked to Witness*, 4.

168. "You know, my mother always said that anybody who didn't share things with people would die. Well, Rose was getting too good for us, she wasn't one of the dirty Indians—she died of cancer." See Mooney, "Social Distance and Exchange," 327.

169. Harmon, *Indians in the Making*, 175.

170. Harmon, *Indians in the Making*, 177–78.

171. Bierwert, *Brushed by Cedar*, 33. When political reforms were brought to Puget Sound communities, they were viewed through this lens: did they promote self-sufficient, autonomous communities? When the Indian Reorganization Act was introduced, for instance, local communities did not strongly oppose the measure because they already viewed themselves as self-governed, autonomous communities. Harmon, *Indians in the Making*, 198. Federal termination policies of the 1950s and 1960s (which sought to terminate tribal status as a path toward assimilating Native communities into the general population) were met with mixed responses. On the one hand, western Washington tribes already saw themselves as competent and self-sufficient, not needing government assistance, and those opposing the measure tended to portray Native people as helpless victims. But western Washington tribes were also not interested in abandoning their own histories or giving up connections with their ancestors. Nor were they interested in relocation: western Washington Natives were already mobile, moving throughout the region for seasonal employment and returning to reservation communities during off-work times of year. Harmon, *Indians in the Making*, 207, 212.

172. Collins, *Valley of the Spirits*, 81. See also Weber, *Protestant Ethic*.

173. Jay Miller, *Lushootseed Culture*, 45. See also Harmon, *Indians in the Making*, 35.

174. Swinomish Tribal Mental Health Project, *A Gathering of Wisdoms*, 211.

175. Swinomish Tribal Mental Health Project, *A Gathering of Wisdoms*, 159.

176. Guilmet and Whited, *People Who Give More*, 70.

177. Marino, "History of Western Washington since 1846," 175. The allotment of lands in 1874 on the Squaxin Island and Skokomish reservations and during the 1880s at Nisqually, Puyallup, and Tulalip, and Nisqually was part of this overall effort.

178. Carlson, *You Are Asked to Witness*, 102. In British Columbia residential schools were made mandatory in 1884. The policy was strictly enforced beginning in 1920, and schools began closing down in the 1950s, following reports of abuse, neglect, and inefficiency. In the United States boarding schools began with President Grant's 1869 "Peace Policy," which placed missionaries in charge of American Indian reservations and encouraged the formation of church-run boarding schools. U.S. boarding schools have continued to the present but began a precipitous decline following the Indian Self-Determination and Education Assistance Act of 1975, which encouraged (but did not necessarily fund) the formation of local reservation schools operated under tribal control. Peak enrollment was in the

1970s, with an estimated 60,000 students. By 2007, enrollment in Native boarding schools was estimated at 9,500.

8. The Healthy Self

Portions of this chapter provided the basis for my article "Salmon as Sacrament: The Revival of First Salmon Ceremonies in the Pacific Northwest," in *Religion, Food, and Eating in North America*, ed. Benjamin Zeller (forthcoming, Columbia University Press).

1. Elmendorf and Kroeber, *The Structure of Twana Culture*, 266.

2. American Friends Service Committee, *Uncommon Controversy*, 6.

3. Schaepe, "Sto:lo Identity and the Cultural Landscape," 255. In Jay Miller's analysis of Lushootseed culture he makes a parallel argument, suggesting that cedar trees provide an apt metaphor for thinking about Coast Salish sense of place. For Miller, cedar trees, longhouses, and canoes serve as the central symbols in Lushootseed culture. Cedar trees symbolize a powerful sense of being rooted in a place as well as the "covering" that such a place provides for its people. See Jay Miller, *Lushootseed Culture*, 1–2. These ancient trees reflect a keen sense "of localization," as he puts it, reflected in the "security of a house and the stability of a canoe," both of which are made from cedar trees, "the very rootedness of which epitomizes" a profound connection to place.

4. Jay Miller, *Lushootseed Culture*, 20. Deur and Turner, *Keeping It Living*. This book makes a compelling argument for the cultivation of gardens prior to the arrival of Europeans, as families maintained garden plots of native plants over many generations.

5. Charles Hill-Tout, in Maud, *The Salish People*, 117.

6. Bierwert, *Brushed by Cedar*, 231–32.

7. American Friends Service Committee, *Uncommon Controversy*, 71.

8. American Friends Service Committee, *Uncommon Controversy*, 187.

9. Pavel et al., "Too Long, Too Silent," 60.

10. Harris, *Resettlement of British Columbia*, 75.

11. Tweddell, "A Historical and Ethnological Study of the Snohomish," 553. By contrast, Suttles argues that within Coast Salish traditions ancestors "had always had human form," that they were originally dropped from the sky at the world's beginning or created by Transformer. Stories describe instances where animals are related to animal people by marriage, or are the descendents of people, but "people are not descendents of animals." He argues that the more common myth is that Transformer "transformed some of the First People into animals but left others, who pleased him, to become founding ancestors of villages." Suttles, *Coast Salish Essays*, 104, 105.

12. Charles Hill-Tout, in Maud, *The Salish People*, 22; Boyd, *Coming of the Spirit of Pestilence*, 55. See also Lee and Frost, *Ten Years in Oregon*, 299–301.

13. Charles Hill-Tout, in Maud, *The Salish People*, 22.

14. Wilkinson, *Messages from Frank's Landing*, 29.

15. Kew, "Salmon Availability," 178.

16. Kew, "Salmon Availability," 179.

17. First salmon ceremonies are described in Jay Miller, *Lushootseed Culture*, 98–99; Amoss, *Coast Salish Spirit Dancing*, 20; Suttles, *Coast Salish Essays*, 163, 188, 468; Crawford, *Native American Religious Traditions*; and Seaburg and Miller, "Tillamook," 564.

18. See Charles Hill-Tout, in Maud, *The Salish People*, 116. Myron Eells writes that salmon were required to be cut lengthwise, with the head and backbone removed as one piece. Cutting a fish crosswise could result in dire consequences. By way of example, he records an oral narrative in which the first Thunderbird was born from a fish improperly cut. See Castile, *Indians of Puget Sound*, 254. Charles Wilkes noted in 1838 that "they had no desire to sell the fish, as they had a superstitious objection to dispose of the fish to strangers, even if induced to sell it, they will always take the heart out and roast if for themselves; for they believe that if the heart of the fish were eaten by a stranger at the first of the season, their success would be destroyed and they would catch no more fish. To prevent this, they consider it requisite that a certain number of 'sleeps' or days should pass before anymore are sold." He noted that when pressed to sell salmon, they offered them for the impossible price of $1.25 each, rather than the usual ten cents, a tactic that successfully put off European traders. See Wilkes, *Narrative of the U.S. Exploring Expedition*. As Sean Connors has noted (unpublished paper delivered to the American Academy of Religion, San Francisco, November 1997), such tactics among the Yurok of Northern California worked effectively to preserve future salmon runs, by ensuring that a necessary number of spawning adults were able to navigate the river, thus ensuring future salmon generations.

19. Amoss, *Coast Salish Spirit Dancing*, 20. Suttles notes that some twentieth-century first salmon ceremonies incorporated prayers to a Supreme Deity, though this was unusual. See Suttles, *Coast Salish Essays*, 161.

20. Hill-Tout describes one such story of four brothers named Qais, who visit a village of salmon people. Salmon die, are eaten by brethren, ritually returned to water, and reborn. Qais request that salmon will come to the human world to feed their people, and they agree, in return for ritual care, so that they can return to life. See Charles Hill-Tout, in Maud, *The Salish People*, 60–62.

21. Elmendorf and Kroeber, *Twana Culture*, 531. The first salmon ceremony is described in greater detail in Elmendorf, *Twana Narratives*, 254–55.

22. Ross, *Adventures of the First Settlers*, 105. See also Dunn, *History of the Oregon Territory*, 121; Cox, *Adventures on the Columbia River*, 171.

23. Charles Wilson, in Stanley, *Mapping the Frontier*, 29. See also Meany, *Diary of Wilkes in the Northwest*, 45. Charles Wilkes recorded an incident in which a young boy in their party was tormenting river eels, throwing stones at them. This, he noted, "excited the wrath of the Indians, as they said they should catch no more fish if he continued his sport. They have many superstitions connected with salmon, and numerous practices growing out of these are religiously observed. Thus, if any one dies in their lodges during fishing season, they stop fishing for several days, if

a horse crosses the ford, they are sure no more fish will be taken." See Wilkes, *Narrative of the U.S. Exploring Expedition*, 366.

24. Charles Hill-Tout, in Maud, *The Salish People*, 116. William Fraser Tolmie reports a similar experience, dated May 13, 1833: "10 a.m. arrived at Kuhelamit village. . . . They had six fine salmon, in a canoe, but superstitiously refused to sell any, because they were the first caught this season, and it is their firm belief that if the first caught salmon are not roasted in a particular manner, the fish will desert the river. Tantalizing as it was, had to proceed without any." Large, *Journals of William Fraser Tolmie*, 167.

25. Hilbert and Bierwert, *Ways of the Lushootseed People*, 14.

26. American Friends Service Committee, *Uncommon Controversy*, 4.

27. As Kew has noted, first salmon ceremonies are public, while spirit dancing is intensely private. Kew, "Central and Southern Coast Salish," 480.

28. Suttles, *Coast Salish Essays*, 188.

29. For a description of the legal battle for fishing rights and the Boldt Decision, see Wilkinson, *Messages from Frank's Landing*. See also Wilkinson, *Blood Struggle*, 150–76.

30. Thrush, *Native Seattle*, 189. As Thrush aptly describes it, the conflict over fishing rights began with Washington statehood in 1889, granting a privileged status to private fisheries, which soon overran native fishers. Federal courts tended to side with Indian rights, while the state consistently opposed them. In the early 1900s state fish and game authorities limited native fishing and failed to protect native fishing sites. The Makah were first to sue for fishing rights, as early as the 1950s. When fish populations decreased in the 1960s, many commercial fishers blamed tribes, despite their relatively small impact on fishing runs. As the state curtailed tribal fishing yet further, tribes became "increasingly defiant about the state-sponsored repression of fishing rights." Thrush, *Native Seattle*, 189. Native people protested, staging fish-ins, which one individual described as "12, 18 ornery old Indian people, standing up for what they firmly believed in." Thrush, *Native Seattle*, 190. The movement was supported by "progressive churches, civil-rights organizations and other groups" and gained national media attention. In 1974 the Boldt Decision was handed down, ensuring "half the harvestable salmon to treaty tribes." Thrush, *Native Seattle*, 190. The decision initially applied only to treatied or "landed" tribes. Over time "landless tribes" were also included in the decision: the Nooksack, Upper Skagit, Sauk-Suiattle, Stillaguamish; in 1981 the Jamestown Klallum; in 1988 six other tribes had pending petitions: Snohomish (denied 2004), Snoqualmie (granted 1997, again in 1999), Cowlitz (received 2000), Chinook (under consideration 2009), Steilacoom (denied 2008), Duwamish (granted federal status in 2001 by Clinton, rescinded by Bush two days later, still petitioning in 2010).

31. McHalsie, "We Have to Take Care," 103.

32. McHalsie, "We Have to Take Care," 104.

33. McHalsie, "We Have to Take Care," 105–6.

34. Carlson, *You Are Asked to Witness*, 55.

35. Schaepe, in Bruce Granville Miller, *Be of Good Mind*, 253.

36. McHalsie, "We Have to Take Care," 105.

37. Please note that at times I use the past tense in this chapter because I am trying to reconstruct Native views of the self as they existed in the nineteenth and early twentieth centuries. This should not be taken as a sign that these views are no longer held—indeed the great majority of them are still held by traditional Native people throughout the Northwest.

38. For additional examples, see Reverend Eells's discussion of "finding tamahnous," in Castile, *Indians of Puget Sound*, 395–97. For information on traditions of the guardian spirit complex, see Spier, *Prophet Dance*, 25–29; Benedict, *Concept of the Guardian Spirit*; and Suttles, *Coast Salish Essays*. A Chinook tradition describes a young man who, during a winter spirit dance, received a spirit power and fell to the floor unconscious. The young man's father, skeptical of his sincerity, accused him of merely being overwhelmed by the sight of an attractive young woman. To prove his point, the father put a hot coal on his son's hand. The coal burned completely through the son's hand before he woke. Seeing this, the father was humbled and became a believer in the traditional faith. Jacobs, *Clackamas Chinook Texts*, 2:245–46, 467.

39. For more on this see Zenk, "Kalapuyans," 550; Suttles and Lane, "Southern Coast Salish," 497; and Amoss, *Coast Salish Spirit Dancing*, 13, regarding the Nooksack.

40. Castile, *Indians of Puget Sound*, 395–98.

41. Elmendorf and Kroeber, *Twana Culture*, 492. Tweddell notes that Snohomish youths sought such spirit powers in the high country, near Lake Getchel and what is now Stevens Pass. Tweddell, "A Historical and Ethnological Study of the Snohomish," 551.

42. Smith, *Puyallup-Nisqually*, 58.

43. Jacobs, *Coos Narrative and Ethnologic Texts*, 98.

44. Jacobs et al., *Kalapuya Texts*, 341–42.

45. Swan, *The Northwest Coast*, 172; and Castile, *Indians of Puget Sound*, 395.

46. Jacobs et al., *Kalapuya Texts*, 346–47. The account continued:

> Well now when we wanted to become a shaman, and a wealthy bondsman, and a hunter, they did not just become so. They would go to the hills (mountains) and (or) to the lakes, that is where they got their power from. All sorts of things (guardian spirit-powers) were in the hills, which was why they became powerful, what they call spirit-power. That is what they obtained. Rattlesnake was there, and grizzly, and wolf. We went for all sorts of things in the hills. A whale lived in the water. They called (another water dwelling spirit-power) sea lion, and they (also) named a large snake. All sorts of things lived in the water. That is what was made into spirit-power. The people did not merely become strong (have power to do certain things). We went to the hills and to the water, and in consequence (of the acquisition there of spirit-powers) we were transformed into shamans, and wealthy headmen, and hunters. That is how we did. Not all the people were shamans, or wealthy headmen, or were hunters. Only

a few of the people were of that sort. They would be swimming five days and nights in a lake, and they worked out in the hills (piling rocks, brush, etc.). They worked for that length of time, they ate nothing, for that long a time they would work at the water and in the hills. The old men and women were always telling about that to the children. That is the reason why they learned to do their work, when they went to the water, to a lake, and to the hills. No matter even if the place (were) very far away, they would still go work (for a spirit-power acquisition) in the hills. All the hills where spirit-powers were (obtainable), that was where wealth was (to be gotten). And in the same way there was wealth (to be had) in the lakes.

47. Jacobs, *Coos Narrative and Ethnologic Texts*, 90.

48. Spirit dancing continues throughout the Northwest today and has seen a significant revival of practice since the 1970s. See for example Suttles, *Coast Salish Essays*; Jacobs, *Clackamas Chinook Texts*; Jacobs, "Indications of Mental Illness"; and Jacobs et al., *Kalapuya Texts*. Spirit quest traditions among the Chinook and Nisqually can be found in Ray, *Lower Chinook Ethnographic Notes*, 78–80; and Smith, *Puyallup-Nisqually*, 58. As Eells has noted, failing to participate in such spirit dances could in fact cause sickness. See Castile, *Indians of Puget Sound*, 400.

49. For another example of a very similar guardian spirit tradition, see Goulet, *Ways of Knowing*.

50. Jacobs, *Coos Narrative and Ethnologic Texts*, 28–29.

51. Smith, *Puyallup-Nisqually*, 57, 59.

52. Smith, *Puyallup-Nisqually*, 68–75.

53. Elmendorf and Kroeber, *Twana Culture*, 488; Elmendorf, *Twana Narratives*, 169.

54. Elmendorf and Kroeber, *Twana Culture*, 480–81. In Twana the distinction was made between *swa'daš* (doctoring power) and *c'ša'lt* (any other type of spirit power). Elmendorf, *Twana Narratives*, 199. The term for the act of spiritual doctoring was *yawa'd·ab*. The Puyallup and Nisqually referred to doctoring power as *tudáb*. See Smith, *Puyallup-Nisqually*, 75.

55. For a similar discussion of wealth as spiritual abilities and strengths, see Thomas Buckley, "Menstruation and the Power of Yurok Women."

56. Collins, *Valley of the Spirits*, 146.

57. Jay Miller, *Lushootseed Culture*, 119.

58. Hajda, "Southwestern Coast Salish," 512.

59. Jay Miller, *Lushootseed Culture*, 45.

60. Amoss, *Coast Salish Spirit Dancing*, 229.

61. Bierwert, *Brushed by Cedar*, 178.

62. Bierwert, *Brushed by Cedar*, 174–75; Jilek, *Indian Healing*; Amoss, *Coast Salish Spirit Dancing*.

63. Bierwert, *Brushed by Cedar*, 178.

64. Kew and Kew, "People Need Friends," 31.

65. Bierwert, *Brushed by Cedar*, 7.

66. Bierwert, *Brushed by Cedar*, 69.

67. Bierwert, *Brushed by Cedar*, 277. "Similarly, the songs of the longhouse, while embodied, are also figures that Coast Salish people understand to have autonomy . . . [these are] presences that not only make themselves known but continue to do so over the course of life and generations."

68. Bierwert, *Brushed by Cedar*, 63–64.

69. Hunn et al., *N'ch'i-Wana, "The Big River,"* 230.

70. Collins, "Religious Change," 26.

71. Collins, *Valley of the Spirits*, 4. See also Hajda, "Southwestern Coast Salish," 512.

72. Seaburg and Miller, "Tillamook," 566.

73. Amoss, *Coast Salish Spirit Dancing*, 12–13.

74. Amoss, *Coast Salish Spirit Dancing*, 62.

75. Collins, *Religious Change*, 173.

76. Collins, *Valley of the Spirits*, 183.

77. Suttles, "Central Coast Salish," 467. "Dancers with songs classed as sqə'yəp used red paint, wore cedar bark, and (according to tradition) danced with knives piercing their flesh. Dancers with skwəníəc songs could cause cedar boards or hoops to become animated and reveal past events and things not visible to ordinary people."

78. Elmendorf and Kroeber, *The Structure of Twana Culture*, 311.

79. Bierwert, *Brushed by Cedar*, 281.

80. Seaburg and Miller, "Tillamook," 566.

81. Bruce Granville Miller, "Rereading the Ethnographic Record," 314.

82. Harmon, *Indians in the Making*, 23–24.

83. Jay Miller, *Lushootseed Culture*, 21.

84. Suttles, "Central Coast Salish," 467. Jay Miller *Lushootseed Culture*, 58–61, lists several categories of spirits and the beings they are often associated with, suggesting that such associations may still exist: hunting and fishing (badger, pheasant, clam, duck); basketry, weapon making, crafts, gambling, preventing diseases from spreading (appear as woman from east or man from west); warfare (monsters, loon, raccoon, grizzly, black bear, cougar, wild cat); wealth (manlike beings who lived in large houses with slaves); undertakers (wolf); traveling to land of the dead (Little Earths); shamanic powers require four or more (otter, beaver, mountain lion, hawk, eagle, shark, whale, salmon, trout, dog, snake, lizard, owl, bear, redheaded woodpecker, kingfisher).

85. Collins, *Religious Change*, 13–14.

86. Bierwert, *Brushed by Cedar*, 195.

87. Kew, "Central and Southern Coast Salish," 478. As he goes on to explain: "Spirit dancers use such places for ritual bathing when they feel a need for strengthening and renewing their powers."

88. The oldest trees in Northwest old growth forests are often cedars; Coast Salish communities were historically aware of this, which was part of why they called cedar "grandmother." Forests in older successional stages, developed after long periods of forest stability, provide a range of tree ages and species and hence a range of habitats, supporting especially rich biodiversity.

89. Gerald B. Miller, "Statement of the Twana Seowin Society" (unpubl.), and Pavel et al., "Too Long, Too Silent," 64.

90. Pavel et al., "Too Long, Too Silent," 78–79.

91. Pavel et al., "Too Long, Too Silent," 54–55.

92. Amoss, *Coast Salish Spirit Dancing*, 229.

93. See also Pavel et al., "Too Long, Too Silent."

94. Amoss, *Coast Salish Spirit Dancing*, 241.

95. Yoder, *Dxwʔdal taqʷšəblu*, 65.

96. Of course it is important to remember that all religious beliefs and practices are variable. Within the Coast Salish context, traditions are often tied to particular families—and can differ from family to family and generation to generation. While the resources cited here provide the most reliable information that we have in print about these historical traditions, it is important to keep in mind that not all Coast Salish people agree with them. Many may agree with them in general but point out that particulars would have varied within their own community or family.

9. "A Power Makes You Sick"

1. Jay Miller, *Lushootseed Culture*, 35; and Elmendorf and Kroeber, *Twana Culture*, 506–7. The Nisqually term for tamanawas healing was *sho'nahm*, or *sho'mahb*. Clark, "George Gibbs' Account of Indian Mythology" (1956), 127–31.

2. Ross, *Adventures of the First Settlers*, 105.

3. Elmendorf and Kroeber, *Twana Culture*, 500.

4. Jacobs, *Coos Myth Texts*, 93.

5. Jacobs, *Clackamas Chinook Texts*, 518.

6. Hilbert and Bierwert, *Ways of the Lushootseed People*, 22.

7. Hilbert and Bierwert, *Ways of the Lushootseed People*, 22. See Suttles and Lane, "The Southern Coast Salish," 498, who describe the *sgwədilič* as "a guarding power." Other healers might also use the *túStəd*, "animated fir poles with a bag tied at one end" that empowered them with second sight. See Collins, *Valley of the Spirits*, 164.

8. Smith, *Puyallup-Nisqually*, 78.

9. Sampson, *Indians of Skagit County*. See also Smith, *Puyallup-Nisqually*, 114–15.

10. Jacobs, *Coos Narrative and Ethnologic Texts*, 91.

11. For instance, one Clackamas Chinook healer described his mode of practice: "I shall not eat. My spirit power would not become strong. We go all full (of our spirit power at its strongest). We put (throw) our breath into it." This same individual described his father's brother, Si'lik'wa, who used to say, "Eat! Humph. No. Why should I eat? I have come all full, my heart has come (at maximal strength). First I shall examine, when I have finished, before you should think of giving me food. . . . My spirit power is still at its strongest now. Its strength goes all full; it goes on ahead of me. That is the way with me." Jacobs, *Clackamas Chinook Texts*, 520.

12. Jacobs et al., *Kalapuya Texts*, 184.

13. Jacobs, *Coos Myth Texts*, 94. See also Barnett, *Indian Shakers*; Kelm, *Colonizing Bodies*.

14. Elmendorf, *Twana Narratives*, 165.

15. Smith, *Puyallup-Nisqually*, 60.

16. Jacobs, *Coos Narrative and Ethnologic Texts*, 91.

17. Jacobs, *Clackamas Chinook Texts*, 544.

18. Daniel Lee and Joseph Frost describe their observation of healing practices during the 1830s: "The people believe that they hold intercourse with spirits that they can see the disease, which is some extraneous thing, as a small shell, or a pipe, or a piece of tobacco, or some other material substance, which they (the doctors) describe. It is firmly believed that they can send a bad 'tam-an-a-was' into a person, and make him die, unless it is cast out by some other 'medicine man.' . . . Several poles are tied together at the ends, and from six to ten men are arranged along them in sitting posture, each having a stick with which he beats on the poles; and thus a loud jarring noise is produced, which may be heard a long distance. This is accompanied with a kind of singing, in which the 'medicine man' leads, while he kneels near his patient on the other side of the poles, making horrid contortions and grimaces, as if some demoniac was raging within. The chant is not long, and then, after a few minutes, is renewed again, and thus repeated several times. The way being now prepared, he approaches his patient, and, after a painful and persevering effort, with his mouth applied as a cupping-glass, he transfers the 'skokom' [malevolent spirit, or spirit of the dead, in Chinook *wawa*] or 'tam-an-a-was' or disease, wholly or in part from the patient to himself!" Lee and Frost, *Ten Years in Oregon*, 179–80.

19. Elmendorf, *Twana Narratives,* 165.

20. Jacobs, *Clackamas Chinook Texts*, 526. Lee and Frost describe a dance they witnessed at the Dalles: "The nights among the Dalles Indians were spent in singing and dancing, and their carousals could be heard a mile. One, and then another of the medicine men, would open his house for a dance, where it was generally kept up five nights in succession; men, women and children or both, danced on a large elk-skin spread down on one side of the fire, that blazed in the center of the group, keeping time to the loud-measured knocking of a large pole suspended horizontally, and struck endwise against a wide cedar-board—the dancer jumping, and invoking his 'tamanawas' or familiar spirit, until, exhausted, he falls as one dead, by the overpowering influence of his 'familiar.' To arouse him from this deep slumber requires the skill of a medicine man, or 'Mesmerizer,' who going around him peeps, and mutters and hoots at his toes, fingers, and ears, and wakes his tamanawas; when he shudders, groans, opens his eyes, and lives again!" Lee and Frost, *Ten Years in Oregon*, 163. The family who had put up the dance to seek healing for a family member or to honor an individual with a naming or memorial ceremony would 'pay' those who came to dance or sing, in return for their offering of their spirit-power. Traditionally, such payments might take the form of horses, blankets, dentalia, or clamshell beads. See Jacobs et al., *Kalapuya Texts*, 184, 340.

21. See Beckham et al., *Native American Religious Practices*; Boyd, *Coming of the Spirit of Pestilence*, and Boyd, *People of the Dalles*. See also Jacobs, *Coos Narrative and*

Ethnologic Texts; Jacobs, *Coos Myth Texts*, 127–260; Jacobs, *Clackamas Chinook Texts*, 258–59; Jacobs, *Content and Style of an Oral Literature*; Jacobs, "Indications of Mental Illness"; Jacobs et al., *Kalapuya Texts*; Bierwert, *Brushed by Cedar*; and Elmendorf, *Twana Narratives*, 165.

22. Bruce Granville Miller, "The Individual, the Collective," 113.

23. "Like a potlatch, a winter dancer required the concerted help of the sponsor's family." Collins, *Valley of the Spirits*, 188. See also Collins, "Religious Change," 33.

24. Amoss, *Coast Salish Spirit Dancing*, 39–40.

25. Amoss, *Coast Salish Spirit Dancing*, 40.

26. Amoss, *Coast Salish Spirit Dancing*, 40. Amoss also identifies a fourth type of relational bond formed within spirit dancing, the bond between non-kin "created by the reciprocal exchanges of money or goods," as part of the potlatch element of the ceremony. Amoss, *Coast Salish Spirit Dancing*, 40.

27. Winter spirit dancing, however, was more likely to emphasize the individualism of Coast Salish cultural life, while Shakers more often emphasized "togetherness rather than independence." Amoss, "Symbolic Substitution," 238. Amoss argues that both the Shaker Church and spirit dancing are very individualistic, and both honor personal autonomy. Within both traditions kinship is highly valued, and for both, the ceremonial system simply could not work without the support of the kin network: sponsoring ceremonial gatherings and feeding and accommodating guests is expensive and complicated. Amoss also argues, however, that spirit dancing has experienced a greater renaissance, growing while the Shaker Church and once popular Pentecostal churches have waned, because spirit dancing serves individual emotional needs while working to preserve the social group in ways that the other two do not. Amoss, *Coast Salish Spirit Dancing*, 145–47.

28. Amoss, *Coast Salish Spirit Dancing*, viii, 41, 149.

29. Amoss, *Coast Salish Spirit Dancing*, 55.

30. Wayne Suttles has made a similar argument regarding contemporary spirit dancing, seeing within the modern integration of potlatch "work" and spirit dancing, an "uneasy sort of alliance. . . . Interest in religious expression through dancing and interest in improving status through gift-giving are at times clearly in competition, as when dancers become possessed and interrupt the 'work' or when the 'work' drags on until the dancers are too weary to dance, or when a dancer will not dance because he cannot afford to." Suttles, *Coast Salish Essays*, 206. Sergei Kan's work offers an interesting comparison with the Coast Salish material. The Tlingit mortuary complex tends to emphasize "hierarchy and competition" at the same time that it affirms "equality, unity and cooperation between matrikin as well as balanced reciprocity between members of the two moieties." There is a "contrast between everyday life where conflicts and disagreements between matrilineal relatives were common and ritual in which they tried to achieve maximum cooperation and present a unified front to members of the opposite moiety." The ritual domain becomes the place where "these contradictory principles of hierarchy and equality, competition and cooperation were reconciled." Kan, *Symbolic Immortality*, 10.

31. Jacobs, *Content and Style of an Oral Literature*, 515. See also Jacobs and Jacobs, *Nehalem Tillamook Tales*.

32. Jacobs, *Content and Style of an Oral Literature*, 510.

33. Elmendorf, *Twana Narratives*, 17.

34. Amoss, *Coast Salish Spirit Dancing*, 19–20.

35. Collins, "Religious Change," 42.

36. Eells, *Indians of Washington Territory*, 675.

37. Jacobs, *Content and Style of an Oral Literature*, 511–12.

38. Jacobs, *Content and Style of an Oral Literature*, 522.

39. Elmendorf and Kroeber, *Twana Culture*, 524. Such understandings help shed light on historical decisions to undergo last rites and baptism, as discussed in chapter 2. If new diseases came from Euroamericans, then they would be best suited to offer a ritual means of combating the disease-causing spirit power.

40. Smith, *Puyallup-Nisqually*, 60–61, 79.

41. Bruce Granville Miller, "The Individual, the Collective," 113.

42. Harmon, *Indians in the Making*, 23. See also Bruce Granville Miller, "Rereading the Ethnographic Record," 313–14; Amoss, *Coast Salish Spirit Dancing*; and Jenness, *The Faith of a Coast Salish Indian*.

43. "The argument so far is that current notions of the individual, personal secrecy, and obligations owed first and foremost to non-human beings create culturally sanctioned autonomy." Bruce Granville Miller, "The Individual, the Collective," 114–15. See also Swinomish Tribal Mental Health Project, *A Gathering of Wisdoms*, 135.

44. John Scouler records an instance regarding the death of Futilifum, a Chinook warrior: "As the case was obviously hopeless it was judged improper to give any active medicine. Before he died he vomited an entire bulb of the phalangium esculentum (camas). . . . After Futilifum's death it was recollected that six months previously, while in good health, he had eaten a quantity of camas at the house of a Kowlitch (Cowlitz) chief who was famed for his skill in medicine. The superstitious fancy of the Indians immediately took fire; they believed that their favorite warrior F. had been charmed to death by the Kowlitch chief; while their resentments were yet warm a party was sent off and unfortunately succeeded in shooting the devoted chief." Scouler, "Journal of a Voyage to N.W. America," 278–79.

45. Jacobs et al., *Kalapuya Texts*, 274.

46. Jacobs and Jacobs, *Nehalem Tillamook Tales*, 158.

47. Jacobs and Jacobs, *Nehalem Tillamook Tales*, 142–43. See also Thompson and Egesdal, *Salish Myths and Legends*, 3–59.

48. Other myths likewise remind Native peoples of the origin of illness in cultural and social conflict, such as a story told by George Gibbs documenting the arrival of smallpox. In this instance Scotam, a female chief living on the sun's road in the west, and Smee-ow, a male chief living on the sun's road in the east, were at war. Scotam sent smallpox to Smee-ow, and Smee-ow responded by creating a herb effective against the smallpox. See Clark, "George Gibbs' Account of Indian Mythology," 125–67.

49. Jacobs, *Content and Style of an Oral Literature,* 515.

50. Jacobs, *Clackamas Chinook Texts,* 513.

51. Jacobs, *Clackamas Chinook Texts,* 516–17.

52. Occasionally, attempting to remove a disease-causing spirit power might be dangerous. A healer could remove a patient's own spirit power, taking it for his or her own if it appeared like a good one. Exchanging it for another, healers had the ability to sing spirit powers in and out of ailing individuals. As one Clackamas Chinook commented: "They said that a shaman might extract it, he would exchange spirit powers. He had seen that his (the patient's spirit power) was a good spirit-power. He extracted it, he inserted a different one." Jacobs, *Clackamas Chinook Texts*, 517.

53. Elmendorf, *Twana Narratives*, 221; Elmendorf and Kroeber, *Twana Culture,* 505.

54. Jacobs, *Coos Narrative and Ethnologic Texts*, 53.

55. For a similar discussion see Schwarz, *Molded in the Image of Changing Woman*; and, among the Dene Tha, see Goulet, *Ways of Knowing*.

56. Guilmet and Whited, *People Who Give More*, 25.

57. Guilmet and Whited, *People Who Give More*, 29.

58. Guilmet and Whited, *People Who Give More*, 29.

59. Elmendorf and Kroeber, *Twana Culture*, 513.

60. Suttles and Lane, "The Southern Coast Salish," 496

61. Suttles, "Central Coast Salish," 467.

62. Armstrong, *Oregon*, 134.

63. See Suttles, *Coast Salish Essays;* Amoss, *Coast Salish Spirit Dancing*; Boyd, *People of the Dalles*, 80. See also Elmendorf and Krober, *Twana Culture,* 516. Smith notes that the elderly, the sick, and small children, those lacking power and a clear sense of self-identity are particularly vulnerable to soul loss. Smith, *Puyallup-Nisqually*, 86.

64. Amoss, *Coast Salish Spirit Dancing*, 44. "Anger, social tensions, sudden shocks or scares, soul loss, bad thoughts or wrong actions, ghosts, use of alcohol and drugs, dreaming of the dead, witchcraft or having something 'put on you,' failure to follow spiritual rules, eating the wrong food, coming into contact with a power which is too strong for you, being near dangerous things, or simply being too non-traditional are often thought to be the primary cause of imbalance, illness, and disorder. Severe emotional and psychological disturbance may be attributed to soul loss, spirit possession, loss of the breath of life or to evil 'work' by an enemy." Swinomish Tribal Mental Health Project, *A Gathering of Wisdoms*, 139–40. See also Jay Miller, *Lushootseed Culture*, 130–31.

65. Amoss, *Coast Salish Spirit Dancing,* 45.

66. "Soul" is a problematic term, not to be understood as identical in meaning with the soul of the Christian tradition. See for example Voss et al., "Tribal and Shamanic-Based Social Work Practice," 228.

67. Jacobs, *Content and Style of an Oral Literature*, 516.

68. Jay Miller, *Lushootseed Culture,* 130–31.

69. Boas, "Doctrine of Souls and Disease," 39.

70. See Castile, *Indians of Puget Sound*, 400. For discussions of the Spirit Canoe Ceremony, one of the most important examples of this mode of healing, see Jay Miller, *Lushootseed Culture*; Bierwert, *Brushed by Cedar*; Hultkrantz, *Shamanic Healing and Ritual Drama*, 65–70.

71. Eells, *Indians of Washington Territory*, 677.

72. Boas, "Doctrine of Souls and Disease," 40.

73. Sampson, *Indians of Skagit County*, 11. Such traditions of soul loss, and the possibility of traveling to the spirit world and retrieving a lost soul, exist in virtually all Northwest tribal communities along the Pacific coast from southeast Alaska to southern Oregon and east to the Plateau. Benedict, *Concept of the Guardian Spirit*; Spier, *Prophet Dance*, 25–29; Beckham et al., *Native American Religious Practices*; Hunn et al., *N'ch'i-Wana, "The Big River."*

74. Elmendorf, *Twana Narratives*, 213. Smith describes a similar event: "He then sent his power along the paths which had been traveled by the patient during the last few days until the lost soul was encountered. His power brought the soul back and replaced it in the patient, who was immediately cured. This cure was done in a manner similar to that of all shamanic curing." And again: "So that time they caught on and brought the soul back from high up, making downward motions, and spread it carefully over the child. As they took their hands from above him, he opened his eyes and smiled. From that moment he nursed and was perfectly well." Smith, *Puyallup-Nisqually*, 87. See also Elmendorf, *Twana Narratives*, 221–37, for additional descriptions of soul recovery ceremonies.

75. This ceremony is described in careful detail in Jay Miller, *Lushootseed Culture*, 135–38. See also Smith, *Puyallup-Nisqually*, 95–99.

76. "The most striking examples of wood sculpture in the Puget Sound region were power figures in the shape of anthropomorphic beings . . . [which were] made by shamans of the central Puget Sound tribes and were part of the equipment of the Spirit Canoe ceremony." See Holm, "Art," 621.

77. Waterman, "The Paraphernalia of the Duwamish Spirit Canoe Ceremony."

78. Suttles and Lane, "Southern Coast Salish," 498.

79. Elmendorf, *Twana Narratives*, 233. For a description of a similar ceremony among the Tillamook see Seaburg and Miller, "Tillamook," 566.

80. Boas, "Doctrine of Souls and Disease," 39.

81. Subiyay (Gerald Bruce Miller) and CHiXapKaid (D. Michael Pavel), *Soul Recovery Ceremony* (Seattle Art Museum, 2005), http://www.seattleartmuseum.org/exhibit/interactives/sabadeb/flash/index.html, viewed June 5, 2012.

82. Jay Miller, *Lushootseed Culture*, 132.

83. Collins, *Valley of the Spirits*, 200. See also Jay Miller, *Lushootseed Culture*, 121.

84. Boas, "Doctrine of Souls and Disease," 40–41. Leslie Spier also argues that communities throughout the Northwest share such traditions of multiple healers working together, and enacting a drama of their spirits' journeys to the underworld, as recorded vividly in studies of the Salish spirit canoe ceremony. Spier records instances of the phenomena among the Tlingit, Bella Coola, Tsimshian,

Haida, Kawkiutl (Kwak'waka'wakw), Nootka, Cowichan, Chilliwack, Klallam, Twana, Skokomish, other Salish tribes (including the Klallam, Snohomish, Puyallup, Nisqually, Snoqualmie, Duwamish, Suquamish, Samamish), the Quileut, Quinalt, Chinook, Chehalis, Carrier, Shuswap, Lillooet, Thompson, southern Okanagan, and Flathead nations. Disease etiologies of soul loss and shamanic abilities to retrieve such wayward souls are also found among Oregon coastal tribes, such as the Tillamook, Alsea, Coos, Lower Umpqua, and Kalapuya. See Spier, *Prophet Dance*, 14–15. See also Dawson, *Notes and Observations on the Kwakiool*, 63–98; Boas, *Mythology of the Bella Coola Indians*; Boas, *First General Report on the Indians of British Columbia*.

85. Kew and Kew, "People Need Friends," 29.

86. Kew and Kew, "People Need Friends," 33–34.

87. Kew and Kew, "People Need Friends," 33–34.

88. Kew and Kew, "People Need Friends," 35.

89. Kew and Kew, "People Need Friends," 35.

90. Amoss, "Memories of Vi," 3.

Conclusion

1. Myron Eells, in Castile, *Indians of Puget Sound*, 419–20.

2. As two groups vie for control over the interpretation of one girl's illness we see more clearly how notions of self and wellness are the product of cultural location. The Skokomish and Squaxin with whom Eells spoke seemed entirely aware of this. Consider for instance that when Eells asked why "white men" were not susceptible to the same diseases as Indians, they explained: "They say that a white man's heart is hard like a stone, so that the invisible stone which they shoot cannot affect it, while the Indian's heart is soft like mud, and thus is easily affected. They also say that a cause of this is that the Indian swims very much, and often times has his clothes off while at home, and so his heart is susceptible to the influence of the tamahnous, while the white man's customs are different, and so his heart is different." White men were seen as being ontologically different, shaped by their imperviousness to the world around them and their existence outside of the network of relationships that defined Coast Salish people and that constituted a healthy working identity. Indeed, as Native persons took on Euroamerican ways, Eells describes local Coast Salish as believing that they also became impervious to Native illnesses and cures, because "they professed to believe that his heart had become hard like a white man's and so rejected the tamahnous." If Ellen Gray was to "become white," which Eells was working diligently to achieve, her embodied self must change as well; her heart must, in the Coast Salish perspective, "become hard like a white man's." Castile, *Indians of Puget Sound*, 421.

3. Eells, "The Decrease of the Indians," 147.

4. As Emily Martin, Susan Bordo, and Margaret Lock have argued, the body is formed, inscribed, experienced in ways shaped by our cultural experience. But the specific gendered *terrain* of that body plays an enormous role in how that cultural experience is played out. The body itself, with all its comings and goings, its ex-

changes and expressions, interacts with these cultural expectations. See Lock, *Encounters with Aging*; and Martin, *Flexible Bodies*.

5. See "Canoe Way: The Sacred Journey," Bainbridge WA: Islandwood Films, 2009.

6. Kan, *Symbolic Immortality*, 8.

7. Bruce Granville Miller, "The Individual, the Collective," 107–8.

8. Bruce Granville Miller, "The Individual, the Collective," 111. Alexandra Harmon uses her analysis of Coast Salish ceremonialism to come to interpret 1855 treaty-making gatherings that reflect this relational sensibility. She argues that because ritualized gatherings "established and symbolized bonds of friendship—prestigious bonds—with illustrious men," such gatherings would have been proof that "the American chief had acknowledged their prestige and the value of having their respect." Harmon, *Indians in the Making*, 80–84. The use of kinship language within treaties would have appealed to Coast Salish sensibilities, because from their perspective the making of treaties was about establishing kin-like relationships. Referring to the president as "Great Father," to his aides as "elder brothers," and to Native people as "children" would have been a form of paternalism for whites, but for Native Americans at such gatherings the phrases may instead have evoked a sense of kinship. Kinship requires exchange of gifts, and that is what occurred at such gatherings. Native resources and land were given in exchange for access to natural resources, doctors, and financial assistance. Harmon, *Indians in the Making*, 83. She also points out that this kinship relationship would quickly have proven itself false, when American officials failed to honor their role as provider. Hence, "most native people saw no reason to defer to them" thereafter. Harmon, *Indians in the Making*, 97. In a similar vein, the nature of treaties would have been understood differently. Native Americans felt that Euroamericans ("Bostons") did not honor their treaties. From a Salish perspective being "good" meant being "prosperous and honored," and so receiving the wealth promised in the treaties would *make* them "good." From a Euroamerican perspective, however, for treaties to make Native Americans "good" would necessitate cultural conversion, a complete assimilation to white culture. Harmon, *Indians in the Making*, 110–11.

9. Harmon, *Indians in the Making*, 240. See also Wilkinson, *Messages from Frank's Landing*.

10. See, for example, Burhansstipanov et al., "American Indian and Alaska Native Cancer Data Issues"; Health Promotion Resource Center, Stanford Center for Research in Disease Prevention, and the Indian Health Service, *Restoring Balance*; Hodge and Casken, "American Indian Breast Cancer Project"; Johnson and Tomren, "Helplessness, Hopelessness, and Despair"; Noren et al., "Challenges to Native American Health Care"; Olson, "Applying Medical Anthropology"; Swinomish Tribal Mental Health Project, *A Gathering of Wisdoms*; Taylor, "Health Problems and Use of Services"; Tom-Orme, "Native American Women's Health Concerns."

Bibliography

Unpublished Works

Beaver, Herbert. "Further Information Respecting the Aborigines; Containing Reports of the Committee on Indian Affairs at Philadelphia, New York, New England, Maryland, Virginia, and Ohio," 1842. *Oregon Historical Society Typescript Copy of Manuscript 372*. Portland: Oregon Historical Society.

Beaver, HMS. *Medical Officers Journal*, 1863. Mf67. Portland: Oregon Historical Society.

Boyd, Robert. "The Introduction of Infectious Diseases among the Indians of the Pacific Northwest, 1774–1874." Unpublished PhD diss., University of Washington, Seattle, 1985.

Buchanan, Charles. "Some Medical Customs, Ideas, Beliefs and Practices of the Snohomish Indians of Puget Sound." *St. Lewis Courier of Medicine* 21. Typescript of original, Special Collections, University of Washington Libraries. Seattle, 1889.

Center for Disease Control and Prevention. "EPI-AID E99–29 Executive Summary Report." October 14, 1999.

Chirouse, Casimir. *Letters of 6 May, 14 July, and 6 August.* Oblates of Marie Immaculate, 1862. MSS 1581. Portland: Oregon Historical Society.

De Smet, Pierre. *Letters.* Excerpts from Unidentified Periodicals, 1850. Multnomah County Library Special Collections.

Donnelly, Joseph P. "Selections from the U.S. Department of Justice Archives Regarding Liquor Traffic among the Indians in the Territories of Washington, and Oregon 1849–1860." Manuscript 765, Joseph P. Donnelly, JJ, Collection. Portland: Oregon Historical Society.

Henry, Anson. *Monthly Medical Reports, Grand Ronde Reservation. Records of the Oregon Superintendency of Indian Affairs, 1848–73.* National Archives, Washington, 1856–58.

Howard, Augustine. "Special Needs of the American Indian." Paper presented at conference on Death and the Individual, *How Can We Provide Better Care?* St. Elizabeth Hall, St. Elizabeth Hospital, Yakima Washington, June 29–30, 1977.

Huggins, Edward. "Journal of Occurrences: 1833–39," *Fort Niqually Records, March, 1836*. Manuscripts and University Archives, 1839. University of Washington Libraries, Seattle.

Johnson, H. H. "*Report to United States Commissioner of Indian Affairs*, September 9, 1909." *Jason Lee Papers.* Manuscript 936. Portland: Oregon Historical Society, undated.

Lee, Jason. "Journal of Jason Lee." Typescript copy of manuscript, Clarence Booth Bagley Miscellaneous Selections of Historical Writings, AIA 2/6, Box 22, Suzzalo Library, U of W, Seattle, undated.

McWhorter, Lucullus Virgil. "The First White Man among the Klickitats." Collected from William Charley, 10 March. MS 1528. McWhorter Collection, Holland Library, Washington State University, Pullman, 1910.

Miller, Gerald B. "Statement of the Twana Seowin Society." Shelton WA: Twana Seowin Society, 1981.

Neilson, Helen. "Focus on the Chehalis Indians 1800–1900," unpublished master's thesis, Pacific Lutheran University, Tacoma WA, 1970.

Sullivan, Nellie (Sister Mary Louise, O.P.). "Eugene Casimir Chirouse, O.M.I. and the Indians of Washington," Unpublished Master's Thesis. Seattle: University of Washington, 1932.

Published Works

Aberle, David. "The Prophet Dance and Reactions to White Contact." *Southwestern Journal of Anthropology* 15, no. 1 (1989): 74–83.

Abram, David. *The Spell of the Sensuous: Perception and Language in a More-Than-Human World*. New York: Vintage Books, 1997.

Adair, John, Durth W. Deuschle, and Clifford R. Barnett. *The People's Health: Medicine and Anthropology in a Navajo Community*. Albuquerque: University of New Mexico Press, 1988.

Adams, David Wallace. *Education for Extinction: American Indians and the Boarding School Experience, 1875–1928*. Lawrence: University Press of Kansas, 1995.

Adams, Diane L. *Health Issues for Women of Color: A Cultural Diversity Perspective.* Thousand Oaks CA: Sage, 1995.

Adamson, Thelma. *Folk-Tales of the Coast Salish*. Memoirs of the American Folk-Lore Society 27. New York: G. E. Stechert, 1934.

Adelman, Penina. "A Drink from Miriam's Cup: Invention of Tradition among Jewish Women." In *Active Voices: Women in Jewish Culture*, ed. Maurie Sacks. Urbana: University of Illinois Press, 1995.

Aitken, Larry. *Two Cultures Meet: Pathways for American Indians to Medicine.* Duluth: University of Minnesota Press, 1990.

American Friends Service Committee. *Uncommon Controversy: Fishing Rights of the Muckleshoot, Puyallup and Nisqually Indians*. Seattle: University of Washington Press, 1970.

Ames, Roger T. "The Meaning of the Body in Classical Chinese Philosophy." In *Self as Body in Asian Theory and Practice*, ed. Thomas Kasulis and Roger Ames. Albany: SUNY Press, 1993.

Amoss, Pamela. *Coast Salish Spirit Dancing: The Survival of an Ancestral Religion*. Seattle: University of Washington Press, 1978.

———. "The Indian Shaker Church." In *Handbook of North American Indians*, vol. 7: *The Northwest Coast*, ed. Wayne Suttles, 633–39. Washington DC: Smithsonian Institution Press, 1990.

———. "Memories of Vi." In *Dxwʔdal taqʷšəblu tulʔal ti syeyaʔyaʔs: Writings about Vi Hilbert, by Her Friends*, ed. Janet Yoder. Seattle: Lushootseed Research, 1992.

———. "Resurrection, Healing, and 'the Shake': The Story of John and Mary Slocum." In *Charisma and Sacred Biography*, Thematic Studies 48, ed. Michael A. Williams, 87–109. Chambersburg: American Academy of Religious Studies, 1982.

———. "Symbolic Substitution in the Indian Shaker Church" *Ethnohistory* 25, no, 3 (1978): 225–49.

Amoss, Pamela, and William Seaburg. *Badger and Coyote Were Neighbors: Melville Jacobs on Northwest Indian Myths and Tales.* Corvallis: Oregon State University Press, 2000.

Amundson, Ronald, and Darrel Numbers. *Caring and Curing: Health and Medicine in Western Religious Traditions.* Baltimore: Johns Hopkins University Press, 1998.

Anderson, Judith Altruda, ed. "Foreword." *Summertime in Georgetown: A Collection of Short Stories by Women and Girls of the Shoalwater Bay Tribal Community*, 15. Tokeland WA: Shoalwater Bay Tribal Publication, 1998.

Anderson, Judith Altuda, ed. *Summertime in Georgetown: A Collection of Short Stories by Women and Girls of the Shoalwater Bay Tribal Community.* Tokeland WA: Shoalwater Bay Tribal Publication, 1998.

Angelo, C. Aubrey. *Sketches of Travel in Oregon and Idaho*. 1858; Repr. Fairfield, WA: Ye Galleon Press, 1988.

Anzaldua, Gloria. *Borderlands/La Frontera*. Consortium–Aunt Lute Books, 1999.

Appleby, Geraldine. *Tsawwasssen Legends*. Ladner BC: Dunning Press, 1961.

Armstrong, A. N. *Oregon: Comprising a Brief History and Full Description of the Territories of Oregon and Washington*. Chicago: Chas. Scott and Company, 1857.

Arnold, David. *Colonizing the Body: State Medicine and Epidemic Disease in 19th Century India*. Berkeley: University of California Press, 1993.

Axtell, James. *The Invasion Within: The Contest of Cultures in Colonial North America*. New York: Oxford University Press, 1985.

Bagley, Clarence B. *Early Catholic Missions in Old Oregon, and Travels Over the Rocky Mountains in 1845–6*. 2 vols.. Seattle: Lowman and Hanford Company, 1932.

Bair, Barbara, and Susan F. Cayleff. *Wings of Gauze: Women of Color and the Experience of Health and Illness*. Detroit: Wayne State University Press, 1993.

Baldridge, Dave. "The Elder Indian Population and Long Term Care." In *Promises to Keep: Public Health Policy for American Indians and Alaska Natives in the 21st Century*, ed. Mim Dixon and Yvette Roubideaux. Washington DC: American Public Health Association, 2001.

Balshem, Martha. *Cancer in the Community: Class and Medical Authority*. Washington DC: Smithsonian Institution Press, 1993.

Barbeau, Marius. *Medicine Men on the North Pacific Coast.* Portland: Department of Northern Affairs and National Resources, 1958.

Barnett, Homer G. *Indian Shakers: A Messianic Cult of the Pacific Northwest.* Carbondale: Southern Illinois University Press, 1957.

———. *The Coast Salish of British Columbia*. Eugene: University of Oregon Press, 1955.

Barney, Garold. *Mormons, Indians and the Ghost Dance.* Carham MD: University Press of America, 1986.

Barry, J. Nielson. "Ko-Come-Ne-Pe-Ca, the Letter Carrier." *Washington Historical Quarterly* 20 (1929): 201–3.

Bartky, Sandra Lee. "Foucault, Femininity, and the Modernization of Patriarchal Power." In *Writing on the Body: Female Embodiment and Feminist Theory*, ed. Katie Conboy, Nadia Medina, and Sarah Stanbury. New York: Columbia University Press, 1997.

Basso, Keith. *Wisdom Sits in Places: Landscape and Language Among the Western Apache.* Albuquerque: University of New Mexico Press, 1993.

Battersby, Christine. "Her Body/Her Boundaries." In *Feminist Theory and the Body*, ed. Janet Price and Margrit Shildrick. New York: Routledge, 1999.

Beck Kehoe, Alice. *The Ghost Dance: Ethnohistory and Revitalization.* Chicago: Holt Rinehart and Winston, 1989.

Beckham, Stephen Dow. *Requiem for a People: The Rogue Indians and the Frontiermen*. Norman: University of Oklahoma Press, 1971.

Beckham, Stephen Dow, Kathryn Anne Toepel, and Rick Minor. *Native American Religious Practices and Uses in Western Oregon*. University of Oregon Anthropological Papers no. 31. 1984.

Benedict, Ruth. *The Concept of the Guardian Spirit in North America*. American Anthropological Association Memoir 29. Menasha WI: George Banta, 1923.

Berkhofer, Robert. *Salvation and the Savage: An Analysis of Protestant Missions and American Indian Response 1787–1862.* 1965; repr. Westport CT: Greenwood Press, 1977.

———. *The White Man's Indian: Images of the American Indian from Columbus to the Present*. New York: Random House, 1978.

Bermudez, Jose Luiz, Anthony Marcel, and Naomi Eilan, eds. *The Body and the Self.* Cambridge MA: MIT Press, 1998.

Bierwert, Crisca. *Brushed by Cedar, Living By the River: Coast Salish Figures of Power.* Tucson: University of Arizona Press, 1999.

———. "I Can Lift Her Up: Fred Ewen's Narrative Complexity." In *Be of Good Mind: Essays on the Coast Salish*, ed. Bruce Granville Miller. Vancouver: University of British Columbia Press, 2007.

———. *Lushootseed Texts: An Introduction to Puget Salish Narrative Aesthetics*. Lincoln: University of Nebraska Press, 1996.

Bigwood, Carol. "Renaturalizing the Body (With the Help of Merleau Ponty)," in *Body and Flesh: A Philosophical Reader*. Malton MA: Blackwell Publishers, 1998.

Biolsi, Thomas, and Larry Zimmerman. *Indians and Anthropologists: Vine Deloria Jr. and the Critique of Anthropology*. Tucson: University of Arizona Press, 1997.

Blackfeather, Judith. "Cultural Beliefs and Understanding Cancer." *American Indian Culture and Research Journal* 16, no. 3 (1992): 140.

Blanchet, Francis Norbert. *Historical Sketches of the Catholic Church in Oregon for the Past Forty Years*. Portland, 1878. Oregon Historial Society, Portland, PNW Reel 3, Microfilm History of the PNW, Sketch VIII, 220–22.

Boas, Franz. *Chinook Texts*. Washington DC: Smithsonian Institution Bureau of Ethnology, 1894.
———. "The Doctrine of Souls and Disease among the Chinook Indians." *Journal of American Folk Lore* 6 (January 1893): 20.
———. *First General Report on the Indians of British Columbia.* Report, Fifty-ninth Meeting, British Association for the Advancement of Science for 1889–1890 (1890): 801–99.
———. *Folk-Tales of Salishan and Sahaptin Tribes*. Collected by James A. Teir, Livingston Farrand, Marian K. Gould, and Herbert K. Spinden. Memoirs of the American Folklore Society 11. New York: G. E. Stechert, 1917.
———. *Kathlamet Texts*. Bureau of American Anthropology Bulletin 26. Washington, 1901.
———. *The Mythology of the Bella Coola Indians*. Memoirs of the American Museum of Natural History 2, pt 2. New York, 1898.
———. "Notes on the Tillamook." *University of California Publications in American Archaeology and Ethnology* 20 (1923): 3–16.
Bolduc, Jean-Baptiste. *Mission of the Columbia*. Trans. Edward Kowrich. Fairfield WA: Ye Galleon Press, 1979.
Bonney, W. P. "Puyallup Indian Reservation." *Washington State Historical Quarterly* 19, no. 5 (1928): 202–5.
Bordewich, Fergus M. *Killing the White Man's Indian: Reinventing Native Americans at the End of the Twentieth Century*. New York: Doubleday, 1996.
Bordo, Susan. "Bringing Body to Theory." In *Body and Flesh: A Philosophical Reader*, ed. Donn Welton. Malden MA: Blackwell Publishers, 1998.
———. "'Material Girl': The Effacements of Modern Culture." In *Body and Flesh: A Philosophical Reader*, ed. Donn Welton. Malden MA: Blackwell Publishers, 1998.
———. *Unbearable Weight: Feminism, Western Culture, and the Body*. Berkeley: University of California Press, 1995.
Bosse, Jean, ed. *Memoirs d'un Grand Brainois: Monseigneur Adrien Croquet, le Saint de l'Oregon*. Braine-L'Alleud, Belgium: Association du Musée de Braine-L'Alleud, 1977.
Boufford, Jo Ivey, and Philip R. Lee. "Federal Programs and Indian Country: A Time for Reinvention." *Public Health Reports* 113, no. 1 (1998): 34–35.
Bourdieu, Pierre. *The Logic of Practice*. Cambridge: Polity Press, 1990.
———. *Outline of a Theory of Practice.* Cambridge: Cambridge University Press, 1997.
Bowden, Henry Warner. *American Indians and Christian Missions: Studies in Cultural Conflict*. Chicago: University of Chicago Press, 1981.
Boxberger, Daniel. "The Not So Common." In *Be Of Good Mind: Essays on the Coast Salish*, ed. Bruce Granville Miller. Vancouver: University of British Columbia Press, 2007.
Boyd, Robert. *People of the Dalles: The Indians of Wascopam Mission*. Lincoln: University of Nebraska Press, 1996.

———. *The Coming of the Spirit of Pestilence: Introduced Infectious Diseases and Population Decline among Northwest Coast Indians, 1774–1874*. Seattle: University of Washington Press, 1999.

Browne, J. Ross. *Indian Affairs in the Territories of Oregon and Washington*. Fairfield WA: Ye Galleon Press, 1977.

Buchanan, James. *Indian Affairs in Oregon and Washington Territories: A Message from the President of the United States*. Fairfield WA: Ye Galleon Press, 1987.

Buckley, Cornelius. *Nicholas Point, SJ: His Life and Northwest Indian Chronicles.* Chicago: Loyola University Press, 1989.

Buckley, Thomas. "Menstruation and the Power of Yurok Women: Methods in Cultural Reconstruction." *American Ethnologist* 9, no. 1 (1982): 47–60.

———. "The Shaker Church and the Indian Way in Native Northwestern California." *American Indian Quarterly* 21, no. 2 (1997): 1–14.

———. *Standing Ground: Yurok Indian Spirituality, 1850–1990*. Berkeley: University of California Press, 2002.

Bucko, Raymond. *The Lakota Ritual of the Sweat Lodge: History and Contemporary Practice*. Lincoln: University of Nebraska Press, 1990.

Buerge, David M., and Junius Rochester. *Roots and Branches: The Religious Heritage of Washington State*. Seattle: Church Council of Greater Seattle, 1988.

Burhansstipanov, Linda. "Cancer: A Growing Problem among American Indians and Alaska Natives." In *Promises to Keep: Public Health Policy for American Indians and Alaska Natives in the 21st Century*, ed. Mim Dixon and Yvette Roubideaux. Washington DC: American Public Health Association, 2001.

Burhansstipanov, Linda, James W. Hampton, and Martha J. Tenney. "American Indian and Alaska Native Cancer Data Issues." *American Indian Culture and Research Journal* 23, no. 3 (1999): 217–42.

Butler, Judith. *Bodies That Matter*. New York: Routledge, 1993.

———. "Contingent Foundations: Feminism and the Question of 'Postmodernism.'" In *Feminists Theorize the Political*, ed. Judith Butler and Joan W. Scott. New York: Routledge, 1992.

———. "Sexual Inversions." In *Feminist Interpretations of Michel Foucault*, ed. Susan Hekman, 59–76. University Park: University of Pennsylvania Press, 1996.

Carey, Charles, ed. "The Mission Record Book of the Methodist Episcopal Church, Willamette Station, Oregon Territory." *Oregon Historical Quarterly* 23, no. 3 (1922): 230–66.

Carlson, Keith Thor. *You Are Asked to Witness: The Sto:lo in Canada's Pacific Coast History*. Chilliwack BC: Sto:lo Heritage Trust, 1997.

Castile, George Pierre. "The Half-Catholic Movement: Edwin and Myron Eells and the Rise of the Indian Shaker Church," *Pacific Northwest Quarterly* 73, no. 4 (1982): 165–74.

Castile, George Pierre, ed. *The Indians of Puget Sound: The Notebooks of Myron Eells*. Seattle: University of Washington Press, 1985.

Castillo, Edward D. "Blood Came from Their Mouths: Tongva and Chumash Re-

sponses to the Pandemic of 1801," *American Indian Culture and Research Journal* 23, no. 3 (1999): 47–62.
Chandler, Michael J., Christopher E. Lalonde, Bryan W. Sokol, and Darcy Hallet. *Personal Persistence, Identity Development, and Suicide: A Study of Native and Non-Native North American Adolescents*. Monograph series no. 273, Monographs of the Society for Research in Child Development 68, no. 2 (2003).
Charney, Israel, ed. *Encyclopedia of Genocide*. Santa Barbara: ABC-CLIO, 1999.
Child, Brenda J. *Boarding School Seasons: American Indian Families 1900–1940*. Lincoln: University of Nebraska Press, 2000.
Churchill, Clare Warner. *Slave Wives of Nehalem*. Portland OR: Metropolitan Press, 1933.
Churchill, Ward. *A Little Matter of Genocide: Holocaust and Denial in the Americas, 1492 to the Present*. San Francisco: City Lights Publishers, 2001.
Clark, Ella, ed. "George Gibbs' Account of Indian Mythology in Oregon and Washington Territories." *Oregon Historical Quarterly* 56, no. 4 (1955): 293–326.
———. "George Gibbs' Account of Indian Mythology in Oregon and Washington Territories." *Oregon Historical Quarterly* 57, no. 2 (1956): 125–67.
———. "The Mythology of the Indians of the Pacific Northwest." *Oregon Historical Quarterly* 54 (1953): 293–326.
Clark, Lynn Anderson. "Irene Shale." In *Summertime in Georgetown: A Collection of Short Stories by Women and Girls of the Shoalwater Bay Tribal Community*. Tokeland WA: Shoalwater Bay Tribal Community Publication, 1998.
———. "The Spirit's Judgment." In *Summertime in Georgetown: A Collection of Short Stories by Women and Girls of the Shoalwater Bay Tribal Community*. Tokeland WA: Shoalwater Bay Tribal Community Publication, 1998.
Clifford, James. *Routes: Travel and Translation in the Late Twentieth Century*. Cambridge MA: Harvard University Press, 1997.
Cline, Walter. "Religion and Worldview." In *The Sinkaietk, or Southern Okanagan of Washington*, ed. Leslie Spier. Menasha WI: George Banta, 1938.
Coakley, Sarah, ed. *Religion and the Body*. Cambridge: Cambridge University Press, 1997.
Cole, Douglas, and Ira Chaikin. *An Iron Hand upon the People: The Law against the Potlatch on the Northwest Coast*. Vancouver: Talon Books, 1990.
Collins, Carey C. "Oregon's Carlisle: Teaching 'America' at Chemawa Indian School," *Columbia: The Magazine of Northwest History*, Tacoma: Washington State Historical Society, 1998.
———. "Through the Lens of Assimilation: Edwin L. Chalcraft and Chemawa Indian School." *Oregon Historical Quarterly* 98, no. 14 (1997–98): 390–425.
Collins, June McCormick. "The Influence of White Contact on Class Distinctions and Political Authority among the Indians of Northern Puget Sound." In *Coast Salish and Western Washington Indians*, vol. 2. New York: Garland Publishing, 1974.
———. "A Study of Religious Change among the Skagit Indians of Western Washington." In *Coast Salish and Western Washington Indians*, vol. 4. New York: Garland Publishing, 1974.

———. *Valley of the Spirits: The Upper Skagit Indians of Western Washington*. Seattle: University of Washington Press, 1974.

Conboy, Katie, Nadia Medina, and Sarah Stanbury, eds. *Writing on the Body: Female Embodiment and Feminist Theory*. New York: Columbia University Press, 1997.

Condit, Celeste. "Women's Reproductive Choices and the Genetic Model of Medicine." In *Body Talk: Rhetoric, Technology and Reproduction*, ed. Mary Lay, Laura J. Gurak, Clare Gravon, and Cynthia Myntti. Madison: University of Wisconsin Press, 2000.

Cooey, Paula. *Religious Imagination and the Body: A Feminist Analysis*. Oxford: Oxford University Press, 1994.

Cook, S. F. *The Epidemic of 1830–3 in California and Oregon*. University of California Publications in American Archaeology and Ethnology 18, no. 3. Berkeley: University of California Press, 1955.

Coues, Elliott, ed., *New Light on the Early History of the Greater Northwest: The Manuscript Journals of Alexander Henry, Fur Trader of the Northwest Company, and of David Thompson, Official Geographer and Explorer of the Same Company, 1799–1814*. New York: Francis and Harper, 1897.

Couture, Anita. "Agnes James, a Beautiful Woman." In *Summertime in Georgetown: A Collection of Short Stories by Women and Girls of the Shoalwater Bay Tribal Community*. Tokeland WA: Shoalwater Bay Tribal Community Publication, 1998.

Cox, Ross. *Adventures on the Columbia River, Including the Narrative of a Residence of Six Years on the Western Side of the Rocky Mountains, among Various Tribes of Indians Hitherto Unknown; Together with a Journey across the American Continent*, ed. Edgar Stewart and Jane Stewart. London, 1831 (2 vols.); Norman: University of Oklahoma Press, 1955.

———. *The Columbia River: Or Scenes and Adventures during a Residence of Six Years on the Western Side of the Rocky Mountains among Various Tribes of Indians Hitherto Unknown*. Ed. Edgar I. Stewart and Jane R. Stewart. Norman: University of Oklahoma Press, 1957.

Coy, Ron Hilbert. "My Mom's Spirit Power." In Janet Yoder ed. *Dxwʔdal taqʷšəblu tulʔal ti syeyaʔyaʔs: Writings About Vi Hilbert, by Her Friends*. Seattle: Lushootseed Research, 1992.

Cronon, William. *Changes in the Land: Indians, Colonists and the Ecology of New England*. 1983; New York: Hill and Wang, 2003.

Crosby, Alfred. *The Columbian Exchange: The Biological and Cultural Consequences of 1492*. Westport CT: Praeger, 1972.

———. "Virgin Soil Epidemics in the Aboriginal Depopulation of America." *William and Mary Quarterly*, 3d ser., 33 (1976): 289–99.

Crow Dog, Mary. *Lakota Woman*. New York: Harper Collins, 1990.

Crawford, Cromwell. "Ayurveda: The Science of Long Life in Contemporary Perspective." In *Eastern and Western Approaches to Healing: Ancient Wisdom and Modern Knowledge*, ed. Anees A. Sheikh and Katharina S. Sheikh. New York: John Wiley and Sons, 1989.

Crawford, Suzanne J. *Native American Religious Traditions.* Saddle Back NJ: Prentice Hall, 2007.
Crawford O'Brien, Suzanne, ed., *Religion and Healing in Native America: Pathways For Renewal.* Westport CT: Praeger, 2008.
Crawford O'Brien, Suzanne, and Dennis Kelley, eds., *American Indian Religious Traditions: An Encyclopedia.* Santa Barbara: ABC-CLIO, 2005.
Csordas, Thomas. *Embodiment and Experience: The Existential Ground of Culture and Self.* Cambridge: Cambridge University Press, 1994.
———. *The Sacred Self: A Cultural Phenomenology of Charismatic Healing.* Berkeley: University of California Press, 1994.
———. "The Navajo Healing Project." *Medical Anthropology Quarterly* 14, no. 4 (2000): 463–75.
———. *Ritual Healing in Navajo Society.* Theme issue, *Medical Anthropology Quarterly* 14, no. 4 (2000).
Curtis, Edward. "The Chinookan Tribes." In *The North American Indian* 8 (1911): 116–23.
Daniels, Cynthia. *At Women's Expense: State Power and the Politics of Fetal Rights.* Cambridge MA: Harvard University Press, 1993.
Davenport, T. W. *Recollections of an Indian Agent.* Oregon Historical Quarterly 8. 1907.
Davies, Wade. *Healing Ways: Navajo Health Care in the Twentieth Century.* Albuquerque: University of New Mexico Press, 2009.
Davis, Betty Ann. "Heeding Warnings from the Canary, the Whale, and the Inuit: A Framework for Analyzing Competing Types of Knowledge about Childbirth." In *Childbirth and Authoritative Knowledge: Cross Cultural Perspectives,* ed. Robbie Davis-Floyd and Carolyn Sargent, 471–73. Berkeley: University of California Press, 1995.
Davis-Floyd, Robbie. *Birth as an American Rite of Passage.* Berkeley: University of California Press, 1992.
Davis-Floyd, Robbie, and Carolyn Sargent, eds. *Childbirth and Authoritative Knowledge: Cross Cultural Perspectives.* Berkeley: University of California Press, 1997.
Dawson, George M. "Notes and Observations on the Kwakiool People of Vancouver Island." *Transactions, Royal Society of Canada* (Montreal), vol. 5, sec. 2 (1888): 63–98.
De Laguna, Frederica. *Under Mount Elias: The History and Culture of the Yakutat Tlingit,* vol. 2. Smithsonian Contributions to Anthropology no. 7. Washington DC: Smithsonian Institution Press, 1972.
Deloria, Philip. *Playing Indian.* New Haven: Yale University Press, 1999.
Deloria, Vine. *Custer Died for Your Sins: An Indian Manifesto.* Norman: University of Oklahoma Press, 1988.
———. *God Is Red: A Native View of Religion.* Golden CO: Fulcrum Publishing, 2003.
———. "Indians, Archaeologists, and the Future." *American Antiquity* 57, no. 4 (1992): 595.
DeMallie, Raymond. "The Lakota Ghost Dance: An Ethnohistorical Account." *Pacific Historical Review* 51 (1984): 385–405.
Demers, Modeste. *Chinook Dictionary, Catechism, Prayers and Hymns, Composed in 1838 and 1839 by Rt. Rev. Modeste Demers; Rev., Cor. and Completed in 1867 by*

Most Rev. F. N. Blanchet, with Modifications and Additions by Rev. L. N. St. Onge, Missionary among the Yakamas and Other Indian Tribes. Montreal, 1871.

Descartes, Rene. *Meditations on the First Philosophy*. Cambridge: Cambridge University Press, 1996.

Deur, Douglas, and Nancy Turner. *Keeping It Living: Traditions of Plant Use and Cultivation on the Northwest Coast of America*. Seattle: University of Washington Press, 2006.

Deveaux, Monique. "Feminism and Empowerment: A Critical Reading of Foucault." In *Feminist Interpretations of Michel Foucault*, ed. Susan Hekman, 211–39. University Park: Pennsylvania State University Press, 1996.

D'Herbomez, Louis. Letter of 11 December 1865. In *Missions de la Congregation des Missionaires Oblates de Marie Immaculee, Quatrieme Annee, 1865*. Marseilles.

Diomedi, Alexander. *Sketches of Modern Indian Life*. Fairfield WA: Ye Galleon Press, 1978.

Dixon, Mim. "The Unique Role of Tribes in the Delivery of Health Services." In *Promises to Keep: Public Health Policy for American Indians and Alaska Natives in the 21st Century*, ed. Mim Dixon and Yvette Roubideaux, 31–60. Washington DC: American Public Health Association, 2001.

Dixon, Mim, and Yvette Roubideaux, eds. *Promises to Keep: Public Health Policy for American Indians and Alaska Natives in the 21st Century*. Washington DC: American Public Health Association, 2001.

Douglas, Mary. *Natural Symbols*. New York: Routledge, 1973.

———. *Purity and Danger*. New York: Routledge, 1993.

Downey, Gary Lee, and Joseph Dumit, eds. *Cyborgs and Citadels: Anthropological Interventions in Emerging Sciences and Technologies*. Santa Fe NM: School of American Research Press, 1997.

Drucker, Philip. "Contributions to Alsea Ethnography." *University of California Publications in American Archaeology and Ethnology* 35 (1939): 81–101.

DuBois, Cora. *The Feather Cult of the Middle Columbia*. General Series in Anthropology 7. Menasha WI: George Banta, 1938.

———. *The 1870 Ghost Dance*. Anthropological Records 3, no. 1. Berkeley: University of California Press, 1939.

Duncan, William. *Metlahkatla: Ten Years' Work among the Tsimshean Indians: From the Journals and Letters of William Duncan.* London: Church Missionary House, 1868.

Dunn, John. *History of the Oregon Territory and British North American Fur Trade, with an Account of the Habits and Customs of the Principal Native Tribes on the Northern Continent.* London, 1846.

Ebert, Teresa. *Ludic Feminism and After: Postmodernism, Desire, and Labor in Late Capitalism*. Ann Arbor: University of Michigan Press, 1996.

Eells, Myron. "The Decrease of the Indians." *American Antiquarian and Oriental Journal* 25, no. 3 (1903): 147.

———. *Indians of Washington Territory*. Washington DC: Smithsonian Anthropological Papers, 1884.

———. "S'kokomish Agency, Washington." *American Missionary* 48, no. 4 (April 1894): 167.

Elliot, William. "Lake Lillooet Tales." *Journal of American Folk-Lore* 44 (1931): 166–81.
Elmendorf, William. Coast Salish Status Ranking and Intergroup Ties. *Southwestern Journal of Anthropology* 27 (1971): 353–80.
———. *Twana Narratives: Native Historical Accounts of a Coast Salish Culture*. Seattle: University of Washington Press, 1993.
Elmendorf, William W., and A. L. Kroeber. *The Structure of Twana Culture: With Comparative Notes on the Structure of Yurok Culture*. Pullman: Washington State University Press, 1960.
———. *Twana Culture*. Pullman: Washington State University Press, 1992.
Engel, George L. "The Need for a New Medical Model: A Challenge for Biomedicine." *Science* 196, no. 4286 (1977): 129–36.
Evans-Pritchard, E. E. *A History of Anthropological Thought*. New York: Basic Books, 1991.
Farella, John. *The Main Stalk: A Synthesis of Navajo Philosophy*. Tucson: University of Arizona Press, 1990.
Farrand, Livingston. Notes on the Alsea Indians of Oregon. *American Anthropologist* 3 (1901): 239–47.
Fenelon, James. *Culturicide, Resistance, and Survival of the Lakota*. New York: Routledge, 1998.
Forquera, Ralph. "Challenges in Serving the Growing Population of Urban Indians." In *Promises to Keep: Public Health Policy for American Indians and Alaska Natives in the 21st Century*, ed. Mim Dixon and Yvette Roubideaux, 121–34. Washington DC: American Public Health Association, 2001.
Foster, Rhonda. "Cultural Resources Management: New Department Established to Protect Cultural Resources." *Klah'Che'Min*, August 2001, 11.
Foucault, Michel. *Birth of the Clinic: An Archaeology of Medical Perception.* New York: Random House, 1973.
———. *Discipline and Punish: The Birth of the Prison.* New York: Random House, 1977.
———. *History of Sexuality: An Introduction*, vol. 1. New York: Random House, 1978.
———. *Madness and Civilization: A History of Insanity in the Age of Reason.* New York: Random House, 1965.
Frachtenberg, Leo. *Alsea Texts and Myths*. Bureau of American Ethnology Bulletin 67. Washington: Government Printing Office, 1920.
———. "Coos." In *Handbook of American Indian Languages*, ed. Franz Boas. *Bureau of American Ethnology Bulletin* 40, no. 2 (1922): 279–430.
———. "Coos Texts." *Columbia University Contributions to Anthropology* 1 (1913): 1–216.
———. "Lower Umpqua Texts and Notes on the Kusan Dialects." *Columbia University Contributions to Anthropology* 4 (1914): 1–156.
Franklin, Susan, and Helena Ragone. *Reproducing Reproduction: Kinship, Power, and Technological Innovation.* Phildelphia: University of Pennsylvania Press, 1997.
Fraser, Gertrude. "Modern Bodies, Modern Minds: Midwifery and Reproductive Change in an African American Community." In*Conceiving the New World Order: The Global Politics of Reproduction*, ed. Faye Ginsburg and Rayna Rapp. Berkeley: University of California Press, 1995.

French, Lindsey. 1994. "The Political Economy of Injury and Compassion: Amputees on the Thai-Cambodia Border." In *Embodiment and Experience: The Existential Ground of Culture and Self*, ed. Thomas Csordas, 69–99. Cambridge: Cambridge University Press, 1994.

Frey, Rodney. "If All These Stories Were Told, Great Stories Will Come!" In *Religion and Healing in Native America: Pathways For Renewal*, ed. Suzanne Crawford O'Brien. Westport CT: Praeger, 2008.

Friedman, Susan Stanford. *Mappings: Feminism and the Cultural Geographies of Encounter.* Princeton: Princeton University Press, 1998.

Frost, Joseph. "Journal, 1840–43." Ed. Nellie Pipes. *Oregon Historical Quarterly* 35 (1934): 359.

Furtwangler, Albert. *Bringing Indians to the Book*. Seattle: University of Washington Press, 2005.

Gallup, Jane. *Thinking through the Body (Gender and Culture).* New York: Columbia University Press, 1988.

Garrand, Victor. *Augustine Laure, SJ, Missionary to the Yakimas*. Fairfield WA: Ye Galleon Press, 1977.

Garrity, John F. "Jesus, Peyote, and the Holy People: Alcohol Abuse and the Ethos of Power in Navajo Healing." *Medical Anthropology Quarterly* 14, no. 4 (2000): 521–42.

Garroute, Eva, and Kathleen Westcott. "'The Stories Are Very Powerful': A Native American Perspective on Health, Illness and Narrative." In *Religion and Healing in Native America: Pathways for Renewal*, ed. Suzanne Crawford O'Brien. Westport CT: Praeger, 2008.

Gary, George. *Diary of Rev. George Gary*. Ed. Charles Carey. Oregon Historical Quarterly 24. 1923.

Gathke, Robert Moulton. *A Document of Mission History, 1833–43*. Oregon Historical Quarterly 36. 1935.

Gayton, A. H. "The Ghost Dance of 1870 in South-Central California." *University of California Publications in American Archaeology and Ethnology* 28, no. 3 (1930): 57–82.

Geertz, Clifford. *The Interpretation of Culture: Selected Essays.* New York: Basic Books, 1973.

Gibbs, George. 1877. "Tribes of Western Washington and Northwest Oregon." *Contributions to North American Ethnology* 1, no. 2 (1877): 157–361.

Gilbert, Madonna. "We Will Remember Survival School: The Women and Children of the American Indian Movement." *MS Magazine*, July 1976, 94.

Glass, Aaron. "The Intention of Tradition: Contemporary Contexts and Contests of the Hamat'sa Dance." In *Coming to Shore: Northwest Coast Ethnology, Traditions and Visions*, ed.Marie Mauze, Michael Harkin, and Sergei Kan, 279–304. Lincoln: University of Nebraska Press, 2000.

Goldsmith, Marsha. "First Americans Face Their Latest Challenge: Indian Health Care Meets State Medicaid Reform." *Journal of the American Medical Association* 275, no. 23 (June 1996): 1786.

Gould, Richard A. *Aspects of Ceremonial Life among the Shakers of Smith River, CA*.

Kroeber Anthropological Society Papers no. 3, 1964; repr. Berkeley: California Indian Library Collections, 1992.

Gould, Stephen Jay. *The Mismeasure of Man*. New York: W. W. Norton, 1996.

Goulet, Jean-Guy. *Ways of Knowing: Experience, Knowledge and Power among the Dene Tha*. Lincoln: University of Nebraska Press, 1998.

Amending the Indian Self Determination and Educational Assistance Act to Provide for Further Self-Governance. Gov. Docs: R-Y 1.1/5: 106–221. Washington DC: Government Printing Office, 1999.

Columbia Basin's American Indians Involved in Hanford Dose Reconstruction. Gov. Docs: OR-Ene/N88.4FII:13. Washington DC: Government Printing Office, 1992.

Griggers, Camilla. *Becoming-Woman*. Theory Out of Bounds, vol. 8. Ann Arbor: University of Michigan Press, 1997.

Grosz, Elizabeth. *Space, Time and Perversion: Essays on the Politics of Bodies*. New York: Routledge, 1995.

———. *Volatile Bodies: Toward a Corporeal Feminism.* Bloomington: Indiana University Press, 1994.

Grounds, Richard, George Tinker, and David Wilkins, eds. *Native Voices: American Indian Identity and Resistance*. Lawrence: University of Kansas Press, 2003.

Guilmet, George, Robert Boyd, David Whited, and Nile Thompson. "The Legacy of Introduced Disease: The Southern Coast Salish." *American Indian Culture and Research Journal* 15, no. 1 (1991): 1–32.

Guilmet, George M., and David L. Whited. *The People Who Give More: Health and Mental Health among the Contemporary Puyallup Indian Tribal Community*. American Indian and Alaska Native Mental Health Research, Journal of the National Center Monograph Series, vol. 2, monograph 2. Denver: University of Colorado Health Sciences Center, 1989.

Gunther, Erna. "Analysis of the First Salmon Ceremony." *American Anthropologist* 28 (1926): 605–17.

———. "A Further Analysis of the First Salmon Ceremony." *University of Washington Publications in Anthropology* 2, no. 5 (1928): 129–73.

———. *Klallam Ethnography.* Publications in Anthropology 1, no. 5. Seattle: University of Washington Press, 1927.

———. "Klallam Folk Tales." *University of Washington Publications in Anthropology* 1, no. 4 (1925): 113–70.

———. "The Shaker Religion of the Northwest." In *Indians of the Urban Northwest*, ed. Marion Smith. 1949; New York: AMS Press, 1969.

Haeberlin, Herman, and Erna Gunther. *The Indians of Puget Sound*. Publications in Anthropology 4, no. 1. Seattle: University of Washington Press, 1930.

Hahn, Robert A. *Sickness and Healing: An Anthropological Perspective.* New Haven: Yale University Press, 1996.

Hajda, Yvonne. "Southwestern Coast Salish." In *Handbook of North American Indians*, vol. 7: *The Northwest Coast*, ed. Wayne Suttles. Washington DC: Smithsonian Institution Press, 1990.

Halkett, John. *Historical Notes Respecting the Indians of North America with Remarks on the Attempts Made to Convert and Civilize Them.* London: Archibald Constable and Company, 1825.

Hanson, Paul, ed. *Visionaries and Their Apocalypses*. Philadelphia: Fortress Press, 1983.

Haraway, Donna. "Cyborg Manifesto: Science, Technology, and Socialist Feminism in the Late Twentieth Century." In *Simians, Cyborgs and Women: The Reinvention of Nature*, 149–81. New York: Routledge, 1991.

———. "Situated Knowledges: The Science Question in Feminism and the Privilege of Partial Perspective." *Feminist Studies* 14, no. 3 (1988): 575–99.

Hare, Jan, and Jean Barman. *Good Intentions Gone Awry: Emma Crosby and the Methodist Mission on the Northwest Coast*. Vancouver: University of British Columbia Press, 2006.

Harjo, Joy. "Three Generations of Native American Women's Birth Experience." *MS Magazine*, July–August 1991, 28–30.

Harjo, Joy, and Gloria Bird, eds. *Reinventing the Enemy's Language: Contemporary Native Women's Writings of North America*. New York: W. W. Norton, 1997.

Harmon, Alexandra. "Coast Salish History." In *Be of Good Mind: Essays on the Coast Salish*, ed. Bruce Granville Miller. Vancouver: University of British Columbia Press, 2007.

———. *Indians in the Making: Ethnic Relations and Indian Identities around Puget Sound*. Berkeley: University of California Press, 1998.

Harris, Cole. *Making Native Space: Colonialism, Resistance, and Reserves in British Columbia*. Vancouver: University of British Columbia Press, 2002.

———. *The Resettlement of British Columbia: Essays on Colonialism and Geographical Change*. Vancouver: University of British Columbia Press, 1997.

———. "Voices of Disaster: Smallpox around the Strait of Georgia in 1782." *Ethnohistory* 41, no. 4 (1994): 591–626.

Hartsock, Nancy. "Postmodernism and Political Change: Issues for Feminist Theory." In *Feminist Interpretations of Michel Foucault*, ed. Susan Helerman, 39–57. University Park: Pennsylvania State University Press, 1996.

Harvey, A. G. "Chief Concomly's Skull." *Oregon Historical Quarterly* 15 (1939): 161–67.

Hassin, Jeanette, and Robert S. Young. "Self-Sufficiency, Personal Empowerment, and Community Revitalization: The Impact of a Leadership Program on American Indians in the Southwest." *American Indian Culture and Research Journal* 23, no. 3 (2000): 265–86.

Health Promotion Resource Center, Stanford Center for Research in Disease Prevention, and the Indian Health Service. *Restoring Balance: Community-Directed Health Promotion for American Indians and Alaska Natives.* Stanford: Stanford University, 1992.

Hekman, Susan J., ed. *Feminist Interpretations of Michel Foucault*. University Park: Pennsylvania State University Press, 1996.

Hennessey, Rosemary. *Materialism, Feminism, and the Politics of Discourse*. New York: Routledge, 1993.

Hilbert, Vi, and Crisca Bierwert. *Ways of the Lushootseed People: Ceremonies and Traditions of Northern Puget Sound Indians*. Seattle WA: United Indians of All Tribes Foundation, 1980.

Hilbert, Vi, and Jay Miller. "Storied Arts: Lushootseed Gifting across Time and Space." In *S'abadeb, The Gifts: Pacific Coast Salish Art and Artists*, ed. Barbara Brotherton. Seattle: University of Washington Press, 2010.

Hines, Gustavus. *Life on the Plains of the Pacific: Oregon, Its History, Conditions and Prospects.* Buffalo, 1851.

Hines, Harvey. *Missionary History of the Pacific Northwest, Containing the Wonderful Story of Jason Lee*. San Francisco: H. K. Hines and J. D. Hammond, 1899.

Hodge, Felicia Schanche, and John Casken. "American Indian Breast Cancer Project: Educational Development and Implementation." *American Indian Culture and Research Journal* 23, no. 3 (2000): 205–16.

Hodgson, Edward R. *The Epidemic of the Lower Columbia*. Pacific Northwesterner 1, no. 4. 1957.

Holdrege, Barbara. "Body Connections: Hindu Discourses of the Body and the Study of Religion.*International Journal of Hindu Studies* 2, no. 3 (1998): 341–86.

Holm, Bill. "Art." In *Handbook of North American Indians*, vol. 7: *The Northwest Coast*, ed. Wayne Suttles. Washington DC: Smithsonian Institution Press, 1990.

Holt, Howard. *Saddlebag Medicine: The Story of Medicine Yakima Valley*. Yakima: H.P. Holt, 1984.

Hoxie, Frederick E. *A Final Promise: The Campaign to Assimilate the Indians*. Omaha: University of Nebraska Press, 1984.

Hoy, David. "Critical Resistance: Foucault and Bourdieu." In *Perspectives on Embodiment: The Intersections of Nature and Culture*, ed. Gail Weiss and Honi Fern Haber, New York: Routledge, 1999.

Huggins, E. L. "Smohalla, the Prophet of Priest Rapids." *Overland Monthly*, 2nd ser., 17 (1891): 208–15.

Hultkrantz, Ake. *Shamanic Healing and Ritual Drama: Health and Medicine in the Native North American Religious Traditions*. New York: Crossroad Publishing Company, 1997.

Hunn, Eugene S., with James Selam and Family. *N'ch'i-Wana, "The Big River": Mid-Columbia Indians and Their Land.* Seattle: University of Washington Press, 1990.

Hymes, Dell. "Folklore's Nature and the Sun Myth." *Journal of American Folklore* 88 (1975): 345–69.

Indian Claims Commission. "The Quileute Indians of Puget Sound." In *Coast Salish and Western Washington Indians*, vol. 2. New York: Garland Publishing, 1974.

Irving, Washington. *Astoria, or Anecdotes of an Enterprise Beyond the Rocky Mountains*. Ed. Edgeley Todd. Norman: University of Oklahoma Press, 1964.

Jackson, Donald. *Letters of the Lewis and Clark Expedition, with Related Documents, 1783–1854*. Urbana: University of Illinois Press, 1962.

Jacob, Michelle. "'This Path Will Heal Our People': Healing the Soul Wound of Diabetes." In *Religion and Healing in Native America: Pathways for Renewal*, ed. Suzanne Crawford O'Brien. Westport CT: Praeger, 2008.

Jacobs, Elizabeth, and Melville Jacobs. *Nehalem Tillamook Tales.* University of Oregon Monographs, Studies in Anthropology 5. 1959.
Jacobs, Melville. *Clackamas Chinook Texts*. 2 vols. Bloomington: University of Indiana, 1958–59.
———. *Content and Style of an Oral Literature: Clackamas Chinook Myths and Tales.* Chicago: University of Chicago Press, 1959.
———. *Coos Myth Texts*. University of Washington Publications in Anthropology 8, no. 2. Seattle: University of Washington, 1940.
———. *Coos Narrative and Ethnologic Texts*. University of Washington Publications in Anthropology 8, no. 1. Seattle: University of Washington, 1939.
———. "Indications of Mental Illness among Pre-Contact Indians of the Northwest States." *Pacific Northwest Quarterly* 50, no. 2 (April 1964): 49–54.
Jacobs, Melville, Leo J. Frachtenberg, and Albert S. Gatschet. *Kalapuya Texts*. University of Washington Publications in Anthropology 11. Seattle: University of Washington, 1945.
Jagger, Alison M., and Susan R. Bordo, eds. *Gender/Body/Knowledge: Feminist Reconstructions of Being and Knowing*. New Brunswick: Rutgers University Press, 1989.
Jaimes Guerrero, M. Annette. "Civil Rights vs. Sovereignty: Native American Women." In *Feminist Genealogies, Cultural Legacies, and Democratic Futures*, ed. Jacqui Alexander and Chandra Mohanty. New York: Routledge, 1992.
———. "Feminism and Tribalism." In *American Indian Religious Traditions: An Encyclopedia*, ed. Suzanne Crawford and Dennis Kelley, 291–300. Santa Barbara: ABC-CLIO, 2005.
———. *The State of Native America: Genocide, Colonization and Resistance*. San Francisco: South End Press, 1992.
Jenkins, Janis H., and Martha Valiente. "Bodily Transactions of the Passions: El Calor among Salvadorean Women Refugees." In *Embodiment and Experience: The Existential Ground of Culture and Self*, ed. Thomas Csordas. Cambridge: Cambridge University Press, 1994.
Jenness, Diamond. *The Faith of a Coast Salish Indian*. Anthropology in British Columbia Memoir no. 3. Victoria: British Columbia Provincial Museum, 1955.
Jilek, W. G. *Indian Healing*. Blaine WA: Big Country Books, 1981.
Johnson, Troy, and Holly Tomren. "Helplessness, Hopelessness, and Despair: Identifying the Precursors to Indian Youth Suicide." *American Indian Culture and Research Journal* 23, no. 3 (1999): 287–301.
Kan, Sergei. *Memory Eternal: Tlingit Culture and Russian Orthodoxy through Two Centuries*. Seattle: University of Washington Press, 1999.
———. *Symbolic Immortality: The Tlingit Potlatch of the Nineteenth Century*. Washington DC: Smithsonian Institution Press, 1993.
Kapsalis, Terri. *Public Privates: Performing Gynecology from Both Ends of the Spectrum*. Durham: Duke University Press, 1997.
Kasulis, Thomas P., Roger T. Ames, and Wimal Dissanayake, eds. *Self as Body in Asian Theory and Practice*. Albany: SUNY Press, 1993.

Kaufert, Patricia, and John O'Neil. "Analysis of a Dialogue on Risks in Childbirth: Clinicians, Epidemiologists, and Inuit Women." In *Knowledge, Power, and Practice: The Anthropology of Medicine and Everyday Life*, ed. Shirley Lindenbaum and Margaret Lock, 32–54. Berkeley: University of California Press, 1993.

Kehoe, Alice Beck. *The Ghost Dance: Ethnohistory and Revitalization*. New York: Holt, Rinehart, and Winston, 1989.

Keller, Jean A. "'In the Fall of the Year We Were Troubled with Some Sickness': Typhoid Fever Deaths, Sherman Institute, 1904." *American Indian Culture and Research Journal* 23, no. 3 (1999): 97–118.

Keller, Robert H. Jr. *American Protestantism and United States Indian Policy, 1869–1882*. Berkeley: University of California Press, 1983.

Kelm, Mary-Ellen. *Colonizing Bodies: Aboriginal Health and Healing in British Columbia, 1900–1950*. Vancouver: University of British Columbia, 1998.

Kew, Michael. "Central and Southern Coast Salish Ceremonies since 1900." In *Handbook of North American Indians*, vol. 7: *The Northwest Coast*, ed. Wayne Suttles, 476–80. Washington DC: Smithsonian Institution Press, 1990.

———. "Salmon Availability, Technology, and Cultural Adaptation in the Fraser River Watershed." In *A Complex Culture of the British Columbia Plateau: Traditional Stl'atl'imx Resource Use*, ed. Brian Hayden, 177–221. Vancouver: University of British Columbia Press, 1992.

Kew, Michael, and Della Kew. "People Need Friends, It Makes Their Minds Strong: A Coast Salish Curing Rite." In *The World Is as Sharp as a Knife: An Anthology in Honor of Wilson Duff*, 29–35. Victoria BC: British Columbia Provincial Museum, 1981.

Killen, Patricia O'Connell. *Religion and Public Life in the Northwest: The None Zone*. Berkeley CA: AltaMira Press, 2004.

King, Cecil. "Here Come the Anthros." In *Indians and Anthropologists: Vine Deloria Jr. and the Critique of Anthropology*, ed. Thomas Biolsi and Larry Zimmerman. Tucson: University of Arizona Press, 1997.

Kleinman, Arthur. *The Illness Narratives*. New York: Basic Books, 1988.

Kondo, Dorinne. *Crafting Selves: Power, Gender, and Discourses of Identity in a Japanese Workplace*. Chicago: University of Chicago Press, 1990.

Kracht, Benjamin R. "The Kiowa Ghost Dance: An Unheralded Revitalization Movement." *Ethnohistory* 39, no. 4 (1992): 452–77.

Krise, Charlene. "Memories of Gathering." *Native Women's Wellness Newsletter*, Summer 2001, 1–3.

Kroeber, Theodora. *Ishi in Two Worlds: A Biography of the Last Wild Indian in North America*. Berkeley: University of California Press, 1967.

Kuklick, Henrika. *The Savage Within: The Social History of British Anthropology, 1885–1945*. Cambridge: Cambridge University Press, 1991.

Kunitz, Stephen J. *Disease Change and the Role of Medicine: The Navajo Experience*. Berkeley: University of California Press, 1983.

Lamb, Kaye, ed. *The Letters and Journals of Simon Fraser, 1806–1808*. Toronto: Macmillan, 1960.

Lamphere, Louise. "Comments on the Navajo Healing Project." *Medical Anthropology Quarterly* 14, no. 4 (2000): 598–602.

Landerholm, Carl. *Notices and Voyages of the Famed Quebec Mission to the Pacific Northwest.* Portland: Oregon Historical Society, 1956.

Large, R. G., ed. *The Journals of William Fraser Tolmie, Physician and Fur Trader*. Vancouver BC: Mitchell Press, 1963.

Larsell, O. *The Doctor in Oregon: A Medical History.* Portland OR: Binfords and Mort, 1947.

———. "Medical Aspects of the Lewis and Clark Expedition." *Oregon Historical Quarterly* 56 (1955): 221–22.

Law, Jane Marie, ed. *Religious Reflections on the Human Body*. Bloomington: Indiana University Press, 1995.

Lawless, Jo Murphy. *Reading Birth and Death: A History of Obstetric Thinking.* Bloomington: Indiana University Press, 1999.

Lay, Mary M., Laura J. Gurak, Clare Gravon, and Cynthia Myntti, eds. *Body Talk: Rhetoric, Technology and Reproduction*. Madison: University of Wisconsin Press, 2000.

Layne, Linda. "Breaking the Silence: An Agenda for a Feminist Discourse of Pregnancy Loss." *Feminist Studies* 23, no. 2 (1997): 289–315.

———. *Motherhood Lost: A Feminist Account of Pregnancy Loss in America.* New York: Routledge, 2002.

———. "Motherhood Lost: Cultural Dimensions of Miscarriage and Stillbirth in America." *Women and Health* 16, nos. 3–4 (Fall 1990): 69–99.

Leder, Drew. 1998. "A Tale of Two Bodies: The Cartesian Corpse and the Lived Body." In *Body and Flesh, a Philosophical Reader*, ed. Donn Welton, 117–29. Malden MA: Blackwell Publishers, 1998.

Lee, Daniel, and Joseph Frost. *Ten Years in Oregon*. New York: J. Collard, 1844.

Lee, Jason. *Diary*. Oregon Historical Quarterly 17. 1916.

———. "Letter of 22 May, 1840." *Christian Advocate*, August 25, 1841.

Lemert, Edwin McCarthy. "The Life and Death of an Indian State." *Human Organization* 13, no. 4 (1954): 23–27.

———. Alcohol *and the NW Coast Indians*. Berkeley: University of California Press, 1954.

Leona, Nichols M. *The Mantle of Elias: The Story of Fathers Blanchet and Demers in Early Oregon.* Portland OR: Binfords and Mort, 1941.

Lesser, Alexander. *The Pawnee Ghost Dance Hand Game: A Study of Cultural Change.* New York: Columbia University Press, 1933.

Levchuk, Bernice. "Leaving Home for Carlisle Indian School." In *Reinventing the Enemy's Language: Contemporary Native Women's Writings of North America*, ed. Joy Harjo and Gloria Bird. New York: W. W. Norton, 1997.

Levi, Jerome M. "The Embodiment of a Working Identity: Power and Process in Raramuri Ritual Healing." *American Indian Culture and Research Journal* 23, no. 3 (1999): 13–46.

Lewton, Elizabeth L., and Victoria Bydone. "Identity Healing in Three Navajo Religious Traditions: Sa'ah Naaghai Bik'eh Hozho." *Medical Anthropology Quarterly* 14, no. 4 (2000): 476–97.

Lloyd, Moya. "A Feminist Mapping of Foucauldian Politics." In *Feminist Interpretations of Michel Foucault*, ed. Susan Hekman, 241–64. University Park: Pennsylvania State University Press, 1996.

Lock, Margaret. "Cultivating the Body: Anthropology and Epistemologies of Bodily Practice and Knowledge." *Annual Review of Anthropology* 22 (1993): 133–55.

———. *Encounters with Aging: Mythologies of Menopause in Japan and North America.* Berkeley: University of California Press, 1995.

Long, Charles. *Significations: Signs, Symbols, and Images in the Interpretation of Religion*. St. Paul MN: Fortress Press, 1986.

Luckert, Karl W. *Coyoteway: A Navajo Holyway Healing Ceremonial.* Tucson: University of Arizona Press, 1979.

Lupton, Deborah. *The Imperative of Health and the Regulated Body.* London: Sage, 1995.

Lyon, M. L., and J. M. Barbalet. "Society's Body: Emotion and the 'Somatization' of Social Theory." In *Embodiment and Experience: The Existential Ground of Culture and the Self*, ed. Thomas J. Csordas, 46–48. Cambridge: Cambridge University Press, 1994.

Marino, Cesare. "History of Western Washington State since 1846." In *Handbook of North American Indians*, vol. 7: *The Northwest Coast*, ed. Wayne Suttles, 169–79. Washington DC: Smithsonian Institution Press, 1990.

Mario, Jacoby. *Longing for Paradise: Psychological Perspectives on an Archetype.* Boston: Sigo Press, 1985.

Marks, Jonathon. "Replaying the Race Card." *Anthropology Newsletter* 39, no. 5 (1998): 1.

Marr, Carolyn J. "Assimilation through Education: Indian Boarding Schools in the Pacific Northwest." University of Washington Digital Collections. http://content.lib.washington.edu/aipnw/marr.html. Accessed June 10, 2011.

Martin, Emily. *Flexible Bodies: Tracking Immunity in American Culture from the Days of Polio to the Age of AIDS.* Boston: Beacon Press, 1994.

———. *The Woman in the Body: A Cultural Analysis of Reproduction*. Boston: Beacon Press, 1987.

Martin, Joel. "Before and Beyond the Ghost Dance: Native American Prophetic Movements and the Study of Religion." *Journal of the American Academy of Religion* 59, no. 4 (Winter 1991): 677–701.

Maud, Ralph, ed. *The Salish People: The Local Contribution of Charles Hill-Tout*, vol. 2: *The Squamish and the Lilloet*. Vancouver: Torchbooks, 1978.

Mauro, Hayes Peter. *The Art of Americanization at Carlisle Indian School*. Albuquerque: University of New Mexico Press, 2011.

Mauss, Marcel. "Les Techniques du Corps." In *Sociologie et Anthropologie*. Paris: Presses Universitaires de France, 1950.

Mauze, Marie, Michael E. Harkin, and Sergei Kan. *Coming to Shore: Northwest Coast Ethnology, Traditions and Visions*. Lincoln: University of Nebraska Press, 2000.

McGuire, Randall. "Why Have Archaeologists Thought the Real Indians Were Dead, and What Can We Do about It?" In *Indians and Anthropologists: Vine Deloria Jr. and the Critique of Anthropology*, ed. Thomas Biolsi. Tucson: University of Arizona Press, 1997.

———. "Archaeology and the First Americans." *American Anthropologist* 94, no. 4 (1992): 827.

McHalsie, Albert (Naxaxalhts'i). "We Have to Take Care of Everything That Belongs to Us." In *Be of Good Mind: Essays on the Coast Salish*, ed. Bruce Granville Miller. Vancouver: University of British Columbia Press, 2007.

McNally, Michael. "The Uses of Ojibwe Hymn Singing at White Earth: Toward a History of Practice." In David D. Hall, ed., *Lived Religion in America: Toward a History of Practice.* Princeton NJ: Princeton University Press, 1997.

McNeley, James K. *Holy Wind in Navajo Philosophy*. Tucson: University of Arizona Press, 1981.

McWhorter, Lucullus Virgil. *The Crime against the Yakimas*. North Yakima: Republic Print, 1913.

———. *Tragedy of the Wahk-Shum*. Yakima: Self Publication, L. V. McWhorter, 1937.

Meany, Edward. *Diary of Wilkes in the Northwest*. Seattle: University of Washington Press, 1926.

Meeker, Ezra. *Pioneer Reminiscences of Puget Sound: The Tragedy of Leschi*. Seattle, 1905.

Neil Maher. "Body Counts: Tracking the Body through Environmental History." In *A Companion to American Environmental History*, ed. Douglas Cazaux Sackman. New York: Wiley Blackwell, 2010.

Meighan, Clement. "Burying American Archaeology." *Archaeology* 47, no. 6 (1994): 64.

Meighnan, Clement M., and Francis R. Riddell. *The Maru Cult of the Pomo Indians: A California Ghost Dance Survival.* Los Angeles: Highland Park SW Museum, 1972.

Merchant, Carolyn. *Ecological Revolutions: Nature, Gender and Science in New England*. Chapel Hill: University of North Carolina Press, 1989.

Merk, Frederick, ed. *Fur Trade and Empire: George Simpson's Journal. Remarks Connected with the Fur Trade: The Course of a Voyage from York Factory to Ft. George and Back to York Factory 1824–1825, Together with Accompanying Documents*. Cambridge MA: Harvard University Press, 1931.

Merleau-Ponty, Maurice. "The Lived Body." In *The Body*, ed. Donn Welton. Malton MA: Blackwell Publishers, 1999.

———. *Phenomenology of Perception*. Trans. James M. Edie. Evanston IL: Northwestern University Press, 1962.

———. *The Primacy of Perception*. Trans. James M. Edie. Evanston IL: Northwestern University Press, 1964.

Meyer, Patricia, ed. *Honore-Timothee Lempfurt, OMI: His Oregon Trail Journal and Letters from the Pacific Northwest, 1848–1853*. Fairfield WA: Ye Galleon Press, 1985.

Mihesuah, Devon. *American Indians: Stereotypes and Realities*. Atlanta, GA: Clarity Press, 1997.

———. *Cultivating the Rosebuds: The Education of Women at the Cherokee Female Seminary, 1850–1909.* Urbana: University of Illinois Press, 1993.
———. *Natives and Academics: Researching and Writing about Academics.* Lincoln: University of Nebraska Press, 1998.
Miller, Bruce Granville, ed. *Be of Good Mind: Essays on the Coast Salish. Vancouver:* University of British Columbia Press, 2007.
———. "The Individual, the Collective, and the Tribal Code." *American Indian Culture and Research Journal* 21, no. 1 (1997): 107–29.
———. "Rereading the Ethnographic Record: The Problem of Justice in the Coast Salish World." In *Coming to Shore: Northwest Coast Ethnology, Traditions and Visions*, ed. Marie Mauze, Michael Harkin, and Sergei Kan, 305–22. Lincoln: University of Nebraska Press, 2000.
Miller, Christopher L. *Prophetic Worlds: Indians and Whites on the Columbia Plateau.* Seattle: University of Washington Press, 1985.
Miller, David Humphreys. *Ghost Dance.* New York: Duell, Sloan and Pearce, 1959.
Miller, Jay. *Lushootseed Culture and the Shamanic Odyssey: An Anchored Radiance.* Lincoln: University of Nebraska Press, 1999.
———. *Mourning Dove: A Salishan Autobiography.* Lincoln, NE: Bison Books, 1994.
Mills, Antonia. *Eagle Down Is Our Law: Witsuwit'en Law, Feasts, and Land Claims.* Vancouver: University of British Columbia Press, 1994.
Milne, Derek, and Wilson Howard. "Rethinking the Role of Diagnosis in Navajo Religious Healing." *Medical Anthropology Quarterly* 14, no. 4 (2000): 543–70.
Minto, John. "The Number and Condition of the Native Race in Oregon When First Seen by White Men." *Oregon Historical Quarterly* 1 (1900): 299–300.
Mittman, Gregg. *Breathing Space: How Allergies Shape Our Lives and Landscapes.* New Haven: Yale University Press, 2007.
———. "Geographies of Hope." In *Landscapes of Exposure: Knowledge and Illness in Modern Environments*, ed. Gregg Mittman, Michelle Murphy, and Christopher Sellers. *Osiris*, 2nd ser., no 19. Chicago: University of Chicago Press, 2004.
Mohanty, Chandra. "Under Western Eyes: Feminist Scholarship and Colonial Discourses." In *Third World Women and the Politics of Feminism*, ed. Chandra Mohanty, Ann Russo, and Lourdes Torres. Bloomington: Indiana University Press, 1992.
Mooney, James. *The Ghost Dance Religion.* Vol. 2, *Fourteenth Annual Report of the Bureau of Ethnology to the Secretary of the Smithsonian Institution, 1892–93.* Washington DC, 1896; Chicago: University of Chicago Press, 1965.
Mooney, Kathleen. "The Effects of Rank and Wealth on Exchange among the Coast Salish." *Ethnology* 17, no. 4 (October 1978): 391–406.
———. "Social Distance and Exchange: The Coast Salish Case." *Ethnology* 15, no. 4 (1976): 326.
Morris, Richard, and Philip Wander. "Native American Rhetoric: Dancing in the Shadows of the Ghost Dance." *Quarterly Journal of Speech* 76, no. 2 (May 1990): 164–91.

Morsink, Johannes. "Cultural Genocide, the Human Rights Declaration and Minority Rights." *Human Rights Quarterly* 21, no. 4 (November 1999): 1009–60.

Moses, Israel. "On the Medical Topography of Astoria, Oregon Territory." *American Journal of Medical Science* 29 (1855): 32–46.

Moss, Madonna. "Shellfish, Gender, and Status on the Northwest Coast: Reconciling Archaeological, Ethnographic, and Ethnohistorical Records of the Tlingit." *American Anthropologist* 95, no. 3 (1992): 631–52.

Mozino, Jose. *Noticias de Nutka.* Seattle: University of Washington, 1970.

Mudge, Zachariah Atwell. *Sketches of Mission Life among the Indians of Oregon.* New York, 1854.

Nash, Linda. *Inescapable Ecologies: A History of Environment, Disease, and Knowledge.* Berkeley: University of California Press, 2007.

Nebelkopf, Ethan, and Mary Phillips, eds. *Healing and Mental Health for Native Americans: Speaking in Red.* Berkeley CA: AltaMira Press, 2004.

Nelson, Richard K. *Make Prayers to the Raven: A Koyukon View of the Northern Forest.* Chicago: University of Chicago Press, 1986.

Nesper, Larry. *The Walleye War: The Struggle for Ojibwe Spearfishing and Treaty Rights.* Lincoln: University of Nebraska Press, 2002.

Noren, Jay, David Kindig, and Audrey Springer. "Challenges to Native American Health Care." *Public Health Reports* 113, no. 1 (1998): 22–33.

Ogden, Peter Skene [Anonymous]. *Traits of American Indian Life and Character by a Fur Trader, 1853.* San Francisco: Grabhorn Press, 1933.

Ohnuki-Tierney, Emiko. *Illness and Culture in Contemporary Japan: An Anthropological View.* Cambridge: Cambridge University Press, 1984.

Oliphant, Orin. *George Simpson and the Oregon Missions.* Portland: Pacific Historical Review, 1937.

Olson, Brooke. "Applying Medical Anthropology: Developing Diabetes Education and Prevention Programs in American Indian Cultures." *American Indian Culture and Research Journal* 23, no. 3 (1999): 185–204.

Olson, Ronald. "The Social Organization of the Haisla of British Columbia." *Anthropological Records* 2, no. 5 (1940): 169–200.

O'Nell, Therese. *Disciplined Hearts: History, Identity and Depression in an American Indian Community.* Berkeley: University of California Press, 1998.

Palmer, Andie. "Taqʷšəblu and Indian Time." In *Dxwʔdal taqʷšəblu tulʔal ti syeyaʔyaʔs: Writings sbout Vi Hilbert, by Her Friends*, ed. Janet Yoder. Seattle: Lushootseed Research, 1992.

Parker, Samuel. *Journal of an Exploring Tour Beyond the Rocky Mountains, under the Direction of the ABCFM, Performed in the Years 1835, 1836, and 1837.* Ithaca NY, 1844.

Parkhill, Thomas. *Weaving Ourselves into the Land: Charles Godfrey Leland, "Indians" and the Study of Native American Religions.* Albany: SUNY Press, 1997.

Pavel, D. Michael, Gerald Miller, and Mary J. Pavel. "Too Long, Too Silent: The Threat to Cedar and the Sacred Ways of the Skokomish." *American Indian Culture and Research Journal* 17, no. 3 (1993): 53–80.

Pearce, Roy Harvey. *Savagism and Civilization: A Study of the Indian and the American Mind.* Berkeley: University of California Press, 1988.

Porter, Midge. "Marie Riddel." In *Summertime in Georgetown: A Collection of Short Stories by Women and Girls of the Shoalwater Bay Tribal Community*, 78–82. Tokeland WA: Shoalwater Bay Tribal Community Publication, 1998.

———. "My Name Is Chinook." In *Summertime in Georgetown: A Collection of Short Stories by Women and Girls of the Shoalwater Bay Tribal Community*. Tokeland WA: Shoalwater Bay Tribal Community Publication, 1998.

———. "Uncle Dave." In *Summertime in Georgetown: A Collection of Short Stories by Women and Girls of the Shoalwater Bay Tribal Community*. Tokeland WA: Shoalwater Bay Tribal Community Publication, 1998.

Powell, Fred Wilbur. *Hall Jackson Kelly: Prophet of Oregon*. Oregon Historical Quarterly 28. 1917.

Price, Janet, and Margrit Shildrick. *Feminist Theory and the Body*. New York: Routledge, 1999.

Prosser, William F. "An Interesting Collection of Indian Relics." *Washington Historian* 1, no. 1 (1899): 27.

Prucha, Francis Paul. *The Churches and the Indian Schools.* Fairfield WA: Ye Galleon Press, 1979.

Raibmon, Paige. *Authentic Indians: Episodes of Encounter from the Late-Nineteenth Century Northwest Coast*. Durham: Duke University, 2005.

Ray, Verne. *Cultural Relations in the Plateau of Northwestern North America.* Los Angeles: Southwest Museum, 1939.

———. "The Historical Position of the Lower Chinook in the Native Culture of the Northwest." *Pacific Northwest Quarterly* 28, no. 4 (October 1937): 363–72.

———. *Lower Chinook Ethnographic Notes.* Publications in Anthropology 7, no. 2. Seattle: University of Washington Press, 1938.

———. *Plateau: Culture Element Distributions XXII*. Anthropological Records 8, no. 2. Berkeley: University of California Press, 1942.

Reagan, Albert, and L. Walters. "Tales from Hoh and Quileute." *Journal of American Folklore*, no. 46 (1933): 297–346.

Reichard, Gladys. *Navajo Religion: A Study of Symbolism*. Princeton University Press, 1963.

Reifel, Nancy. "American Indian Views of Public Health Nursing." *American Indian Culture and Research Journal* 23, no. 3 (1999): 143–54.

Relander, Click. *Drummers and Dreamers*. 1956; repr., Seattle: Northwest Interpretive Association, 1986.

Reyes, Lawney L. *White Grizzly Bear's Legacy: Learning to Be Indian*. Seattle: University of Washington Press, 2002.

Rhoades, Everett R. ed. *American Indian Health: Innovations in Heath Care, Promotion and Policy*. Baltimore: Johns Hopkins University Press, 2000.

Ricoeur, Paul. *Figuring the Sacred: Religion, Narrative, and Imagination*. St. Paul MN: Fortress Press, 1995.

Riley, Carroll L. "Ethnological Field Investigation and Analysis of Historical Material Relative to Group Distribution and Utilization of Natural Resources among Puget Sound Indians." In *Coast Salish and Western Washington Indians*, vol. 2. New York: Garland Publishing, 1974.

Riley, Denise. *"Am I That Name?" Feminism and the Category of 'Women' in History.* Minneapolis: University of Minnesota Press, 1989.

Rivera, Luis. *A Violent Evangelism: The Political and Religious Conquest of the Americas.* Louisville: John Knox Press, 1992.

Roberts, Dorothy. *Killing the Black Body: Race, Reproduction, and the Meaning of Liberty*. New York: Pantheon Press, 1998.

Rogers. Genny. "Sharing the Message at Home: Genny Rogers Shares How She Took Charge of Her Cancer Treatment—and Saved Her Breasts." *Native Women's Wellness*, Fall 2002, 5.

Rose, Wendy. "The Great Pretenders: Further Reflections on White Shamanism." In *The State Of Native America: Genocide, Colonization and Resistance*, ed. M. Annette Jaimes, 403–21. Boston: South End Press, 1992.

Ross, Alexander. *Adventures of the First Settlers on the Oregon or Columbia River*. London, 1849.

Rossi, Louis. *Six Years on the West Coast of America, 1856–1862.* Fairfield WA: Ye Galleon Press, 1983.

Ruby, Robert, and John Brown. *The Chinook Indians: Traders of the Lower Columbia River*. Norman: University of Oklahoma Press, 1976.

———. *Dreamer Prophets of the Columbia Plaetau: Smohalla and Skolaskin.* Norman: University of Oklahoma Press, 1989.

———. *John Slocum and the Indian Shaker Church.* Norman: University of Oklahoma Press, 1996.

Rudine, Robert. "Center of the World." In *Dxwʔdal taqʷšəblu tulʔal ti syeyaʔyaʔs: Writings about Vi Hilbert, by Her Friends*, ed. Janet Yoder, 40–43. Seattle: Lushootseed Research, 1992.

Sacket, Lee. "The Siletz Indian Shaker Church." *Pacific Northwest Quarterly* 64, no. 3 (1973): 120–26.

Said, Edward. *Orientalism.* New York: Random House, 1979.

Sale, Kirkpatrick. *The Conquest of Paradise: Columbus and the Columbian Legacy*. New York: Plume, 1991.

Sampson, Martin. *The Indians of Skagit County.* Mount Vernon: Skagit County Historical Society, 1972.

Sandner, Donald. *Navajo Symbols of Healing*. New York: Harcourt Brace Jovanovich, 1979.

Sandrick, Karen. "The Wisdom of the Old Ways: Lorelei DeCora's Porcupine Clinic on the Pine Ridge Reservation." *Hospitals and Health Networks* 71, no. 4 (February 20 1997).

Sauer, Beverly. "Hot Tomalley: Women's Bodies and Environmental Politics in the State of Maine." In *Body Talk: Rhetoric, Technology and Reproduction*, ed. Mary

Lay, Laura Gurak, Clare Gravon, and Cynthia Myntti. Madison: University of Wisconsin Press, 2000.
Sawicki, Jana. "Feminism, Foucault, and 'Subjects' of Power and Freedom." In *Feminist Interpretations of Michel Foucault*, ed. Susan Hekman, 159–78. University Park: Pennsylvania State University, 1996.
SBIN. *Shoalwater Bay Indian Nation FY2001 Congressional Appropriations Request*, 2000.
———. "The Pregnancy and Infant Mortality Emergency of the Shoalwater Bay Reservation, Washington State: A Joint Report of Findings Issued by the Shoalwater Bay Tribal Council, Indian Health Service, and Washington State Department of Health, October 27, 1994." In *Shoalwater Bay Indian Nation FY2001 Congressional Appropriations Request*, 2000.
———. "Statement of the Shoalwater Bay Indian Tribe Presented before the House Interior Appropriations Subcommittee Regarding the FY2000 Indian Health Service Budget, April 15, 1999." In *Shoalwater Bay Indian Nation FY2001 Congressional Appropriations Request*, 2000.
———. Tom Anderson. "Cultural Assessment Report: A Brief History of the Shoalwater Bay Reservation to Clarify the Issues; Cultural, Environmental and Otherwise." In *Shoalwater Bay Indian Nation, FY2001 Congressional Appropriations Request*, 2000.
———. U.S. Environmental Protection Agency, Office of Environmental Assessment, Region 10. "The Shoalwater Bay Reservation, A Limited Environmental Assessment: 1994–1995." Revision 3.0. January 17, 1997. In *Shoalwater Bay Indian Nation FY2001 Congressional Appropriations Request*, 2000.
Schaepe, David. "Sto:lo Identity and the Cultural Landscape of the S'ólh Téméxw." In *Be of Good Mind: Essays on the Coast Salish*, ed. Bruce Granville Miller. Vancouver: University of British Columbia Press, 2007.
Scheper-Hughes, Nancy. "Social Indifference to Child Death." *Lancet* 337, no. 8750 (1991): 1144–48.
Scheper-Hughes, Nancy, and Margaret M. Lock. "The Mindful Body: Prolegomenon to Future Work in Anthropology." *Medical Anthropology Quarterly* 1, no. 1 (1987): 6–41.
Schoenberg, Wilfred. *A History of the Catholic Church in the Pacific Northwest, 1743–1983*. Washington DC: Pastoral Press, 1987.
Schuster, Helen. *The Yakama*. Indians of North America Series. New York: Chelsea House Publications, 1990.
Schwarz, Maureen Trudelle. "Lightning Followed Me: Contemporary Navajo Therapeutic Strategies for Cancer." In *Religion and Healing in Native America: Pathways for Renewal*, ed. Suzanne Crawford O'Brien, 19–42. Westport CT: Praeger, 2008.
———. *Molded in the Image of Changing Woman: Navajo Views on the Human Body and Personhood*. Tucson: University of Arizona Press, 1997.
Scott, Leslie M. "Indian Diseases as Aids to Pacific Northwest Settlement." *Oregon Historical Quarterly* 29 (1928): 144–61.

———. "Indian Women as Food Providers and Tribal Counselors," *Oregon Historical Quarterly*, 42 (1941): 208–19.

Scouler, John. "Journal of a Voyage to N.W. America." *Oregon Historical Quarterly* 6, nos. 1 and 2 (1905): 54–75.

Seaburg, William, and Jay Miller. "Tillamook." In *Handbook of North American Indians*, vol. 7: *The Northwest Coast*, ed. Wayne Suttles, 560–67. Washington DC: Smithsonian Institution Press, 1990.

Sheikh, Anees A., and Katherine S. Sheikh. *Eastern and Western Approaches to Healing: Ancient Wisdom and Modern Knowledge*. New York: John Wiley and Sons, 1989.

Shelton, Suzanne. "Spiritual Focus Brings People Together." *Providence Health System, Central Washington Area* (newsletter), 1996.

Shipman, Joan. "Separation." In *Summertime in Georgetown: A Collection of Short Stories by Women and Girls of the Shoalwater Bay Tribal Community*, 70–72. Tokeland WA: Shoalwater Bay Tribal Community Publication, 1998.

Shipman, Rosalita. "Memories." In *Summertime in Georgetown: A Collection of Short Stories by Women and Girls of the Shoalwater Bay Tribal Community*, 73. Tokeland WA: Shoalwater Bay Tribal Community Publication, 1998.

"Shoalwater Reservation Centennial: From Carcowan through the Charleys—100 Years." *Sou'Wester* 1, no. 3 (Autumn 1966).

Schoenberg, Wilfred. *A History of the Catholic Church in the Pacific Northwest, 1743–1983*. Washington DC: Pastoral Press, 1987.

Sider, Gerald. "The Walls Came Tumbling Up: The Production of Culture, Class and Native American Societies." *Australian Journal of Anthropology* 17, no. 3 (2006): 276–90.

Sloan, R.P., E. *Bagiella*, L. *VandeCreek*, M. *Hover*, C. *Casalone*, T. *Jinpu Hirsch*, Y. *Hasan*, B. *Kreger*, and P. *Poulos*. "Should Physicians Prescribe Religious Activities?" *New England Journal of Medicine* 342, no. 25 (June 22, 2000): 1913–16.

Smith, Andrea. *Conquest: Sexual Violence and American Indian Genocide.* Cambridge MA: South End Press, 2005.

Smith, Jonathan Z. *To Take Place: Toward Theory in Ritual*. Chicago: University of Chicago Press, 1992.

Smith, M. W. *The Puyallup-Nisqually*. Columbia University Contributions to Anthropology 32. New York: Columbia University Press, 1940.

Smith, Marian W., ed. *Indians of the Urban Northwest*. 1949; New York: AMS Press, 1969.

Smith, Silas B. "Primitive Customs and Religious Beliefs of the Indians of the Pacific Northwest Coast." *Oregon Historical Quarterly* 2 (1901); 255–65.

Snyder, Sally. "Quest for the Sacred: An Interpretation of Potlatch." *Ethnology* 14, no. 2 (1975): 149–61.

Spencer, Herbert. *Principles of Biology*. 1864; Charleston SC: Bibliobazaar, 2009.

Sperlin, O. B. 1930. "Two Kootenay Women Masquerading as Men? Or Were They One?" *Washington Historical Quarterly* 21 (1930)*: 120–30.*

Spier, Leslie. *The Ghost Dance of 1870 among the Klamath of Oregon.* Publications in Anthropology 2, no. 2. Seattle: University of Washington Press, 1927.

———. *Klamath Ethnography.* Publications in American Archaeology and Ethnology 30. Berkeley: University of California Press, 1930.

———. *The Prophet Dance of the Northwest and Its Derivatives: The Source of the Ghost Dance.* General Series in Anthropology 1. Menasha, WI: George Banta, 1935.

Spier, Leslie, and Edward Sapir. *Wishram Ethnography.* Publications in Anthropology 3, no. 3. Seattle: University of Washington Press, 1930.

SPIPA. *South Puget Intertribal Planning Agency Annual Report,* 1999.

———. *South Puget Intertribal Planning Agency Annual Report,* 2000.

———. "South Puget Intertribal Planning Agency's Intertribal Intergenerational Women and Girls' Gathering, Annual Report," 2004.

———. "Tribal Clinic Profiles." *Native Women's Breast and Cervical Health Magazine,* 2000.

Spivak, Gayatri. *A Critique of Postcolonial Reason: Toward a History of the Vanishing Present.* Cambridge MA: Harvard University Press, 1999.

———. *In Other Words: Essays in Cultural Politics.* New York: Routledge, 1988.

Squeoch, Marion Dick. *This Is Our Land: It Has Been Since Time Immemorial—An Overview of the History and Culture of the 14 Confederated Tribes and Bands of the Yakama Indian Nation.* Toppenish: Confederated Tribes and Bands of the Yakama Nation, 1996.

Stanley, George, ed. *Mapping the Frontier: Charles Wilson's Diary of the Survey of the 49th Parallel, 1858–1862, While Secretary of the British Boundary Commission.* Seattle: University of Washington Press, 1970.

St. Clair, Henry Hull, and Leo J. Frachtenberg. "Traditions of the Coos Indians." *Journal of American Folklore* 22 (1909): 25–41.

St. James, Carolyn. "Shoalwater Bay Looks Forward to New Learning Resources Center, Clinic." *South Puget Intertribal News* 3, no. 1 (January–March 2003): 8.

Stewart, T. D. "The Chinook Sign of Freedom: A Study of the Skull of the Famous Chief Concomly." In *Annual Report of the Board of Regents of the Smithsonian Institution Showing the Operations, Expenditures, and Condition of Institution for the Year Ended June 30, 1959.* Publication 4392. Washington DC: Smithsonian Intitution, 1960.

Stocking, George W. *Race, Culture and Evolution: Essays in the History of Anthropology.* New York: Free Press, 1968.

Storck, Michael, Thomas J. Csordas, and Milton Strauss. "Depressive Illness and Navajo Healing." *Medical Anthropology Quarterly* 14, no. 4 (2000): 571–97.

Strickland, W. P. *History of the Missions of the Methodist Episcopal Church, from the Organization of the Missionary Society to the Present Time.* New York: Harper and Brothers, 1849.

Strong, James Clark. *Wah-kee-nah and Her People: The Curious Customs, Traditions and Legends of the North American Indians.* New York: Putnam's Sons, 1893.

Strong, Thomas Nelson. *Cathlamet on the Columbia: Recollections of the Indian People and Short Stories of Early Pioneer Days in the Valley of the Lower Columbia River.* Portland OR: Metropolitan Press, 1930.

Strong, William Duncan. "The Occurrence and Wider Implications of a 'Ghost Cult' on the Columbia River Suggested by Carvings in Wood, Bone, and Stone." *American Anthropologist* 47, no. 2 (April 1945): 244–61.

Sullivan, Lawrence. "Body Works: Knowledge of the Body in the Study of Religion." *History of Religions* 30 (1990): 86–99.

Suttles, Wayne. "The Central Coast Salish." In *Handbook of North American Indians*, vol. 7: *The Northwest Coast*, ed. Wayne Suttles. Washington DC: Smithsonian Institution Press, 1990.

———. *Coast Salish Essays*. Vancouver: Talonbooks, and Seattle: University of Washington Press, 1987.

———. "Recognition of Coast Salish Art." In *S'abadeb, The Gifts: Pacific Coast Salish Art and Artists*, ed. Barbara Brotherton, 50–67. Seattle: University of Washington Press, 2008.

Suttles, Wayne, ed. *Handbook of North American Indians*, vol. 7: *The Northwest Coast*. Washington DC: Smithsonian Institution Press, 1990.

Suttles, Wayne, and Barbara Lane. "The Southern Coast Salish." In *Handbook of North American Indians*, vol. 7: *The Northwest Coast*, ed. Wayne Suttles, 485–502. Washington DC: Smithsonian Press, 1990.

Swan, James G. *The Northwest Coast, or, Three Years' Residence in Washington Territory*. Seattle: University of Washington Press, 1969.

Swinomish Tribal Mental Health Project. *A Gathering of Wisdoms: Tribal Mental Health: A Cultural Perspective*. La Conner WA: Swinomish Tribal Community, 1991.

Szasz, Margaret. *Education and the American Indian: The Road to Self-Determination 1928–1973*. Albuquerque: University of New Mexico Press, 1974.

Taussig, Michael. *Shamanism, Colonialism, and the Wild Man: A Study in Terror and Healing*. Chicago: University of Chicago Press, 1987.

Taylor, Charles. *Sources of the Self: The Making of the Modern Identity*. Cambridge MA: Harvard University Press, 1989.

Taylor, Herbert Jr., and Lester Hoaglin Jr. 1962. "The Intermittent Fever Epidemic of the 1830's on the Lower Columbia River." *Ethnohistory* 9, no. 2 (Spring 1962): 160–78.

Taylor, Timothy L. "Health Problems and Use of Services at Two Urban American Indian Clinics." *U.S. Public Health Service, Public Health Reports* 103, no. 1 (1988): 88–95.

Teit, James. "Mid-Columbia Salish." *University of Washington Publications in Anthropology* 2, no. 4 (1928): 83–128.

———. "Salishan Tribes of Western Plateaus." *Bureau of American Ethnology Annual Report* 45 (1930): 25–396.

Thompson, M. Terry, and Steven M. Egesdal, *Salish Myths and Legends: One People's Stories.* Lincoln: University of Nebraska Press, 2008.

Thomson, J. *Indian Affairs in the Territories of Oregon and Washington.* Secretary of the Interior, House of Represenatives, Executive Document no. 39, 35th Congress, First Session, 1857.

Thornton, J. Quinn. *Oregon and California in 1848*, vol. 1. New York: Harper and Brothers, 1864.
Thornton, Robert. *Being and Place among the Tlingit.* Seattle: University of Washington Press, 2008.
Thornton, Russel. *American Indian Holocaust and Survival: A Population History Since 1492.* Norman: University of Oklahoma Press, 1987.
———. *We Shall Live Again: The 1870 and 1890 Ghost Dance Movements as Demographic Revitalization.* Cambridge: Cambridge University Press, 1986.
Thrush, Coll. *Native Seattle: Histories from the Crossing Over Place.* Seattle: University of Washington Press, 2007.
Thurman, Melburn. "The Shawnee Prophet's Movement and the Origins of the Prophet Dance." *Current Anthropology* 25 (1984): 530–31.
Thwaites, Reuben Gold, ed. *Original Journals of the Lewis and Clark Expedition 1804–1806*, vols. 3–4. New York: Antiquarian Press, 1959.
———. *Travels in the Far Northwest*, vol. 2: *Oregon Missions and Travels over the Rocky Mountains in 1845–46: Pierre Jean De Smet, S.J.* Cleveland: Arthur H. Clark Company, 1906.
Tillich, Paul. *Theology of Culture*. Oxford: Oxford University Press, 1959.
Tinker, George. *Missionary Conquest: The Gospel and Native American Cultural Genocide*. St. Paul: Fortress Press, 1993.
Todorov, Tzvetan. *The Conquest of America: The Question of the Other*. New York: Harper and Row, 1984.
Tom-Orme, Lillian. "Native American Women's Health Concerns: Toward Restoration of Harmony." In *Health Issues for Women of Color: A Cultural Diversity Perspective*, ed. Diane L. Adams, 27–41. Thousand Oaks CA: Sage, 1995.
Trafzer, Clifford E. 1997. *Death Stalks the Yakama: Epidemiological Transitions and Mortality on the Yakama Indian Reservation, 1888–1964*. East Lansing: University of Michigan Press, 1997.
———. "Infant Mortality on the Yakama Indian Reservation." *American Indian Culture and Research Journal* 23, no. 3 (1999): 77–96.
Trennert, Robert A. *White Man's Medicine: Government Doctors and the Navajo 1863–1955.* Albuquerque: University of New Mexico Press, 1998.
Tuan, Yi-Fu. *Space and Place: The Perspective of Experience.* Minneapolis: University of Minnesota Press, 1977.
Turner, Bryan. *The Body and Society: Explorations in Social Theory*. Thousand Oaks CA: Sage, 1996.
Turner, Terrence. "Bodies and Anti-Bodies: Flesh and Fetish in Contemporary Social Theory." In *Embodiment and Experience: The Existential Ground of Culture and the Self*, ed. Thomas J. Csordas, 27–47. Cambridge: Cambridge University Press, 1994.
Tweddell, Colin E. "A Historical and Ethnological Study of the Snohomish Indian People." In *Coast Salish and Western Washington Indians*, vol. 2. New York: Garland Publishing, 1974.

Tyrell, J. B., ed. *David Thompson's Narrative of His Explorations in Western America, 1784–1812*. Publications of the Champlain Society, 12. Toronto: Champlain Society, 1916.

Valencius, Conevery. *The Health of the Country: How American Settlers Understood Themselves and Their Land*. New York: Basic Books, 2002.

Valory, Dale. *The Focus of Indian Shaker Healing*.Kroeber Anthropological Society Papers 35. 1966; Berkeley: California Indian Library Collections Project, 1989.

Van Krieken, Robert. "The Stolen Generations and Cultural Genocide: The Forced Removal of Australian Indigenous Children and Its Implications for the Sociology of Childhood." *Childhood,* no. 6 (August 1999): 297–311.

Verano, John, and Douglad Ubelaker. *Disease and Demography in the Americas.* Washington DC: Smithsonian Institution Press, 1992.

Vecsey, Christopher. "The Lord's Prayer." In *Dxwʔdal taqʷšəblu tulʔal ti syeyaʔyaʔs: Writings about Vi Hilbert, by Her Friends*, ed. Janet Yoder, 50–52. Seattle: Lushootseed Research, 1992.

Verne, Ray. *Lower Chinook Texts.* Publications in Anthropology 7. Seattle: University of Washington Press, 1938.

Vestal, Stanley. *New Sources of Indian History: 1850–1891. The Ghost Dance: The Prairie Sioux, A Miscellany.* Norman: University of Oklahoma Press, 1934.

Vibert, Elizabeth. "'The Native Peoples Were Strong to Live': Reinterpreting Early Nineteenth Century Prophetic Movements in the Columbia Plateau." *Ethnohistory* 42, no. 4 (1995): 197–229.

Vizenor, Gerald. "Native American Critical Metaphors of the Ghost Dance." *World Literature Today* 66, no. 2 (Spring 1992): 223–27.

Voss, Richard W., Victor Douville, Alex Little Soldier, and Gayla Twiss. "Tribal and Shamanic-Based Social Work Practice: A Lakota Perspective." *Social Work* 44, no. 3 (May 1999): 228–45.

Waldram, James B. "The Efficacy of Traditional Medicine: Current Theoretical and Methodological Issues." *Medical Anthropology Quarterly* 14, no. 4 (2000): 603–25.

Walker, Deward. "New Light on the Prophet Dance Controversy." *Ethnohistory* 16 (1969): 245–55.

Wallace, Anthony F. C. "Revitalization Movements." *American Anthropologist* 58 (1956): 264–81.

———. *Revitalizations and Mazeways: Essays on Culture Change*, vol. 1. Lincoln: University of Nebraska Press, 2003.

Waterman, T. T. "The Paraphernalia of the Duwamish Spirit Canoe Ceremony." *Indian Notes* 7 (April 1930): 129–48; (July): 295–312; (October): 535–61.

———. "The Shake Religion of Puget Sound." *Smithsonian Institution Annual Report for 1922*. Washington DC: Smithsonian Institution, 1924.

Waters, Alysha. "Native American Food Production Systems, a Historic Perspective: Their Link to Healthy Communities." *Native Women's Wellness Newsletter*, Summer 2001, 6–7.

Weber, Max. *The Protestant Ethic and the Spirit of Capitalism*. New York: Penguin, 2002.

Weiss, Gail. *Body Images: Embodiment as Intercorporeality*. New York: Routledge, 1999.
Weiss, Gail, and Honi Fern Haber, eds. *Perspectives on Embodiment: The Intersections of Nature and Culture*. New York: Routledge, 1999.
Welton, Donn. *The Body: Classic and Contemporary Readings*. Malden MA: Blackwell Publishers, 1999.
———. *Body and Flesh: A Philosophical Reader*. Malden MA: Blackwell Publishers, 1998.
White, Richard. *The Organic Machine: The Remaking of the Columbia River*. New York: Hill and Wang, 1995.
Whitener, Barbara. "Language Program." *Klah'Che'Min*, August 2001, 9.
Wilkes, Charles. *Narrative of the U.S. Exploring Expedition: 1838, 1839, 1840, 1841, 1842*. Philadelphia: Lea and Blanchard, 1845.
———. *Columbia River to Sacramento, 1839–1942*. Oakland: Biobooks, 1958.
Wilkinson, Charles. *Blood Struggle: The Rise of Modern Indian Nations*. New York: W. W. Norton, 2006.
———. *Messages from Frank's Landing: A Story of Salmon, Treaties, and the Indian Way*. Seattle: University of Washington Press, 2000.
Wolf, Diane L. *Feminist Dilemmas in Fieldwork*. Boulder CO: Westview Press, 1996.
Wyeth, Nathaniel. "Correspondence and Journals." In *Sources of Oregon History*, vol. 1, ed. Frederick Young. Eugene: University of Oregon, 1899.
Yoder, Janet, ed. *Dxwʔdal taqʷšəblu tulʔal ti syeyaʔyaʔs: Writings about Vi Hilbert, by Her Friends*. Seattle: Lushootseed Research, 1992.
Young, Iris. "Pregnant Embodiment." In *Body and Flesh: A Philosophical Reader*, ed. Donn Welton. Malden MA: Blackwell Publishers, 1998.
Zenk, Henry. "Kalapuyans." In *Handbook of North American Indians*, vol. 7: *The Northwest Coast*, ed. Wayne Suttles, 547–53. Washington DC: Smithsonian Institution Press, 1990.

Index

Illustrations follow p. 194 and are indexed by figure number.

Also by the author

American Indian Religious Traditions: An Encyclopedia (3 vols.)

Native American Religious Traditions

Religion and Healing in Native America: Pathways for Renewal

Articles and chapters by the author have appeared in *Columbia Guide to Religion in American History*; *Encyclopedia of Religion*; *Journal of Ritual Studies*; *Material Religion: The Journal of Objects, Art, and Belief*; *Teaching Religion and Healing*; *Teaching Theology and Religion*; and *The Repatriation Reader: Who Owns Native American Remains?*